O A P L
OXFORD AMERICAN PAIN LIBRARY

Opioid Therapy in the 21st Century
Second Edition

O A P L
OXFORD AMERICAN PAIN LIBRARY

Opioid Therapy in the 21st Century

Second Edition

Edited by

Howard S. Smith, M.D.

Professor of Anesthesiology, Internal Medicine, and Physical
    Medicine and Rehabilitation
Director of Pain Management
Albany Medical College
Department of Anesthesiology
Albany, NY

Executive Series Editor

Russell K. Portenoy, MD

Chairman of the Department of Pain Medicine and Palliative Care
Beth Israel Medical Center
New York, NY

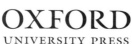

OXFORD
UNIVERSITY PRESS

OXFORD
UNIVERSITY PRESS

Oxford University Press is a department of the University of Oxford.
It furthers the University's objective of excellence in research, scholarship,
and education by publishing worldwide.

Oxford   New York
Auckland   Cape Town   Dar es Salaam   Hong Kong   Karachi
Kuala Lumpur   Madrid   Melbourne   Mexico City   Nairobi
New Delhi   Shanghai   Taipei   Toronto

With offices in
Argentina   Austria   Brazil   Chile   Czech Republic   France   Greece
Guatemala   Hungary   Italy   Japan   Poland   Portugal   Singapore
South Korea   Switzerland   Thailand   Turkey   Ukraine   Vietnam

Oxford is a registered trademark of Oxford University Press in the UK
and certain other countries.

Published in the United States of America by
Oxford University Press
198 Madison Avenue, New York, NY 10016

Library of Congress Cataloging-in-Publication Data

Opioid therapy in the 21st century / edited by Howard S. Smith. -- 2nd ed.
p. ; cm. — (Oxford American pain library)
Includes bibliographical references and index.
ISBN 978-0-19-984497-5 (alk. paper)
I. Smith, Howard S., 1956- II. Series: Oxford American pain library.
[DNLM: 1. Analgesics, Opioid—therapeutic use—Handbooks.   2. Analgesics,
Opioid—adverse effects—Handbooks.   3. Opioid-Related Disorders—prevention &
control—Handbooks.   4. Pain—drug therapy—Handbooks. QV 39]
LC Classification not assigned

615'.7822—dc23
2012039782

9 8 7 6 5 4 3 2 1

Printed in the United States of America
on acid-free paper

Disclosures

Andres F. Carrion has nothing to disclose.

Stanley Martin Cohen has been on speakers bureaus from Bristol-Meyers Squibb, Gilead, Genentech, and Vertex; on advisory boards for BMS, Gilead, and Vertex; and a consultant for BMS and Gilead.

Leslie Dawvaroo has nothing to disclose.

Archita P. Desai has nothing to disclose.

Michael W. Fried has received research grants from Genentech, Merck, Vertex, Tibotec, Gilead, Bristol-Meyers Squibb, Anadys, Contaus, and Abbott; has been a consultant for Genentech, Tibotech, Vertex, Merck Pharmasset, Glaxo, Novartis, Abbott, and Gilead; and has received research grants from the NIH.

Christin M. Giordano has nothing to disclose.

Shriram Jakate has nothing to disclose.

Donald M. Jensen is on the Consulting and Advisory Boards for Abbott, Boehringer-Ingelheim, Genentech/Roche, Johnson & Johnson/Tibotec, Merck, Pharmasset/Gilead, Vertex; has received research grants from Abbott, Boehringer-Ingelheim, Genentech/Roche, Johnson & Johnson/Tibotec, Merck, Pharmasset/Gilead, Vertex; has spoken at Consensus Medical Communications, Projects in Knowledge, Clinical Care Options; and has had a publication for SLACK, Inc.

Leila Kia has nothing to disclose.

Arthur Y. Kim has served as consultant to Vertex Pharmaceuticals and has received research funding from the National Institutes of Health (NIAID and NIDA).

Josh Levitsky is on the Speaker Bureau for Genentech and Vertex.

Paul Martin served as a consultant for Vertex, Genetech, Abbott, and Merck.

Kristina A. Matkowskyj has nothing to disclose.

Christopher E. McGowan has nothing to disclose.

Anjana A. Pillai is a speaker for Merck and Otsuka.

Nancy Reau has served on the advisory boards of BMS, Vertex, Gilead, and Genetech/Roche and as a consultant to Merck. She has received research support from Vertex and Gilead.

Dedication

I would like to dedicate this book in memory of my mother Arlene and my father Nathan, to my wife Joan, and our children Alyssa, Joshua, Benjamin, and Eric.

Acknowledgments

I would like to acknowledge the enormous efforts of Pya Seidner in the preparation of this text as well as the efforts of Russell K. Portenoy MD, Yvonne Honigsberg, Andrea Seils, and the Oxford University Press team.

Foreword

In 1986, I came to the United States from the United Kingdom to practice anesthesiology. My mentor at the time absorbed me into his interest in pain medicine, and so began what has been a long career looking after people in pain. Unlike in the United Kingdom, "opiophobia" was something that came into every US practitioner's consciousness in the 1980s, and strong efforts were afoot to redress the balance. The excitement that surrounded our efforts to widen pain practice, and in particular to make opioids available for a wider range of pain diagnoses, was tied up in our conviction that patients were suffering unnecessarily, and that we could help reduce their suffering. To some extent we have, but we did not calculate that despite our best efforts to educate young clinicians within our sphere, there was a huge shortfall in training community clinicians to use these complicated drugs for complex chronic pain patients. It is a tragedy, actually, that the message ever got out that there is a simple answer to chronic pain, because instead of helping we have added a new layer of distress into the lives of many chronic pain patients: dependence on drugs that are often dangerous and often not helping pain.

Does all this suggest that we should not use opioids, or at least not use opioids for chronic pain? Absolutely not. Opioids are—and are likely to remain—the only class of drugs we know capable of relieving serious pain. It is imperative that these drugs remain in use, and more imperative than ever that we understand how to use them. Howard Smith has edited (and in large part written) a book that will be enormously helpful in filling the knowledge gap. The book provides a very thorough exploration of many of the fundamental aspects necessary to understanding opioids, and how to use them effectively and safely. Contributing authors include some of the best known and experienced in the field, and they have provided a trustworthy exposition. In particular, there are detailed chapters on opioid pharmacology, a necessary basis for clinical practice that optimizes efficacy while maintaining safety. The pharmacology is presented under chapters that have relevance to the clinic use of opioids, including chapters on route selection, managing side effects, and utilizing opioid rotations. A chapter on the pre-opioid prescribing period provides a wealth of helpful algorithms and practice tools that can help the less experienced practitioner with one of the most important decisions to be made: whether to start someone on chronic opioid therapy or, by implication, stop therapy if it would not be advisable to let acute treatment become chronic. There are several chapters on screening for potential abuse risk—which is, of course, relevant mostly for patients with chronic noncancer pain—and this concentration on screening makes the book of particular value for the management of noncancer pain. There are also chapters on managing cancer pain, and pain in other special populations, so this book can be a resource for anybody using opioids as pain medication.

If we have gone wrong at all, it is in underestimating the complexity of opioid pain management. Howard Smith's book goes a long way towards correcting whatever deficit in knowledge made us believe that opioid management would ever be simple.

Jane C. Ballantyne

Preface

Chronic pain is one of the most common and debilitating health care conditions, and among the most notoriously challenging to treat. It often compromises quality of life and is an under-recognized and undertreated disabling condition. Many patients suffering from chronic pain could arguably be helped by the appropriate administration of opioid therapy; however, opioids remain likely underutilized due to controversies and misconceptions surrounding their use. Despite the effectiveness of opioid analgesics in providing significant pain relief, the entire class of therapeutics is sometimes disregarded altogether as a feasible option for alleviating chronic pain, without weighing the risk benefit ratio of opioid therapy versus alternative treatment options.

This book is designed to provide clinicians with up-to-date, evidence-based information about appropriate opioid use, including the potential benefits of therapy as well as the potential adverse effects that can occur. It is intended to aid physicians in making informed, rational decisions for optimal patient care, and to provide guidance on appropriate and safe prescribing practices regarding opioids. I hope that this book helps to dispel misconceptions surrounding opioids and improves the comfort level of physicians considering their use.

Part of the Oxford American Pain Library, this concise guide serves as a practical, user-friendly reference for physicians across the range of primary care and medical specialties. It includes an overview of appropriate clinical applications of opioids, covering such topics as opioid pharmacology, route selection, and individualization of therapy, as well as strategies for managing and mitigating the risk of abuse, addiction, and diversion. There are also special sections dedicated to the unique needs of pediatric, geriatric, and palliative care patient populations.

I am indebted to all of the book's contributors for their support and willingness to share their expertise. As is often the case, there will likely be some aspects of opioid therapy that may have been omitted, or under-overemphasized. The subject matter sometimes elicits strong opinions, and I have done my best to ensure that the topic has been covered thoroughly, appropriately, and conscientiously, in the best interest of patient care. I believe that the approach and scope of the book will help readers gain greater insights into the appropriate use of opioid therapy, and to encourage consideration of all appropriate options for treating chronic pain. I am happy to be able to provide readers a current second edition of the book.

Howard S. Smith
October 2012

Contents

Contributors

Janet L. Abrahm, MD
Chief, Division of Adult Palliative
Care
Department of Psychosocial
Oncology and Palliative Care
Dana-Farber Cancer Institute
Professor of Medicine
Harvard Medical School
Cambridge, MA

Charles E. Argoff, MD
Professor of Neurology
Albany Medical College
Director, Comprehensive Pain
Center
Albany Medical Center
Albany, NY

Lucy Chen, MD
Assistant Professor
MGH Center for Translational Pain
Research
Department of Anesthesia, Critical
Care and Pain Medicine
Massachusetts General Hospital,
Harvard Medical School
Boston, MA

**Mellar P. Davis MD, FCCP,
FAAHPM**
Professor of Medicine, Cleveland
Clinic Lerner School of Medicine
Case Western Reserve University
Director, Clinical Fellowship
Program
Palliative Medicine and Supportive
Oncology Services
Division of Solid Tumor
Taussig Cancer Institute
The Cleveland Clinic
Cleveland, OH

Andrew Dubin, MD, MS
Associate Professor of Physical
Medicine & Rehabilitation
Department of Physical Medicine &
Rehabilitation
Albany Medical College
Albany NY

Kenneth L. Kirsh, PhD
Director of Behavioral Medicine
Pain Treatment Center of
Bluegrass
Lexington, KY

**Kenneth C. Jackson II,
PharmD, CPE**
Professor and Chair
Department of Pharmacy Practice
Maier Foundation Chair in Pharmacy
School of Pharmacy
University of Charleston
Charleston, WV

Jianren Mao, MD, PhD
Vice Chair for Research
Director, MGH Center for
Translational Pain Research
Richard J. Kitz Professor of
Anesthesia Research
Department of Anesthesia, Critical
Care and Pain Medicine
Massachusetts General Hospital,
Harvard Medical School
Boston, MA

Bill H. McCarberg, MD
Founder, Chronic Pain
Management Program
Kaiser Permanente San Diego
Adjunct Assistant Clinical Professor

University of California San Diego
San Diego, CA

Gary McCleane, MD
Consultant Pain Management
Rampark Pain Centre
Lurgan
Northern Ireland, UK

Amy L. Mitchell, PharmD
Neonatal/Pediatric Clinical
Pharmacy Specialist
The Children's Hospital at Albany
Medical Center
Assistant Professor, Department of
Pediatrics
Albany Medical College
Adjunct Assistant Professor,
Department of Pharmacy Practice
Albany College of Pharmacy
Albany, NY

Lida Nabati, MD
Division of Adult Palliative Care
Department of Psychosocial
Oncology and Palliative Care
Dana-Farber Cancer Institute
Instructor in Medicine
Harvard Medical School
Cambridge, MA

Steven D. Passik, PhD
Department of Psychiatry and
Anesthesiology
Vanderbilt University Medical
Center
Psychosomatic Medicine
Nashville, TN

Howard S. Smith, MD
Professor of Anesthesiology,
Internal Medicine, and Physical
Medicine and Rehabilitation
Director of Pain Management
Albany Medical College
Department of Anesthesiology
Albany, NY

Gary Thompson, MB
Consultant Anesthetist
Lagan Valley Hospital
Lisburn
Northern Ireland, UK

Lynn R. Webster, MD
Medical Director
CRILifetree
Salt Lake City, UT

Chapter 1

Introduction to Opioids

Howard S. Smith

Opioids are among the most versatile and potent analgesics currently available, yet incomplete knowledge, societal views, and irrational fears continue to impede their optimal use. Health care providers should be comfortable employing opioid therapy in treatment plans when appropriate. Additionally, clinicians should be familiar with risk management strategies for assessing drug-taking behaviors, adverse effects of opioids, and analgesic and functional therapeutic outcomes. It is hoped that clinical activities embodying the concept of balance (i.e., providing medical availability and instructions as to the appropriate use of opioids, as well as risk management plans designed to prevent the abuse or misuse of these agents) will lead to optimal patient outcomes.

Opioids remain one class of pharmacologic agent among a vast armamentarium of therapeutic approaches to the management of pain. It is essential that opioids not be just reflexively used with pain problems as sole therapy, but rather be utilized in an appropriate and thoughtful manner. After completing a patient's history and physical examination, the clinician should diligently pursue a discrete etiology for the pain and attempt to target a specific treatment to match the pathophysiologic mechanisms. Gonzales et al. (1991) performed a survey revealing that pain consultation identified a previously undiagnosed etiology for the pain in 64% of cancer patients, which led to the use of primary therapy (i.e., antineoplastics or antibiotics) in almost 20% of cases. Furthermore, opioids should generally be utilized as part of a multimodal strategy that may include other pharmacologic agents (i.e., anti-inflammatory agents, antiepileptic drugs, antidepressants, α-2 agonists), lifestyle/postural changes, complementary and alternative medicine approaches, physical and behavioral medicine approaches, interventional techniques, neuromodulation techniques, and surgical approaches.

The importance of using a multidisciplinary approach, performing a thorough history and physical examination when dealing with persistent pain, and utilizing multiple modalities and strategies (rather than just opioids) in the management of persistent pain cannot be overemphasized. However, this book focuses on chronic opioid therapy (COT).

The use of COT to treat persistent noncancer pain (PNCP) is growing, based in part on evidence from clinical trials and a growing consensus among pain specialists (Urban et al. 1986; Zenz et al. 1992; Portenoy 1996a, b; Collett 1998; McCleane and Smith 2007). Appropriate use of these drugs requires skills in opioid prescribing, knowledge of the principles of addiction medicine, and a commitment to performing and documenting a comprehensive assessment repeatedly over time. Inadequate assessment can lead to undertreatment, compromise the effectiveness of therapy when implemented, and prevent an appropriate response when problematic drug-related behaviors occur (JCAHO 1999; Max et al. 1999; Katz 2002).

The abuse of opioid analgesics has increased (Compton and Volkow 2006), but a significant portion of the supply of opioids available for abuse appears to be obtained through pharmacy, hospital, and residential burglary thefts and not, for the most part, from prescriptions written by health care providers (Joranson and Gilson 2007; Inciardi et al. 2007). Strategies to diminish the abuse and diversion of prescription opioids include prescription monitoring programs, supply-chain interventions, individual patient management interventions, educational programs, and abuse-deterrent formulations (Katz et al. 2007). Investigations have looked at opioids that are less easily extracted for intravenous abuse (Katz et al. 2006) and those that seem less attractive to abusers according to the Opioid Attractiveness Scale (Butler et al. 2006).

Not only do various opioids differ in attractiveness, but individual patients differ as well (Smith 2008a); with a significant part being genetic in nature. Angst and colleagues conducted a randomized, double-blind and placebo-controlled trial with 121 twin pairs, measured pain sensitivity before and after an infusion of alfentanil, assessed the analgesic response, and compared variations in opioid side effects. Heritability was found to account for 59% of the variability for nausea, 38% for itchiness, 36% for drug disliking, 30% for respiratory depression, 32% for dizziness, and 26% for drug-liking. In a prior study, the team concluded that genetics accounted for 60% of the drugs' variability in relieving pain (Angst et al. 2012).

Regulatory agencies, state medical boards, and various peer review groups (among others) not only expect appropriate medical care, but also require proper documentation. In cases of COT for PNCP, aside from the usual subjective/objective/assessment/plan (SOAP) format of medical progress notes, various other issues require documentation. Although no explicit requirements are spelled out as far as what and how to document in relation to COT, some feel that the use of specific tools or instruments in the chart on some or all visits may boost adherence to documentation expectations, as well as the consistency of such documentation (Passik et al. 2005). Assessment tools may also be helpful in the analysis of persistent pain (Wincent et al. 2003).

Opioids: Background

Opioids are broad-spectrum analgesics utilized for the treatment of nociceptive and neuropathic pain. Although no ideal analgesics exist, and while opioids are far from perfect, they may be among the best broad-spectrum analgesics currently available for many patients.

Exogenous opioids act by activating the body's endogenous opioid receptors in the pain modulating systems, which may dampen nociceptive input. Almost all clinically useful opioid analgesics are μ opioid receptor (MOR) agonists.

Opioid agonists produce effects by binding to membrane-bound opioid receptors and initiating activation of G protein–coupled receptors (GPCRs). It appears that both full and partial agonists induce the same active conformational states of the receptor, and it is the number of active receptors that governs the rate of G protein activation (Traynor et al. 2002). The rate-limiting step in this activation is the dissociation of guanosine diphosphate (GDP), which is bound to the G_α subunit of the G protein under resting conditions. Subsequent guanosine triphosphate (GTP) binding and dissociation of G_α–GTP and β_γ subunits— with resultant interaction of these subunits with downstream effectors—lead to opioid effects (Figure 1.1).

Perhaps the ablity of opioids to produce analgesic effects in a wide variety of painful conditions is in part related to the multiple mechanisms of opioids and the many locations at which opioids may enhance antinociceptive processes.

The sites where opioids may act to achieve analgesia include the following.

1. Peripheral

Although opioid receptors are expressed by primary sensory neurons (Chen et al. 1997), they are functionally inactive under most basal conditions. However, with tissue injury/inflammation, the action of bradykinin on the B2 receptor improves efficiency of MOR coupling to G and promotes MOR signaling (Berg et al. 2007).

There are multiple ways in which endogenous opioids can access peripheral sites of tissue insult to activate peripheral MORs (Smith 2008b; Sehgal et al. 2011). Cannabinoid (CB) agonists' binding to peripheral CB(2) receptors results in CB(2) activation, with subsequent stimulated release of β endorphin from keratinocytes (Ibrahim et al. 2005).

Alternatively, peripheral endogenous opioids may be released from immune cells at the site of tissue insult after stimulation by stress or corticotropin-releasing hormone (Mousa 2003). Intercellular adhesion molecule-1, which is expressed by the endothelium, mediates adhesion and extravasation of leukocytes and may be crucial to the accumulation of opioid-releasing immunocytes at the site of tissue insult (Machelska et al. 2002).

One of the cardinal features of inflammation is pain; however, leukocytes that accumulate at inflammatory sites may counteract inflammatory pain by releasing opioid peptides which may bind to opioid receptors on peripheral sensory neurons. Chemokines such as CXCL 1/2 generated from inflammatory processor or from TNF-α may have important dual roles involved in the release of opioid peptides from leukocytes. One role of CXCL 1/2 is likely that of leukocyte recruitment (Brack et al. 2004) by promoting increased L-selectin, P-selectin, and/or integrins alpha (4) and beta (2) and/or intercellular adhesion molecule-1 (ICAM-1) that contribute to leukocyte adherence and extravasation from the circulation (e.g., out of blood vessels) as well as chemotaxis to the site of inflammation (Mousa et al. 2000; Machelska et al. 2002; Machelska et al. 2004). The second role of CXCL 1/2 is to induce calcium-regulated p38MAPk-dependent translocation in the leukocyte leading to opioid peptide release (Rittner et al. 2006; Rittner et al. 2007).

Pro-opiomelanocortin (POMC) processing begins as the nascent polypeptide chain enters the endoplasmic reticulum (ER) directed by the signal peptide (Loh et al. 2002), and POMC cleavage begins in the *trans*-Golgi network (TGN) (Tanaka et al. 1991; Tanaka and Kurosumi 1992). The POMC prohormone

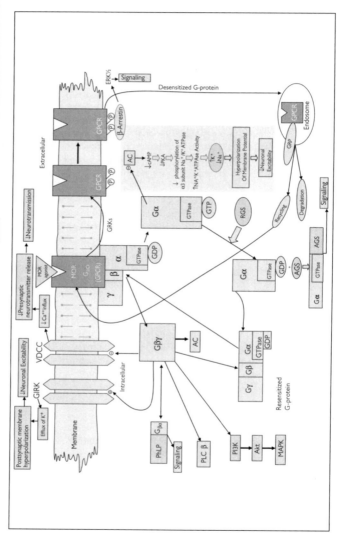

Figure 1.1 Acute MOR agonist-mediated signaling

is directed to the regulated secretory pathway at the TGN by binding to a sorting receptor, identified as (membrane-bound) carboxypeptidase E (CPE) (Cool et al., 1997; Mousa et al. 2004). Prohormone convertase 1 (PC1) mediates the initial processing of pro-opiomelanocortin (POMC) into corticotropin (ACTH) and β-lipotropic hormone (β-LPH). PC2 ProPC2, the immature form of PC2, binds to its chaperone protein 7B2 which helps facilitate PC2 transport as well as contribute to the maturation and activation of PC2.

In the prevailing model of PC2 and 7B2 trafficking in the secretory pathway, free PC2 tends to misfold and to be retained in the ER, whereas free 7B2 or 7B2±PC2 complexes are more readily transported through the downstream compartments into secretory granules (SG) (Mbikay et al. 2001). Affinity between the two molecules is influenced by, among other factors, the pH and the calcium concentration in the successive compartments of the secretory pathway. The pro7B2-proPC2 complex is formed in the alkaline and calcium-poor ER. It is enzymically inactive. Under the mildly acidic, calcium-richer conditions of the TGN and the immature secretory granules (ISG), pro7B2 is cleaved by furin (Mbikay et al. 2001) and leading to mature, activated PC2 in secretory granuales. PC2 mediates the conversion of β-LPH to β-endorphin and of ACTH to α-MSH (Figure 1.2). Additionally, aside from CXCL 1/2, it appears that interleukin-1β (IL-1β), corticotropin-releasing factor (CRF)—particularly locally expressed CRF in the inflamed tissue site (Schafer et al. 1996)—and/or norepinephrine (NE) may also contribute to leukocyte release of β-endorphin (Cabot et al. 1997; Schäfer et al. 1994; Binder et al. 2004; Rittner et al. 2005). The autocatalytic conversion of proPC1 occurs in the ER and its activation takes place in the TGN and immature secretory granules (ISGs) through secondary cleavages within the pro-segment and the C-terminal domain (Mbikay et al. 2001).

2. Spinal

The MOR-expressing neurons in the dorsal horn of the spinal cord appear to be significantly involved in opioid analgesia (Kline and Wiley 2008).

a. They activate opioid receptors at the central terminals of C-fibers in the spinal cord.
b. They activate opioid receptors on the second-order pain transmission cells, thus inhibiting ascending transmission of the pain signal.
c. Systemically administered morphine leads to an opioid-induced increase in spinal acetylcholine (Ach), and the opioid-induced increase in spinal Ach—via activation of the spinal cholinergic systemappears to contribute to opioid-mediated antinociception via modulation of both muscarinic and nicotinic receptors (Chen and Pan 2001), Also, it is conceivable that gamma-amino butyric acid (GABA) receptors may be involved in the regulation of the intrapsinal Ach release (Kommalage and Höglund 2005).

Heinke and colleagues suggested that binding of opioids to MORs reduces nociceptive signal transmission at central Aδ- and C-fiber synapses mainly by inhibition of presynaptic N-type VDCCs (Heinke et al. 2011). P/Q-type VDCCs and the transmitter release machinery are targets of opioid action as well (Heinke et al. 2011). The conventional idea is that GPCRs inhibit neurotransmitter

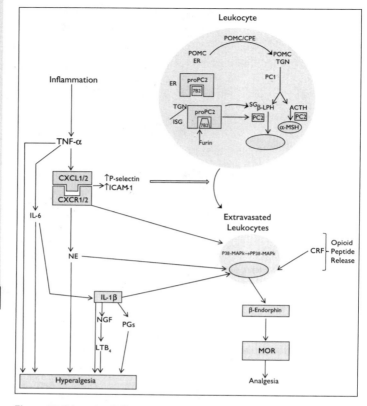

Figure 1.2 Schematic of inflammation-induced opioid peptide release from leukocytes

release through the inactivation of voltage-gated Ca2+ [Ca(V)] channels by the binding of G protein bc subunits (Gbc), which is voltage-dependent (Dolphin 2003; Evans and Zamponi 2006; Dai et al. 2009). However, recent evidence suggests that some GPCRs may activate other signaling pathways. In primary afferents, Ca(V)2.1 (P/Q-type) and Ca(V)2.2 (N-type), channel control neurotransmitter release and are the ones inhibited by MORs (Rusin and Moises 1995; Evans and Zamponi 2006; Dai et al. 2009). Primary afferents contain a unique splice variant of Ca(V)2.2 channels having the 37a exon instead of the 37b exon (Bell et al. 2004; Castiglioni et al. 2006). The 37a exon contains a consensus site for tyrosine phosphorylation by Src family kinases (SFKs) that is absent in the 37b exon, and this makes these channels susceptible to a voltage-independent inhibition by MORs receptors (Diverse-Pierluissi et al. 1997; Strock and Diverse-Pierluissi 2004; Raingo et al. 2007).

Agonist stimulation of the mu opioid receptor (MOR) results in the Gβγ release, which can activate Src family tyrosine kinases. Activated Src then promotes phosphorylation of STAT5A, which is found to associate physically with the putative docking motif YXXL present at the C-terminal tail of MOR. Phosphorylated STAT5A then dimerizes and translocates to the nucleus where it binds to specific DNA sequences and alters gene transcription (Mazarakou and Georgoussi 2005). It is conceivable that high-dose opioid administration via activation of calcium-dependent signaling pathways with subsequent activation of protein phosphatase-1 (PP1), at potential synapses, may normalize the phosphylation state of GluR1 at Ser^{831} and that of GluR2 at Ser^{880} with resultant depotentiation of synaptic strength in C fibers and reversal of long term potentiation and hyperanalgesia (Drdla-Schutting et al. 2012) (Figure 1.3).

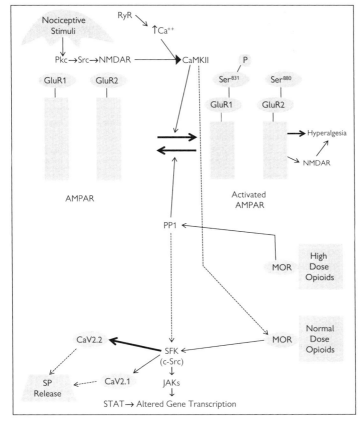

Figure 1.3 Schematic of opioid signaling effects on nociceptive processes

3. Supraspinal

Opioids may bind to MORs in the periventricular-periaqueductal gray regions, as well as some intralaminar and midline thalamic nuclei, some lateral reticular nuclei (Pert and Yaksh 1974), and various cortical areas. However, a major mechanism of supraspinally mediated opioid analgesia involves activating opioid receptors in the midbrain and turning on the descending inhibitory systems, and perhaps also inhibiting the descending nociceptive facilitative systems (Figure 1.4).

Potent Mu opioid receptor agonists act both pre- and postsynaptically in the Rostral ventromedial medulla (RVM), predominantly via two major mechanisms: (1) activating "OFF-cells" (which promote antinociceptive activity), and (2) suppressing "ON-cells" (which promote nociceptive activity) (Heinricher and Ingram 2008; Heinricher et al. 2010a). Opioids inhibit the tonic GABAergic inhibitory activity which normally keeps OFF-cells at a low level of activity; opioid-induced disinhibition leads to OFF-cell activation. Studies with P450-deficient mice and a variety of pharmacologic have demonstrated that P450 epoxygenase activity is required for opioid antinociception (Conroy et al. 2010; Heinricher et al. 2010b) (Figure 1.5). It is conceivable that since NSAIDs inhibit cyclooxygenase (COX) activity, NSAIDs may enhance the epoxygenase (EPO) pathway via hunting of arachidonic acid to the EPO pathway and in this manner contribute to augmented analgesia when NSAIDs and opioids are co-administered.

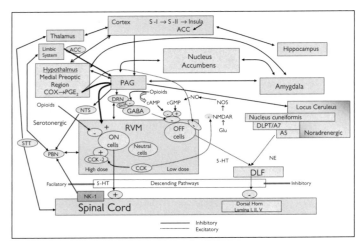

Figure 1.4 Potential Supraspinal/Spinal Modulation of Nociception

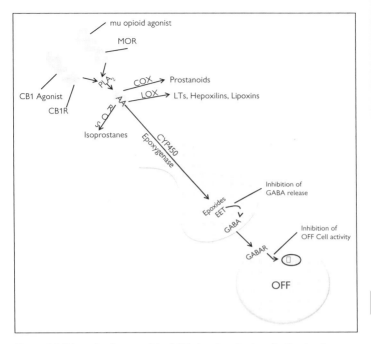

Figure 1.5 Schematic of a potential opioid-induced mechanism of antinociception (Adapted from Heinricher et al. 2010b)

Summary

Opioids are potent broad-spectrum analgesics that may act via multiple mechanisms and may possess antinociceptive qualities in the periphery as well as spinal and supraspinal regions. Opioids have been utilized for nociceptive pain (Altman and Smith 2010), and neuropathic pain (Smith and Argoff 2011). Increases in opioid misuse have made it all the more crucial to perform due diligence when assessing and documenting issues that surround the prescription of chronic opioid therapy (Smith and Kirsh 2007; Smith et al. 2009). Also, chronic opioid therapy may be associated with a variety of adverse effects as well as diminished efficacy over time. It is hoped in the future that combination opioid analgesics (Smith 2008c) [e.g. opioids plus peripheral opioid antagonists, opioid plus opioid (morphine/oxycodone) (de la Iglesia et al. 2012; Webster 2012), opioid plus chemokine antagonists (Wilson et al. 2011), opioid plus cannabinoid (Portenoy et al. 2012), opioid plus TLR4 anatgonist (Hutchinson et al. 2010), opioid plus CCK antagonists or both actions within one molecule (Hanlon et al. 2011)] may maximize analgesia while minimizing adverse effects.

References

Altman RD, Smith HS. Opioid therapy for osteoarthritis and chronic low back pain. *Postgrad Med.* 2010;122(6):87–97.

Angst MS, Lazzeroni LC, Phillips NG, et al. Aversive and Reinforcing Opioid Effects: A Pharmacogenomic Twin Study. *Anethesiology.* 2012;117(1):22–37.

Bell TJ, Thaler C, Castiglioni AJ, et al. Cell-specific alternative splicing increases calcium channel current density in the pain pathway. *Neuron.* 2004;41(1):127–138.

Berg KA, Patwardhan AM, Sanchez TA, et al. Rapid modulation of (micro)-opioid receptor signaling in primary sensory neurons. *J Pharmacol Exp Ther.* 2007;321(3):839–847.

Binder W, Mousa SA, Sitte N, et al. Sympathetic activation triggers endogenous opioid release and analgesia within peripheral inflamed tissue. *Eur J Neurosci.* 2004;20(1):92–100.

Brack A, Rittner HL, Machelska H, at al. Control of inflammatory pain by chemokine-mediated recruitment of opioid-containing polymorphonuclear cells. *Pain.* 2004;112(3):229–38.

Butler SF, Benoit CM, Budman SH, et al. Development and validation of an opioid attractiveness scale: a novel measure of the attractiveness of opioid products to potential abusers. *Harm Reduct J.* 2006;3:5.

Cabot PJ, Carter L, Gaiddon C, et al. Immune cell-derived beta-endorphin. Production, release, and control of inflammatory pain in rats. *J Clin Invest.* 1997;100(1):142–148.

Castiglioni AJ, Raingo J, Lipscombe D. Alternative splicing in the C-terminus of CaV2.2 controls expression and gating of N-type calcium channels. *J Physiol.* 2006;576(Pt 1):119–134.

Chen JJ, Dymshitz J, Vasko MR. Regulation of opioid receptors in rat sensory neurons in culture. *Mol Pharmacol.* 1997;51(4):666–673.

Chen SR, Pan HL. Spinal endogenous acetylcholine contributes to the analgesic effect of systemic morphine in rats. *Anesthesiology.* 2001;95(2):525–530.

Collett BJ. Opioid tolerance: the clinical perspective. *Br J Anaesth.* 1998;81(1):58–68.

Compton WM, Volkow ND. Major increases in opioid analgesic abuse in the United States: concerns and strategies. *Drug Alcohol Depend.* 2006;81(2):103–107.

Conroy JL, Fang C, Gu J, et al. Opioids activate brain analgesic circuits through cytochrome P450/epoxygenase signalling. *Nat Neurosci.* 2010;13(3):284–286.

Cool DR, Normant E, Shen F, et al. Carboxypeptidase E is a regulated secretory pathway sorting receptor: genetic obliteration leads to endocrine disorders in Cpe(fat) mice. *Cell.* 1997;88(1):73–83.

Dai S, Hall DD, Hell JW. Supramolecular assemblies and localized regulation of voltage-gated ion channels. *Physiol Rev.* 2009;89(2):411–452.

de la Iglesia FA, Pace GW, Robinson GL, Huang NY, Stern W, Richards P. Tolerability and efficacy of two synergistic ratios of oral morphine and oxycodone combinations versus morphine in patients with chronic noncancer pain. *J Opioid Manag.* 2012;8(2):89–98.

Diverse-Pierluissi M, Remmers AE, Neubig RR, Dunlap K. Novel form of cross-talk between G protein and tyrosine kinase pathways. *Proc Natl Acad Sci USA.* 1997;94(10):5417–5421.

Dolphin AC. G protein modulation of voltage-gated calcium channels. *Pharmacol Rev.* 2003;55(4):607–627.

Drdla-Schutting R, Benrath J, Wunderbaldinger G, Sandkühler J. Erasure of a spinal memory trace of pain by a brief, high-dose opioid administration. *Science*. 2012;335(6065):235–238.

Evans RM, Zamponi GW. Presynaptic Ca2+ channels – integration centers for neuronal signaling pathways. *Trends Neurosci*. 2006;29(11):617–624.

Gonzales GR, Elliott KJ, Portenoy RK, et al. The impact of comprehensive evaluation in the management of cancer pain. *Pain*. 1991;47(2):141–144.

Hanlon KE, Herman DS, Agnes RS, et al. Novel peptide ligands with dual acting pharmacophores designed for the pathophysiology of neuropathic pain. *Brain Res*. 2011;1395:1–11.

Heinke B, Gingl E, Sandkühler J. Multiple targets of μ-opioid receptor-mediated presynaptic inhibition at primary afferent Aδ-and C-fibers. *J Neurosci*. 2011;31(4):1313–1322.

Heinricher MM, Martenson ME, Nalwalk JW, et al. Neural basis for improgan antinociception. *Neuroscience*. 2010a;169(3):1414–1420.

Heinricher MM, Maire JJ, Lee D, et al., Physiological basis for inhibition of morphine and improgan antinociception by CC12, a P450 epoxygenase inhibitor. *J Neurophysiol*. 2010b;104(6):3222–3230.

Heinricher MM, Ingram SL. The brainstem and noceiptive modulation. In: Bushnell MC, Basbaum AI, eds. *The Senses. A Comprehensive Reference; Pain*. San Diego, CA: Academic Press; 2008:593–626.

Hutchinson MR, Lewis SS, Coats BD, et al., Possible involvement of toll-like receptor 4/myeloid differentiation factot-2 activity of opioid inactive isomers causes spinal proinflammation and related behavioural consequences. *Neuroscience*. 2010;167(3):880–893.

Ibrahim MM, Porreca F, Lai J, et al. CB2 cannabinoid receptor activation produces antinociception by stimulating peripheral release of endogenous opioids. *Proc Natl Acad Sci U S A*. 2005;102(8):3093–3098.

Inciardi JA, Surratt HL, Kurtz SP, et al. Mechanisms of prescription drug diversion among drug-involved club- and street-based populations. *Pain Med*. 2007;8(2):171–183.

Joint Commission on the Accreditation of Healthcare Organizations (JCAHO). Patient Rights and Organization Ethics. Referenced from the Comprehensive Accreditation Manual for Hospitals, Update 3, 1999. Walter Reed Army Medical Center Web site. www.wramc.army.mil/JCAHO/Division.cfm?D_Id 1. Accessed July 5, 2007.

Joranson DE, Gilson AM. A much-needed window on opioid diversion. *Pain Med*. 2007;8(2):128–129.

Katz N. The impact of pain management on quality of life. *J Pain Symptom Manage*. 2002;24(Suppl 1):S38–S47.

Katz NP, Buse DC, Budman SH, et al. Development and preliminary experience with an ease of extractability rating for prescription opioids. *Drug Dev Ind Pharm*. 2006;32(6):727–746.

Katz NP, Adams EH, Benneyan JC, et al. Foundations of opioid risk management. *Clin J Pain*. 2007;23(2):103–118.

Kline RH 4th, Wiley R. Spinal mu-opioid receptor-expressing dorsal horn neurons: role in nociception and morphine antinociception. *J Neurosci*. 28(4):904–913.

Kommalage M, Höglund AU. Involvement of spinal GABA receptors in the regulation of intraspinal acetylcholine release. *Eur J Pharmacol*. 2005;525(1–3):69–73.

Loh YP, Maldonado A, Zhang C, et al. Mechanism of sorting proopiomelanocortin and proenkephalin to the regulated secretory pathway of neuroendocrine cells. *Ann NY Acad Sci.* 2002 ;971:416–425

Max MB, Payne R, Edwards WT, et al. *Principles of Analgesic Use in the Treatment of Acute Pain and Cancer Pain*, 4th ed. Glenview, IL: American Pain Society; 1999.

Machelska H, Brack A, Mousa SA, et al. Selectins and integrins but not platelet-endothelial cell adhesion molecule-1 regulate opioid inhibition of inflammatory pain. *Br J Pharmacol.* 2004;142(4):772–780

Machelska H, Mousa SA, Brack A, et al. Opioid control of inflammatory pain regulated by intercellular adhesion molecule-1. *J Neurosci.* 2002;22(13):5588–5596.

Mazarakou G, Georgoussi Z. STAT5A interacts with and is phosphorylated upon activation of the mu-opioid receptor. *J Neurochem.* 2005;93(4)918–931.

Mbikay M, Seidah NG, Chrétien M. Neuroendocrine secretory protein 7B2: structure, expression and functions. *Biochem J.* 2001;357(Pt 2):329–342.

McCleane G, Smith HS. Opioids for persistent noncancer Pain. *Med Clin North Am.* 2007;91(2):177–197.

Mousa SA, Shakibaei M, Sitte N, et al.. Subcellular pathways of beta-endorphin synthesis, processing, and release from immunocytes in inflammatory pain. *Endocrinology.* 2004;145(3):1331–1341.

Mousa SA. Morphological correlates of immune-mediated peripheral opioid analgesia. *Adv Exp Med Biol.* 2003;521:77–87.

Mousa SA, Machelska H, Schäfer M, Stein C. Co-expression of beta-endorphin with adhesion molecules in a model of inflammatory pain. *J Neuroimmunol.* 2000;108(1-2):160–170.

Passik SD, Kirsh KL, Whitcomb L, et al. Monitoring outcomes during long-term opioid therapy for noncancer pain: results with the Pain Assessment and Documentation Tool. *J Opioid Manage.* 2005;1(5):257–266.

Pert A, Yaksh T. Sites of morphine induced analgesia in the primate brain: relation to pain pathways. *Brain Res.* 1974;80(1):135–140.

Portenoy RK. Opioid therapy for chronic nonmalignant pain: a review of critical issues. *J Pain Symptom Manage.* 1996a;11(4):203–217.

Portenoy RK. Opioid therapy for chronic nonmalignant pain. *J Law Med Ethics.* 1996b;24(4):296-309.

Portenoy RK, Ganae-Motan ED, Allende S, et al. Nabiximols for opioid-treated cancer patients with poorly-controlled chronic pain: a randomized, placebo-controlled, graded-dose trial. *J Pain.* 2012;13(5):438–449.

Raingo J, Castiglioni AJ, Lipscombe D. Alternative splicing controls G protein-dependent inhibition of N-type calcium channels in nociceptors. *Nat Neurosci.* 2007;10(3):285–292.

Rittner HL, Labuz D, Richter JF, et al. CXCR1/2 ligands induce p38 MAPK-dependent translocation and release of opioid peptides from primary granules in vitro and in vivo. *Brain Behav Immun.* 2007;21(8):1021–1032.

Rittner HL, Labuz D, Schaefer M, et al. Pain control by CXCR2 ligands through Ca2+-regulated release of opioid peptides from polymorphonuclear cells. *FASEB J.* 2006;20(14):2627–2629.

Rittner HL, Machelska H, Stein C. Leukocytes in the regulation of pain and analgesia. *J Leukoc Biol.* 2005;78(6):1215–1222.

Rusin KI, Moises HC. Mu-Opioid receptor activation reduces multiple components of high-threshold calcium current in rat sensory neurons. *J Neurosci.* 1995;15(6):4315–4327.

Schafer M, Mousa SA, Zhang Q, et al. Expression of corticotropin-releasing factor in inflamed tissue is required for intrinsic peripheral opioid analgesia. *Proc Natl Acad Sci USA.* 1996;93(12):6096–6100.

Schäfer M, Carter L, Stein C. Interleukin 1 beta and corticotropin-releasing factor inhibit pain by releasing opioids from immune cells in inflamed tissue. *Proc Natl Acad Sci USA.* 1994;91(10):4219–4223.

Sehgal N, Smith HS, Manchikanti L. Peripherally acting opioids and clinical implications for pain control. *Pain Physician.* 2011; 14(3):249–258.

Smith HS. Variations in opioid responsiveness. *Pain Physician.* 2008a;11(2):237–248.

Smith HS. Peripherally-acting opioids. *Pain Physician.* 2008b;11(2 Suppl):S121–132.

Smith HS. Combination opioid analgesics. *Pain Physician.* 2008c;11(2):201–214.

Smith HS, Argoff CE. Pharmacological treatment of diabetic neuropathic pain. *Drugs.* 71(5):557–589.

Smith HS, Kirsh KL. Documentation and potential tools in long-term opioid therapy for pain. *Med Clin North Am.* 2007;91(2):213–228.

Smith HS, Kirsh KL, Passik SD. Chronic opioid therapy issues associated with opioid abuse potential. *J Opioid Manag.* 2009;5(5):287–300.

Strock J, Diverse-Pierluissi MA. Ca2+ channels as integrators of G protein-mediated signaling in neurons. *Mol Pharmacol.* 2004;66(5):1071–1076.

Tanaka S, Kurosumi K. A certain step of proteolytic processing of proopiomelanocortin occurs during the transition between two distinct stages of secretory granule maturation in rat anterior pituitary corticotrophs. *Endocrinology.* 1992;131(2):779–786.

Tanaka S, Nomizu M, Kurosumi K. Intracellular sites of proteolytic processing of pro-opiomelanocortin in melanotrophs and corticotrophs in rat pituitary. *J Histochem Cytochem.* 1991;39(6):809–821.

Traynor JR, Clark MJ, Remmers AE. Relationship between rate and extent of G protein activation: comparison between full and partial opioid agonists. *J Pharmacol Exp Ther.* 2002;300(1):157–161.

Urban BJ, France RD, Steinberger EK, et al. Long-term use of narcotic/antidepressant medication in the management of phantom limb pain. *Pain.* 1986;24(2):191–196.

Webster L. Efficacy and safety of dual-opioid therapy in acute pain. *Pain Med.* 2012;13 Suppl 1:S12–20.

Wilson NM, Jung H, Ripsch MS, Miller RJ, White FA. CXCR4 signaling mediates morphine-induced tactile hyperalgesia. *Brain Behav Immun.* 2011; 25(3):565–573.

Wincent A, Lidén Y, Arnér S. Pain questionnaires in the analysis of long lasting (chronic) pain conditions. *Eur J Pain.* 2003;7(4):311–321.

Zenz M, Strumpf M, Tryba M. Long-term oral opioid therapy in patients with chronic nonmalignant pain. *J Pain Symptom Manage.* 1992;7(2):69–77.

Zhang G, Chen W, Marvizón JC. Src family kinases mediate the inhibition of substance P release in the rat spinal cord by μ-opioid receptors and GABA(B) receptors, but not α2 adrenergic receptors. *Eur J Neurosci.* 2010;32(6):963–973.

Chapter 2

Overview of Opioid-Related Terminology

Kenneth C. Jackson II and Howard S. Smith

Definitions Relevant to Opioid Analgesia

Allodynia: Pain due to a stimulus that does not normally provoke pain (Merskey and Bogduk 1994).

Hyperalgesia: The perception of a painful sensation of abnormal severity, representing an exaggerated response, following a noxious stimulus.

Pain: Defined by the International Association for the Study of Pain as an unpleasant sensory and emotional experience associated with actual or potential tissue damage or described in terms of such damage (Merskey and Bogduk 1994).

The following three definitions are consensus definitions recognized by the American Academy of Pain Medicine, the American Pain Society, and the American Society of Addiction Medicine.

Addiction: A primary, chronic, neurobiologic disease with genetic, psychosocial, and environmental factors influencing its development and manifestations. It is characterized by behaviors that include one or more of the following: impaired control over drug use, compulsive use, continued use despite harm, and craving.

Physical Dependence: A state of adaptation made evident by a drug-class-specific withdrawal syndrome that can be produced by abrupt cessation, rapid dose reduction, decreasing blood level of the drug, or administration of an antagonist.

Tolerance: A state of adaptation in which exposure to a drug induces changes that result in diminution of one or more of the drug's effects over time.

Narcotic: A term historically used to describe opium and its derivatives. The word derives from a Greek word meaning "benumbing." In modern society, the word *narcotic* has become a legal term that includes a wide range of sedating and potentially abused substances; it is no longer limited to opioid analgesics. This term maintains an extremely negative connotation and should be avoided by clinicians in discussing opioid therapy with patients and other clinicians.

Opiate: A term used to describe substances derived from opium. The term *opiate* is often incorrectly used interchangeably with *opioid*.

Opioid: An opium-like substance. In the past, *opioid* was used to describe endogenous opium-like substances, and the term *opiate* described drugs derived from opium. Today *opioid* is the preferred term in both clinical and scientific dialogue for describing this class of analgesic medications.

Natural occurring opioids: Opioid analgesics isolated from the opium poppy plant. Examples include codeine and morphine.

Semi-synthetic opioids: Opioid analgesics chemically modified from substances isolated from the opium poppy plant. Examples include hydrocodone, oxycodone, and oxymorphone.

Synthetic opioids: Opioid analgesics that are completely synthesized from chemical components and do not use a substance from the opium poppy plant as the parent molecule for further modification. Examples include fentanyl, levorphanol, and methadone.

Opiophobia: The irrational fear experienced by clinicians or patients related to the appropriate use of opioid analgesics.

Pseudoaddiction: Drug-seeking behavior for the appropriate purpose of pain relief, rather than abuse or substance misuse (Weissman and Haddox 1989). It is characterized by a demand for more medication for analgesic purposes, as well as by behaviors that appear similar to those seen in addicted patients (e.g., anger, hostility). Pseudoaddiction can be differentiated from drug misuse by increasing the dose by an appropriate amount and determining whether the complaints abate.

Pseudotolerance: A situation in which opioid dose escalation occurs and appears consistent with pharmacological tolerance but, after a thoughtful evaluation, is better explained by a variety of other variables (Pappagallo 1998). These may include increased analgesic requirements due to progressive disease, presence of new pathology, or increased or excessive physical activity. Patients may also become noncompliant, have drug interactions, or even divert medications in a manner that incorrectly produces the appearance of tolerance.

Full Opioid Agonists: Medications that bind to and fully activate the opioid receptors, thereby producing maximal opioid effects.

Partial Opioid Agonists: Medications that partially occupy and activate the opioid receptors. These agents are known to maintain a dose ceiling effect that can limit their potential for dose escalation.

Mixed Opioid Agonist–Antagonists: Medications that block activity at μ opioid receptors and fully occupy and activate the κ region of the opioid receptor. These agents are known to maintain a dose ceiling effect that can limit their potential for dose escalation.

Abuse Deterrent Opioids: Medications that include a mechanism intended to decrease the misuse of opioid analgesics. (Webster et al. 2011) The deterrence mechanism can include multiple facets, including tamper resistant packaging, the addition of another pharmacological agent (e.g., opioid antagonist), or changes to the medication delivery system that can impede the use of the opioid by routes not intended for appropriate medical use.

REMS: Risk Evaluation and Mitigation Strategies. A process where the US Food and Drug Administration can require a pharmaceutical manufacturer to develop an approach that ensures the benefits of a medication outweigh the risks associated with the medication. The REMS program is not specific to opioids, but has become an integral part of the evolving landscape related to regulation of opioid analgesics.

Definitions Related to Opioid Therapy-Based Pain Categorization

Pain may be classified in many ways. One approach is to classify it according to etiology, and another is to categorize it according to its responsiveness to a particular treatment (Smith 2005). Utilizing this approach, pain many be divided into opioid-responsive pain (ORP), moderately opioid-responsive pain (MORP), and poorly opioid-responsive pain (PORP).

Opioid-Responsive Pain (ORP): Pain with a very significant response (e.g., good to excellent analgesia) to opioids (usually with low to moderate doses of opioids).

Moderately Opioid-Responsive Pain (MORP): Pain with a modest response to opioids (usually with moderate to high doses of opioids).

Poorly Opioid-Responsive Pain (PORP): Pain that responds poorly to high-dose opioid therapy.

ORP and MORP may remain as such over many years or may change over time (e.g., ORP becoming MORP or PORP, or MORP becoming PORP). There is no foolproof way to predict which pain will be opioid responsive; therefore, all pain should be assumed to be such. Furthermore, for pain to be considered truly poorly opioid-responsive, the patient should have failed to achieve significant analgesia after an appropriately high titration of multiple opioid analgesics, as there may be wide individual variation in analgesic response to different opioids.

References

Merskey H, Bogduk N. *Classification of Chronic Pain.* 2nd ed. Seattle: IASP Press; 1994.

Pappagallo M. The concept of pseudotolerance to opioids. *J Pharm Care Pain Symptom Control.* 1998;6(2):95–98.

Smith HS. Taxonomy of pain syndromes. In Pappagallo M, ed. *The Neurological Basis of Pain.* New York: McGraw-Hill, 2005; 289–300.

Webster L, St. Marie B, McCarberg B, et al. Current status and evolving role of abuse-deterrent opioids in managing patients with chronic pain. *J Opioid Manage.* 2011;7(3):235–45.

Weissman DE, Haddox JD. Opioid pseudoaddiction—an iatrogenic syndrome. *Pain.* 1989;36(3):363–366.

Chapter 3

Diagnosis and Assessment of Pain

Charles E. Argoff and Andrew Dubin

More than 50 million Americans suffer from chronic pain, including cancer pain, chronic headache, chronic neuropathic painful states (e.g., painful diabetic neuropathy, postherpetic neuralgia [PHN], and complex regional pain syndrome [CRPS]), and chronic musculoskeletal pain, including soft-tissue pain disorders (e.g., chronic myofascial pain and fibromyalgia). On an annual basis, chronic pain increases health care costs and disables more people than do heart disease and cancer combined. However, chronic pain is often viewed as a symptom rather than the chronic disease that it can become.

Early evaluation and assessment are critical to the treatment of pain. Inadequate treatment of acute pain can lead to a progression to chronic pain in some but not all patients. The mechanisms that allow this to happen (e.g., a progression from acute herpetic neuralgia, or shingles, to PHN) are not completely understood; however, anatomic and physiologic changes may occur in the peripheral and/or central nervous system (CNS) and can facilitate the development of chronic pain. This may result in persistent pain beyond the time after healing, as is characteristic of chronic pain states. Since it is not possible to predict with certainty whether acute pain will evolve into chronic pain for any individual patient, each patient must be properly assessed, diagnosed, and assertively treated so that everything that can be done to prevent the development of chronic pain is done.

Pain that is improperly assessed or inadequately managed can result in reductions in functional capacity and diminished quality of life. Untreated pain may have a significant negative impact on a patient's ability to function from both a physical and a cognitive viewpoint. All normal activities—including employment, recreation, and routine activities of daily living—may be adversely affected. Not infrequently, patients with chronic pain may develop or experience exacerbations of depression, anxiety, and sleep disturbances, as well as loss of self-esteem. Lost workdays, impaired job performance, absenteeism, and presenteeism are some of the ways in which employment can be impacted by the presence of chronic pain.

The clinical assessment is the first step in the management of any pain problem. The pain assessment provides the basis for the therapeutic relationship between physician and patient and allows the physician to try to characterize the pain, identify its cause, and develop a treatment plan. Table 3.1 presents a list of specific questions that can be asked during the pain assessment (Argoff 2006).

Table 3.1 Pain Assessment Questions

1. When did the pain start?
2. Was the specific onset of the pain remembered (as for example, with postherpetic neuralgia or trauma)?
3. Was there a specific cause to the pain (e.g., injury, surgery)?
4. Are there already known medical or surgical conditions for the patient (e.g., diabetes, osteoarthritis, osteoporosis, connective tissue disease) that can provide clues regarding the cause of the chronic pain?
5. For how long has the pain existed?
6. Where is the pain?
7. What does the pain feel like—is it sharp, stabbing, dull, throbbing, aching, burning, knife-like, or a combination of these?
8. What impact on physical function is associated with the pain?
9. What makes it better? What makes it worse?
10. Are there past medical, neurologic, or psychosocial factors that help you, the treatment provider, to understand the pain better?
11. What diagnostic testing is required to assist in the assessment?
12. Is there a history of substance abuse?
13. Is there a history of tobacco or alcohol use?

Characterizing the Pain

To determine the appropriate management approach, the pain must be properly characterized. A detailed pain history should include assessment of the following:

- **Location.** The location of the pain should be identified; that is, is the pain generalized, is it experienced at one or more sites (i.e., focal or multifocal), or is it experienced at a site remote from the perceived causative lesion (i.e., referred pain)? It is essential to distinguish between focal, multifocal, and generalized pain in order to target appropriate diagnostic and therapeutic interventions.

- **Temporal characteristics.** The pain's temporal characteristics, such as its onset and duration, its course and daily variation, and whether it is continuous or intermittent, should be identified. The absence or presence of breakthrough pain should be determined.

- **Aggravating or relieving factors.** Is the pain associated with certain types of movements, positions, or activities? What factors relieve the pain?

- **Intensity.** Understanding the intensity of the pain is critical to therapeutic decision making because it influences the selection of analgesic drug, route of administration, and rate of dose titration. What is the average pain, least pain, worst pain, and current pain?

- **Quality.** The quality of the pain can suggest its pathophysiology. For example, neuropathic pain may be described as burning, tingling, or lancinating.

Pathophysiology of the Pain

The success of the assessment and treatment of chronic pain may be enhanced by recognition of the difference between nociceptive, inflammatory, and neuropathic pain. Nociceptors are specialized nerve endings that can respond to typical "normal" pain-producing stimuli (thermal, chemical, mechanical) and other potential causes of tissue damage. An activated nociceptor, through C and Aδ nerve fibers, transmits its pain-producing information from the peripheral nerves to the CNS, where it is processed further at spinal cord and brain levels. Pain does not occur until the appropriate areas of the brain are activated; that is, "there is no such thing as pain without a brain." A person does not experience nociceptive input as pain unless the nociceptive information reaches appropriate areas of the brain. Inflammation may play a major role not only in acute pain, but also in the development of chronic pain. In contrast, neuropathic pain results from injury to the peripheral nervous system or CNS. Ongoing injury is not required for these abnormalities to be expressed. There is actually fairly clear evidence that neuropathic pain results from reorganization of the nervous system following injury. Peripheral and central sensitization are the key mechanisms involved in the development of a neuropathic state. This reorganization of the nervous system may lead to a lowered threshold to the nociceptive processing that may now occur. Stimuli that may not normally be painful now, in the neuropathic pain state, elicit pain (allodynia). Although allodynia may occur following an acute injury as a result of normal nociceptive or inflammatory mechanisms, it is not normal for this to continue indefinitely. Stimuli that are normally painful may be more painful than usual (hyperalgesia). Any sensory stimuli, painful or otherwise, may be perceived in an exaggerated manner (hyperesthesia). These clinical findings are characteristic of neuropathic pain and reflect an altered nervous system that is now able to facilitate pain production to a higher extent, because it is more easily excitable than it would be in a normal state. It must be emphasized that neuropathic pain may therefore be experienced even when the affected individual is not subjected to a tissue-damaging stimulus. Although it is not appropriate to view all chronic pain states as neuropathic, CNS changes that facilitate pain transmission have been postulated in chronic pain as well. The specific mechanisms underlying this transformation are being actively studied; their elucidation may hold the key to the prevention of both acute and chronic pain, as well as best treatments for these conditions. Among the many different chronic pain states for which this could be relevant are PHN, CRPS, chronic headache, chronic pain related to degenerative joint disease, chronic low back pain, and fibromyalgia.

Identifying the Cause of Pain

The goals of the clinical assessment include not only making the pain diagnosis, but also attempting to make the diagnosis as specific as possible. Determining the cause of chronic pain poses certain clinical challenges. Diagnostic strategies that may be effective for acute painful conditions are often of little help in diagnosing chronic pain. When assessing chronic pain it is important to determine the etiology of the pain complaint; however, it may not always be recognizable. Acute pain and cancer-related pain usually have an identifiable physical cause, and in many cases chronic nonmalignant pain results from an identifiable cause as well. In other cases, however, although a true physical cause for the chronic pain exists, it may be difficult to recognize this source. Failure to identify the cause of pain should not preclude its proper treatment. Unfortunately for some patients with chronic pain, when a physical cause cannot be found, the pain, in numerous cases, is attributed to psychological problems. Often, the pain complaint is dismissed or inadequately treated, causing the patient to suffer needlessly. Like other chronic illnesses that do not have a clear etiology, chronic pain should be managed aggressively. For example, despite the fact that hypertension does not have a clear cause in most patients, it is a highly recognized, assertively treated condition. Patients with chronic pain deserve the same level of care.

Pain Assessment Tools

Because pain is a subjective experience, the patient's self-report provides the most valid measure for assessment. Several pain-assessment tools are currently available, and new tools are being developed. Individual patients with chronic pain often report widely different pain levels even for similar conditions and similar degrees of functional impairment. It is important to always assess the intensity of pain, as well as the degree of functional impairment, in a person with chronic pain. As an example, the brief pain inventory addresses not only the pain level but also the impact of that pain on various functional domains. It is a validated tool, takes only minutes to complete, and is a practical way for a doctor in a busy practice to assess not only chronic pain but also the results of its treatment. It was originally developed for patients with cancer-related pain. Unidimensional tools such as the visual analogue scale or the pain intensity scale assess only the intensity of pain, not its effects on function, and are therefore not as desirable as multidimensional tools. Special tools such as the FACES scale may be appropriate for patients who are cognitively impaired. Special tools are available for the assessment of neuropathic pain as well. See Table 3.2 for a list of some of the available assessment tools (Galer and Jensen 1997; Krause and Backonja 2003; Williamson and Hoggart 2005; Resnik and Dobreykowski 2005; Bennett et al. 2006; Jensen 2006).

Physical Examination in Pain Assessment

In addition to characterizing the pain complaint, a comprehensive pain assessment includes a physical examination and, if appropriate, laboratory and radiographic procedures. Diagnostic testing is useful for making as specific a diagnosis as possible, but it must not be used to verify or invalidate the

Table 3.2 Pain Assessment Tools
Unidimensional Tools
Numerical Pain Rating Scale
Visual Analog Scale
Multidimensional Tools
Brief Pain Inventory
Multidimensional Pain Inventory
SF-36
Disability Scales
Sickness Impact Profile
Roland-Morris Disability Scale
Special Scales
Neuropathic Pain Scale (NPS)
Neuropathic Pain Questionnaire (NPQ)
Neuropathic Pain Symptom Inventory (NPSI)

complaint of pain. Unfortunately, the limitations of available diagnostic tests such as magnetic resonance imaging (MRI) and electrophysiological tests (e.g., electromyography/nerve conduction velocity) have often led examiners to tell their patients that there is nothing wrong with them. For example, the degree of structural abnormality of the lumbar spine detected by MRI does not necessarily correlate with the severity of pain experienced by a patient with chronic low back pain. MRI may detect little or no structural abnormality in individuals with severe low back pain, but this modality may show disc herniations or other structural problems in those with no low back pain. Electrophysiological tests may be normal in patients with painful small-fiber neuropathies and other painful conditions. Although a normal test is completely consistent with the pathophysiology of small-fiber neuropathy, a negative test result often prompts some to question the legitimacy of the pain rather than acknowledge the limitations of the test. (Also, electrophysiologic abnormalities may develop three to four weeks after neural insult but be normal immediately after neural insult.)

Chronic pain presents unique challenges. While many times an obvious cause or source for acute pain can be elucidated by performing a detailed yet focused history and physical, the same cannot always be said for chronic pain syndromes. Unfortunately, this all too often results in the practitioners treating chronic pain as a psychological issue, rather than delving into other possible causes. The history and physical examination are vitally important in assessing the patient with chronic pain. Without this, one is unable to develop a plan of care that will allow for optimization of the patient's function, quality of life, and control of his or her pain.

A common chronic pain complaint seen in physiatric as well as orthopedic practices is one of ankle and foot pain. Orthopedic surgeons, by virtue of their unique training, are keenly aware of causes of acute pain syndromes involving the foot and ankle. Chronic pain syndromes present a more problematic issue, and require thorough investigation for treatable causes.

The physical examination of the ankle, foot, and toes should start with inspection, followed by palpation. Obvious bony deformities or malalignment issues should be noted. This can be seen in cases of post traumatic or acquired arthritis, rheumatoid arthritis, neuropathic Charcot joints, or as a manifestation of a chronic crystal induced arthropathy. Synovial hypertrophy at the ankle may be seen in patients with underlying rheumatoid arthritis and can easily be appreciated on palpation.

Palpation of the anterior ankle joint, between the medial and lateral malleoli, may reveal crepitus with plantar flexion and dorsi flexion. This would be consistent with true ankle joint degenerative joint disease (DJD), as the range of motion for the true ankle joint is limited to dorsi and plantar flexion. Crepitus with inversion and eversion of the heel region (hind foot) is found in subtalar joint pathology. Both the true ankle joint and subtalar joint can be involved in arthritis, as well as neuropathic Charcot joint deformity.

The foot is a unique structure. It is designed to interact with a variety of surfaces and tolerate significant cyclical loading. As such it must be able to bear significant weight while maintaining flexibility. Additionally, it serves as the terminal device for the leg and must retain exquisite sensory function to perform this task. Any compromise in mechanical structure or sensory function predisposes the foot to develop chronic pain issues.

Structurally, the foot is composed of the tarsal bones, metatarsal, and phalanges. The tarsal bones include the calcaneous, talus, navicular, cuboid, and the three cuneiform bones.

Functionally the foot can be divided into the hind foot, mid foot, and fore foot. The hind foot is composed of the calcaneous, talus, and subtalar joint. The mid foot is made up of the navicular, cuboid, and three cuneiform bones. The fore foot is composed of the metatarsals and phalanges. The foot has multiple articulations, but three joints of particular interest in regards to pain and associated gait dysfunction. The subtalar joint allows for hind foot inversion and eversion. The Chopart joint, also referred to as the midtarsal joint, is made up of the talo-navicular articulation as well as the calcaneo cuboid articulation. By virtue of its articulations it serves a major role in transmitting load to the mid foot and fore foot during ambulation. The Lis Franc joint refers to the tarsometatarsal articulation, and is important in the gait cycle as weight is transferred over the limb and the body continues through the rollover phase of the gait cycle. Functionally, the tarsometatarsal complex can be divided into three columns. The medial column (the first metatarsal-medial cuneiform joint), the middle column (the second and third tarsometatarsal joints as well as the articulations between the middle and lateral cuneiforms), and the lateral column (the articulations between the fourth and fifth metarsals and the cuboid). All of these joints should be placed thru their ranges of motion and palpated for crepitus during the exam. Pain with range of motion should be noted, as well as restrictions in range compared to the contra lateral foot. Structural issues such as a tarsal coalition can be an unappreciated cause of chronic foot pain. This can present with complaints of hind foot and mid foot pain, with physical exam findings of a fixed planovalgus (flat foot) foot deformity. This may also manifest with a persistently spastic dystonic peroneus longus and brevis muscle group, causing a functional dystonic foot. Imaging with CT scan or MRI will reveal the tarsal coalition if present.

Additional observation of the foot should include assessment of the medial longitudinal arch with and without weight bearing. Loss of the arch with weight bearing, but preservation while not weight bearing, can be seen in ligamentous laxity and a flexible flat foot deformity. Loss of the arch, with and without weight bearing, speaks to a true bony structural deformity requiring additional assessment of the bony foot.

The phalanges should be viewed as well. Obvious hallux valgus or bunion deformities should be made note of. This can be seen in arthritis of the great toe, and will manifest with pain during the push off phase of the gait cycle. Range of motion of the great toe should be assessed with and without weight bearing. Loss of the ability to passively dorsiflex the great toe while the patient is weight bearing can be due to tightness of the flexor hallicus longus tendon as well as the Achilles tendon complex, and is a common source of medial arch pain and a functional hallux rigidus.

Evalauation of the ankle and foot is incomplete without assessment of sensation, pulses, and motor strength for dorsi flexion, plantar flexion, and great toe extension and flexion. Achilles reflexes should be checked and compared side to side. Abnormal sensation in both feet with absent achilles reflexes in a patient with a deformed foot raises the specter of an underlying neuropathy with a neuropathic etiology for the foot deformity. All major sensory modalities should be assessed, including light touch, pin sensation, and appreciation of both hot and cold.

Absent dorsalis pedis and posterior tibial pulses can be seen with peripheral vascular disease (PVD), which can be part of underlying systemic issues such as PVD from diabetes.

Carpal tunnel syndrome (CTS) would appear at first blush to be an easy diagnosis to establish. Unfortunately, like a chameleon, it is a great masquerader. Many things can look like CTS. Numbness of the hand involving the thumb, index, and long fingers can be CTS, but the differential diagnosis can also include cervical radiculopathy, cervical myelopathy, upper trunk/lateral cord level brachial plexopathy, compression at the elbow (ligament of Struthers syndrome), or pronator teres syndrome. Additionally, rotator cuff tendonitis as well as cervical myofascial pain syndromes may produce muscle referral pain patterns that mimic a C 5,6 and even C 7 distribution. Complex regional pain syndromes (CRPS), both neurogenic and soft tissue in etiology, can result in complaints of hand numbness, tingling, and pain. Given the complexity of upper extremity pain complaints and the potential for overlap, the physical examination takes on paramount importance. Initial evaluation should focus on inspection of the involved hand. Observe for atrophy of the thenar eminence. This is not a common finding, but when seen it is highly suggestive of severe CTS, and carries with it a poor prognosis for recovery even with surgical decompression.

If hypothenar and thenar eminence atrophy are noted, CTS becomes less likely as an isolated entity, and a C 8 level radiculopathy, lower trunk brachial plexopathy, or even cervical myelopathy start to increase as possibilities.

Examination must include evaluation of sensory function. Mapping out of median nerve sensory function must be assessed, and should be compared to ulnar and radial sensory function to confirm alteration in median sensation. Care should be taken to document that thenar sensation is retained in the face of decreased median distribution sensation in the fingers. Thenar eminence sensation should be retained in CTS, as the median thenar branch traverses over the transverse carpal ligament rather than thru the carpal tunnel. Loss of thenar mass region sensation in concert with altered radial sensory sensation should raise the specter of a C 6 level radiculopathy versus cervical myelopathy.

Tinels sign, tapping over the median nerve at the wrist, may result in tingling in a median nerve distribution. This finding is neither sensitive nor specific for CTS and can be elicited with percussion over a noncompressed nerve. A positive carpal pressure test, pressure applied for 30 seconds over the distal transverse ligament, may also result in production of numbness and tingling in a median nerve distribution. Once again, this test is neither sensitive nor specific. The Phalens test is also neither sensitive nor specific.

Evaluation of the involved upper extremity must also include assessment of reflexes. A C 6 or C 6, 7 level radiculopathy can mimic CTS in pain and sensory dysfunction distribution. With a C 6 level radiculopathy, however, there will be associated blunting of the wrist extensor reflex. With a C 7 radiculopathy, blunting of the triceps reflex will be noted. Additionally, a positive Spurlings sign may be noted. Spurlings sign is reproduction of radicular symptoms with cervical extension and lateral flexion to the involved side. With a C 6 radiculopathy, an abduction tension release sign may be noted. This will manifest with improvement of symptoms with placement of the involved arm on top of the patients head. The abduction tension release sign will also help differentiate shoulder pain from impingement syndrome from C 5 level radiculopathy with associated shoulder pain. In impingement syndrome the pain will worsen with attempted placement in an abduction tension release sign position. Manual muscle testing is also required to rule out a cervical radiculopathy. Weakness of the biceps and wrist extensors can be seen in a C 6 radiculopathy.

Weakness of the triceps and flexor digitorum superficialis can be seen with a C 7 radiculopathy. A C 8, T 1 level radiculopathy can cause weakness of the thenar muscles, but should not be mistaken for CTS as the sensory disturbances will be along the ulnar border of the hand. Hyperreflexia should also be noted. Loss of a wrist extensor reflex, with brisk triceps patella and achilles reflexes noted, should trigger an investigation for a possible C 6 level radiculomyelopathy. Notation of ankle clonus or Hoffmanns signs in the upper extremity finger flexors adds additional support to the diagnosis. In chronic upper extremity pain syndromes it is critical to realize that cervical myelopathy, radiculopathy, brachial plexopathy, median nerve compression at the elbow or pronator teres or wrist, can overlap in terms of presentation. As such, before accepting the diagnosis of an undifferentiated chronic pain syndrome care must be taken to rule out clearly definable and potentially treatable causes.

Upper extremity pain syndromes present unique challenges. They result in impairments of activities of daily living, impact on quality of life, and can be frustrating to diagnose—but also rewarding to treat. Shoulder region pain is a very common, but nonspecific complaint that can be due to multiple etiologies. An understanding of shoulder anatomy is imperative for understanding the causes of shoulder pain. The shoulder is made up of multiple articulations, including the glenohumeral, acromioclavicular, and sternoclavicular joints, as well as a scapulothoracic articulation. Multiple muscles act at the shoulder joint. These include the deltoid, biceps, triceps, latissimus dorsi, pectoralis major, trapezius, rhomboids levator scapulae, serratus anterior, and the rotator cuff muscle group. Any of these muscles can directly or indirectly cause referral pain to the shoulder area. The deltoid, biceps, triceps pectoralis major, latissmus dorsi, and rotoator cuff muscles (spraspinatus, infrapsinatus teres minor, and subscapularis) are primary movers of the gleno-humeral joint. The trapezius, rhomboids, and serratus anterior are scapular stabilizers. Scapular stabilization is imperative for upper extremity function, loss of which can result in significant shoulder pain and dysfunction.

Functionally, the shoulder is a ball and socket joint. Unlike the hip, which is also a ball and socket joint, the shoulder is not intrinsically stable. The shallow nature of the glenoid cup allows for increased range of motion (ROM) but sacrifices stability. The cup is augmented by a labrum that serves to deepen the glenoid cup. Ultimately, the stability and function of the gleno-humeral joint is dependent upon the surrounding musculature.

Degenerative joint disease of the shoulder can involve the gleno-humeral (GH) joint, as well as the acromoclavicular (AC) joint, either in isolation or in combination. The challenge is trying to determine the source generator for the shoulder pain. Intra-articular, musculo-tendonus, bursal, or neurogenic are all potential causes.

Observation during history taking is imperative. Patients with DJD of the shoulder will subconsciously guard the spontaneous movement of the shoulder. Without realizing it, they will keep all ranges of motion below shoulder height and within a restricted pain free arc.

Additionally, observe for atrophy of the deltoid, supraspinatus, infraspinatus, and biceps muscles. This will require side-to-side comparison, as subtle atrophy can be missed if only the affected extremity is examined. Atrophy involving all of the above muscles could be secondary to cervical root level issues at C 5, 6, or may be secondary to disuse atrophy from pain. Disuse atrophy typically results in decreased muscle volume, but the overall shape and contour of the muscle will be maintained. Neurogenic atrophy typically results in severe loss of muscle volume and alteration in the contour and shape of the involved muscle or muscle groups. Focal atrophy of the deltoid may be secondary to axillary nerve neuropathy. Focal atrophy of rotator cuff musculature can be neurogenic in etiology as well as secondary to rotator cuff tear.

In assessing the shoulder with DJD it is critical to determine if there is an underlying cervical radiculopathy or isolated axillary nerve neuropathy, as this will complicate the management and prognosis.

Range of motion assessment should be done both passively and actively. Elicitation of pain with the examiner ranging the shoulder joint thru internal and external rotation is consistent with shoulder DJD. This is less likely to be seen in a rotator cuff tendonitis, which is typically more painful on volitional patient activation. Crepitus on range of motion testing is also a common feature of shoulder DJD.

Manual muscle testing of the internal and external rotators of the shoulders should be carried out with the arm at the side and with the elbow flexed at 90 degrees. In this way GH rotation can be tested without placing the arm in an abducted position, which will be poorly tolerated if there is DJD involving the GH joint. Shoulder abduction can be assessed in an isometric manner with the arm at the side and having the person attempt active abduction at the GH joint while resistance is applied. Once again, this allows for strength assessment while avoiding painful arcs of motion. Biceps function is assessed by having the person flex the elbow against resistance applied to the volar forearm. Upper muscle fiber subscapularis function can be assessed with the belly press test. This is performed by having the patient press the palm of his or her hand into the belly using the internal rotators of the shoulder. A positive test is noted if the elbow drops to the side or behind the trunk. The lift-off test evaluates the lower fibers of the subscapularis, and is performed by having the patient place the dorsum of the hand at the position of the mid lumbar spine. The test is considered positive if the patient is unable to lift off the hand utilizing internal rotation at the GH joint, and substitutes shoulder extension or elbow extension to perform the maneuver. An incompetent rotator cuff results in superior migration of the humeral head within the glenoid, causing impingement, which in turn further exacerbates the functional deficits of the shoulder with underlying DJD. The grading for strength testing is on the 0 to 5 scale, with 0 being no activation, 1 flicker of activity without motion, 2 full range of motion gravity eliminated, 3 full range of motion against gravity only, 4 full range of motion against greater than gravity resistance, (able to take partial resistance), and lastly 5, which is full range of motion against full resistance.

Critical elements of sensory testing include the axillary patch or sergeants or regimental patch to assess C 5 as well as axillary nerve function. Sensory function to the lateral forearm is via the lateral antebrachial cutaneous nerve. This is the sensory continuation of the musculocutaneous nerve, which in turn supplies motor function to the biceps, coracobrachialis, and brachialis muscles. Sensory function to the thumb and index finger allows for evaluation of C 6 root level function. Detailed evaluation of C 5,6 level root function is imperative as the major nerve supply to the shoulder musculature derives from the C 5,6 roots.

The resolution of shoulder pain with placement of the affected arm on top of the head, a positive abduction tension release sign is highly suggestive of a C 5 level radiculopathy and for all practical purposes rules out GH DJD, subacromial bursitis, or impingement syndrome as the source of the shoulder pain. The complaint of deep gnawing aching type pain at the level of the rhomboid major muscle, just medial to the medial scapular border, is also highly suggestive of C 5 root level involvement.

AC joint pathology can be assessed by the scratch test. The patient is asked to reach across their anterior chest to touch the posterior aspect of the contralateral shoulder, as if they where scratching their shoulder. A positive test will elicit pain over the ipsilateral AC joint with an audible and palpable clunk being appreciated many times. This is classically seen in the face of a history of previous AC joint separation.

Physical examination is the mainstay in the evaluation of the shoulder. Electrodiagnostic testing can have utility if one suspects radiculopathy, brachial plexopathy, or an isolated axillary or suprascapular nerve neuropathy. The diagnosis of complex regional pain syndrome, both neurogenic and soft tissue in etiology, can usually be established by performing a detailed physical. Successful management of upper extremity pain is dependent upon determining the etiology of the pain.

Lower extremity pain can be a vexing problem. It may be structural, neurogenic, muscular, connective tissue, or a combination of the above in etiology. Referral pain is common. Knee region pain is a common location for pain complaints in the lower extremity. The most common cause for knee pain is knee pathology, but referral pain from hip pathology is common. Radicular pain from L 3,4 root compression can also cause knee region pain. It can lead to mobility and activities of daily living (ADL) deficits. Patients may complain of pain with activity. Stair climbing, kneeling, or squatting activities will be poorly tolerated. With aging, the incidence of knee arthritis increases. Arthritis can be as a result of cumulative wear and tear, or secondary to antecedent trauma. Typically it involves the femoral tibial articulation. Less frequently the patellofemoral joint can be involved. The femoral tibial joint is composed of a medial and lateral joint space. The medial joint space is more commonly involved in DJD of the knee. The mechanics and weight bearing thru the medial joint and the medial meniscus cartilage predispose the medial joint space to preferential involvement.

Swelling of the knee region can present diagnostic challenges. Low-grade repetitive trauma is a common cause of pre-patella bursitis. Swelling of the prepatella bursa can cause dramatic distention of the pre patella region. Despite the swelling, significant pain is an uncommon complaint. Pre-patella bursa swelling with associated pain raises the specter of an infected bursa.

The pes anserine bursa serves as a mechanical buffer between the bony medial tibial flare and the attachment of the semitendonosis, sartorious, and grascilis muscles. Pes anserine bursitis will present with pain along the medial tibial flare, below the true knee joint, and typically results from direct blunt trauma to the area.

Patients with knee arthritis will have several common complaints. Pain with weight bearing is a frequent complaint. Additionally, patients will complain of pain transitioning from sit to stand. Not infrequently they will also note a sensation of knee instability or buckling. The buckling sensation can be due to joint instability, or pain inhibition of quadriceps function. Swelling if seen is usually mild, unless there is an underlying inflammatory process such as rheumatoid arthritis, infection, or superimposed acute trauma. As the medial joint space is more commonly involved in DJD, medial joint collapse with varus knee deformity is the hallmark finding in late stage knee DJD. Rheumatoid arthritis typically involves synovial and ligamentous structures early on, and results in ligamentous laxity. This in turn leads to accentuation of the normal anatomic structural valgus at the knee. Therefore, observation of a valgus knee deformity should raise the question of possible underlying rheumatoid arthritis. As the deformity progresses range of motion will be lost. Patients will lose end range terminal extension, which will contribute to the sensation of knee instability or weakness. A loss of flexion will impair the patient's ability to come from sit to stand, and as such patients may note that they avoid soft chairs or chairs without armrests.

Physical examination of the knee starts with visual inspection, and should include observation of overall alignment of the knee as well as any obvious swelling. Observation of gait is also critical to for assess dynamic instability. Analysis of stance time on the involved limb will give information regarding pain with standing. Symmetric lower extremity stance time argues against pain even in the face of deformity. Shortened stance time on the involved limb would be consistent with pain or instability of the limb, now increasing the significance of any structural deformity that might be observed.

Palpation allows for the assessment of swelling as well as possible source generators of pain. Palpation of the medial and lateral joint lines may be painful, depending upon which joint compartment is more involved with DJD. The medial collateral ligament will shorten and the lateral collateral ligament will stretch in the patient with a varus knee deformity. Attempts at stretching the medial collateral ligament by applying a valgus force will elicit pain. The opposite will be seen in the patient with an underlying valgus knee deformity from DJD or more commonly rheumatoid arthritis. Gentle downward pressure over the patella compresses the patello-femoral joint and allows for assessment of retro-patella DJD, a common source of knee pain. Palpation of the pes anserine bursa will be exquisitely painful in an acute traumatic bursitis.

Range of motion should be assessed. Loss of terminal extension or inability to flex the knee beyond 90 degrees has functional implications. Loss of terminal extension increases the patient's sensation of instability and buckling during weight bearing. Loss of flexion beyond 90 degrees can make ascending stairs and transitioning from sit to stand problematic.

Reflexes should always be evaluated. Loss of the patella reflex on the involved side may be secondary to an L 4 radiculopathy or an incomplete femoral nerve neuropathy. Both scenarios complicate the rehabilitation of the patient with a painful knee as weakness and associated instability may persist even after structural deformity issues are addressed.

Psychosocial Factors and Other Comorbidities

Psychosocial factors often play a role in the chronic pain experience, adding to the complexity of the evaluation and treatment of these disorders. Chronic pain rarely occurs without psychological factors such as anxiety, depression, and anger. These factors should be identified early in the assessment, and the patient's attitudes and beliefs about pain should be understood.

Clarifying Expectations of Chronic Pain Management

Beginning with the assessment and throughout the course of treatment, the patient must have a clear understanding of the goals of chronic pain management.

These goals must be realistic; generally, physicians and patients should aim to reduce pain and improve quality of life and functioning to the fullest extent possible. Complete resolution of the pain is much more likely to occur in patients with acute pain than in those with chronic pain. The evaluation and treatment of chronic pain almost never lead to a medication, nerve block, or new exercise that will "cure" the pain. In truth, full resolution of the pain is not likely to occur. The management of chronic pain does involve a detailed assessment of the problem, including both medical and nonmedical aspects, and the development of a comprehensive treatment plan. The patient with chronic pain must have the expectation that the pain will be managed as successfully as possible, and the understanding that it will not be cured. Following a detailed assessment of the problem, medical, physical rehabilitative, and psychosocial treatment strategies may all be appropriate to consider.

Conclusion

The management of pain—and especially chronic pain—should be viewed in the same way as the management of any other chronic disease. The proper diagnosis and assessment of pain are critical for determining the appropriate therapies and evaluating their relative effectiveness. Once a comprehensive evaluation has been completed, a treatment plan can be implemented and monitored. The goal of the treatment plan is to provide acceptable analgesia with an acceptable side-effect profile using pharmacologic, interventional, rehabilitative, and cognitive-behavioral approaches singly or in combination.

References

Argoff CE. Chronic pain management: general principles. In Johnson RT, Griffin JW, McArthur JC, eds. *Current Therapy in Neurologic Disease*. 7th ed. Philadelphia: Mosby Elsevier, 2006; 55–57.

Bennett ML, Smith BH, Terrance N, et al. Can pain be more or less neuropathic? Comparison of symptom assessment tools with ratings of certainty by clinicians. *Pain*. 2006;122(3):289–294.

Galer BS, Jensen MP. Development and preliminary validation of a pain measure specific to neuropathic pain: the Neuropathic Pain Scale. *Neurology*. 1997;48(2):332–338.

Jensen MP. Using pain quality assessment measures for selecting analgesic agents. *Clin J Pain*. 2006;22(1 Suppl):S9–S13.

Krause SJ, Backonja MM. Development of a neuropathic pain questionnaire. *Clin J Pain*. 2003;19(5):306–314.

Resnik L, Dobreykowski E. Outcomes measurement for patients with low back pain. *Orthop Nurs*. 2005;24(1):14–24.

Williamson A, Hoggart B. Pain: a review of three commonly used pain rating scales. *J Clin Nurs*. 2005;14(7):794–804.

Chapter 4

Opioid Pharmacology

Mellar P. Davis and Howard S. Smith

Opioids have a long, rich history in the management of pain and have emerged as the major drug class for the treatment of moderate to severe cancer pain. Opioids have a unique pharmacology. Their oral bioavailability is variable, depending upon the type of opioid. They are metabolized by type I cytochromes and type II conjugase enzymes (Inturrisi 2002). Half-life varies significantly from one agent to another.

Pharmacokinetics

Opioids can be divided into those with good and those with poor oral bio-availability. Opioids with poor oral bioavailability have high first-pass clearance through the liver rather than poor diffusion through the gastrointestinal mucosa (Shand et al. 1975; Bullingham et al. 1984; Chauvin et al. 1986; Callaghan et al. 1993; O'Brien et al. 1996; Tegeder et al. 1999).

The bioavailability of oral morphine ranges from approximately 25% to 35% and demonstrates large interindividual variability. In addition to morphine, several other lipophilic opioids—including fentanyl, sufentanil, alfentanil, and buprenorphine—have 30% or less oral bioavailability (see Table 4.1). Generally, with the exception of morphine, opioids with poor oral bioavailability are delivered by routes that bypass hepatic first-pass clearance (e.g., subcutaneous, transdermal, sublingual).

Opioid clearance is dependent upon the individual expression of certain enzymes (CYP3A4, CYP2D6, UGT2B7) and transporters (e.g., P-glycoprotein) (Smith 2011; Leppert 2011). The expression of hepatocyte enzymes (CYP3A4, CYP2D6, CYP1A2, UGT1A1, UGT2B7) is genetically determined. (Zhang and Benet 2001; Smith 2011; Leppert 2011) (see Table 4.2).

Overall, opioid clearance will depend on (1) the volume of distribution (Vd, which is a theoretical volume; volumes larger than body size actually reflect

Table 4.1 Opioids with 30% or Less Oral Bioavailability
Morphine
Fentanyl
Sufentanil
Alfentanil
Buprenorphine

Table 4.2 Opioids and Enzymes Involved in Metabolism				
Opioid	CYP3A4	CYP2D6	CYP1A2	UGT2B7
Morphine				+
Hydromorphone				+
Oxycodone		+		
Methadone	+	+	+	
Fentanyl	+			
Sufentanil	+			
Alfentanil	+			
Tramadol		+		
Codeine		+		
Hydrocodone		+		

tissue binding) and (2) intrinsic enzyme activity of cytochromes, conjugase enzymes and enzyme expression outside of the liver (CYP3A4 and UGT2B7). Certain enzymes can be induced (CYP3A4) that result in increased drug clearance over time, and others are inhibited by comedications (CYP2D6, CYP3A4) which prolong opioid clearance (Lin and Lu 1998; Tukey and Strassburg 2000; Lamba et al. 2002; Ingelman-Sundberg 2004; Kiang et al. 2005). The half-life of an opioid will, therefore, be a direct function of Vd, inversely related to intrinsic drug clearance (CL_{int}), ($T_{1/2} = Vd/CL_{int}$) and influenced by co-medication and organ failure. Certain drugs (e.g., methadone) have a large Vd and relatively low CL_{int} and as a result will have a long half-life. Hydrophilic drugs with a smaller Vd and greater intrinsic clearance will have a shorter half-life (Lehmann 1997).

There are wide interindividual variabilities in opioid metabolism secondary to pharmacogenetically determined differences in enzyme expression (Wilkinson 2005). Patients with two defective genes (CYP2D6) will not clear certain opioids (e.g., tramadol, codeine) well or may fail to activate an opioid (e.g., codeine, tramadol) that works through a metabolite (e.g., morphine, and o-desmethyltramadol) (Leppert 2011). Codeine is activated to morphine by CYP2D6; therefore, poor metabolizers or intermediate metabolizers with two slow metabolizing genes (CYP2D6 #10 or 17) will not experience adequate pain relief with codeine or tramadol which are activated by CYP2D6 (Wilkinson 2005; Leppert 2011).

Opioid half-life is not dependent on route of administration. Certain delivery systems (oral sustained release, transdermal reservoir, or matrix patch) prolong drug delivery and, as a result, the pharmaceutical preparation extends the time to steady state. Time to steady state and dose intervals are related to the opioid half-life. Dosing intervals that are longer than the half-life lead to the resurgence of pain, while too short an interval causes opioid accumulation and potential toxicity.

Organ failure prolongs drug half-life in accordance to how much drug clearance is dependent upon the damaged organ (Volles and McGory 1999). Glucuronidated opioids (e.g., morphine, hydromorphone, and perhaps buprenorphine) have relatively well preserved pharmacokinetics in hepatic renal failure and are relatively safe, since glucuronidation is well preserved in liver failure and conjugases are expressed in organs outside the liver. However, bioavailability of glucuronidated opioids will be increased due to shunting, since most have high hepatic first-pass clearance.

Certain lipophilic opioids such as fentanyl have significant tissue binding (tissue partition) and will accumulate with around-the-clock (ATC) dosing. Fentanyl accumulates in muscle and fat and redistributes back into circulation, leading to complex multicompartmental kinetics and different slopes to drug half-life (termed α and β) over time (Peng 1999; Scholz 1996). Once the fat and muscle are saturated, fentanyl half-life will be prolonged relative to single doses. Initial clearance and half-life (which reflects fentanyl redistribution from circulation to fat and muscle) is short, but as tissue saturates with fentanyl, clearance will depend on CYP3A4 activity and will be prolonged. Methadone has the most unpredictable pharmacokinetics due to wide individual variability in the expression of CYP2B6, CYP3A4, CYP2D6, as well as a large Vd (Hall and Hardy 2005). Dosing strategies for methadone are quite different from those used with other opioids because the pharmacokinetics more complex (Davis 2005); the risk of delayed toxicity is greater.

Pharmacodynamics

In general, serum levels of opioids do not correlate with the degree of analgesia or toxicity. This is particularly true for hydrophilic opioids which have delayed entrance into the CNS. It appears that opioid receptor interactions are more important than opioid pharmacokinetics in determining the degree of pain relief (Davis and Pasternak 2005). Opioid receptors are found in peripheral nerves, the dorsal horn (where sensory input comes into the central nervous system), medial thalamus, insular cortex, cingulate gyrus, amygdala (which governs the affective component to pain), and, to a lesser extent, within the sensory cortex (Finnegan et al. 2004).

Opioid receptors are classic G protein, coupled receptors that contain a seven-transmembrane helical structure with an intracellular C (COOH) tail and extracellular N (NH_2) tail. The µ opioid receptor (MOR), which is largely responsible for analgesia, is derived from four exons, the last of which is highly variable in expression due to differences in splicing mRNA. Multiple subtypes derived from mRNA splicing are designated by a letter next to the opioid receptor (e.g., splice variants MOR-1, MOR-1A, MOR-1B). Recently, splice variants 5' upstream of exon (exon11) have been described which influence receptor responsiveness to particular opioids.

Recent findings centered on opioid receptor dynamics have altered the classical concept of "all or nothing" receptor response put forth by R. P. Stephenson (Kenakin 2011). The opioid receptor is constantly going through dynamic conformational changes which are stabilized in a particular configuration by a particular opioid. Cellular signals resulting from stabilization of the receptor by the ligand is like a "bar code" that leads to selective activation of several different pathways (G protein, beta-arrestin 2, kinases). An opioid will bias signals along one or more pathway (pluridimensional signaling). As a result opioids will have many different efficacies uniquely derived from the particular receptor conformation formed by the ligand-receptor interaction (Kenakin 2011; Kenakin 2007a; Kenakin 2007b).This accounts for the unique responses to different opioids which activate the same receptor.

Clinically, patients achieve varying degrees of analgesia from different MOR agonists and exhibit incomplete analgesic tolerance when switched from one MOR agonist to another as a result of biased signaling and unique receptor conformation stabilization. It appears that genetic differences in receptors (e.g., genetic polymorphisms) and receptor dimers are partly responsible for the wide range of analgesic sensitivities between individuals. Multiple splice variants of the MOR-1 gene respond differently to different opioids (e.g., morphine is the most potent MOR agonist at the MOR-1A splice variant, and fentanyl is the least potent) (Pasternak 2005). Two other receptors (Δ and κ) also contribute to analgesia.

When bound by a potent opioid, opioid receptors activate certain G proteins that are either pertussis-toxin-sensitive or -insensitive. The end result is hyperpolarization of neurons by (1) blocking cyclic AMP production, (2) stimulating inward-rectifying potassium channels, and (3) blocking calcium channels (Law et al. 2000; Davis and Pasternak 2005; Garzón and Rodr´guez-Muñoz 2005; Surratt and Adams 2005).

Opioids also cause a counter-opioid response through activation of nonopioid receptors. Certain phosphorylases (protein kinase C and protein kinase A) and G proteins (G_s, G_2) will activate pronociceptive (pain-promoting) receptors such as the N-methyl-D-aspartate (glutamate) receptor. In addition, certain kinases activate certain adenylate cyclase subtypes and up-regulate pronociceptive neurotransmitters (substance P and calcitonin-gene-related protein) (Ossipov 2005). Analgesic tolerance may be due to reductions in receptor numbers via internalization, receptor desensitization and down-regulation, activation of counter-opioid receptors and neurotransmitters, or other mechanisms not presently known.

Clinical Pharmacology of Opioids

Side Effects

Side effects from opioids are common; many are related to activation of the opioid receptors (constipation, sedation, and respiratory depression). However, some side effects (myoclonus, hallucination, and confusion) are not reversed by opioid receptor antagonists such as naloxone and naltrexone, but respond to dose reduction or opioid rotation. Opioid side effects add to patients' symptom burden. Certain side effects such as respiratory depression are life-threatening, but fortunately tolerance to respiratory depression develops quickly. Constipation remains a constant problem in the opioid tolerant, as tolerance does not develop to this side effect. Patients on opioids should be prescribed laxatives and stool softeners at the onset of opioid administration. Transient drowsiness frequently occurs with initiation of opioids but resolves after a few days. Sedation over a prolonged period can occur, particularly if there are comorbidities or if sedative medications (e.g., antihistamines, benzodiazepines) are also prescribed. Treatment includes assessing for comorbidities, limiting sedative medications, and, if these fail, opioid rotation, opioid dose reduction (if pain is controlled), or (if pain is only partially controlled) the addition of an adjuvant analgesic with opioid dose reduction. Methylphenidate and donepezil have been used to treat opioid related sedation (Stone 2011). Route conversion to spinal opioids will also reduce sedation. Nausea and vomiting will initially occur in 10% to 40% of patients who are started on an opioid. Most will develop tolerance, but may temporarily require an antiemetic. Phenothiazine, haloperidol, metoclopramide, or serotonin receptor antagonists have been used for nausea and vomiting induced by opioids. The evidence of benefit with these antiemetics is quite weak (Laugsand 2011). There is weak evidence that opioid rotation reduces opioid associated nausea and vomiting. Delirium and myoclonus are dose limiting. Haloperidol, quetiapine, olanzapine, and chlorpromazine have been recommended for the treatment of opioid-induced delirium, though opioid rotation is most often required (Stone 2011). It is important to screen for metabolic abnormalities (hyponatremia, hypercalcemia), brain metastases, and infection before attributing delirium to an opioid (McNicol 2003).

Physical Dependence

Physical dependence and drug tolerance are frequently mistaken for opioid addiction. Physical dependence is the end result of physiological changes due to continuous or frequent drug exposure, which leads to compensatory adaptations in multiple CNS regions. Wise and Bozarth (1984) found a complete double-dissociation between brain substrates for physical dependence and those for addiction. Microinjections of opioids into brain loci near the locus coeruleus and dorsal pontine/mesencephalic border produce classic signs of opioid physical dependence (and withdrawal symptoms upon abrupt opioid cessation) without inducing opioid-seeking behaviour demonstrated by conditioned place preference in animals (Gardner 2008). Conversely, opioids are avidly self-administered when the microinjector tips are inserted in the ventral tegmental area (Bozarth and Wise 1981, 1982), lateral hypothalamus (Stein and Olds 1977; Olds 1979), and nucleus accumbens (Acb) (Olds 1982), without inducing physical dependence or withdrawal (Gardner 2008). Symptoms of withdrawal induced by abrupt cessation of a potent opioid or administration of a receptor antagonist are central neurologic arousal, sleeplessness, irritability, psychomotor agitation, diarrhea, rhinorrhea, piloerection, and neuropathic pain syndrome (Ballantyne and LaForge 2007; Chang et al. 2007). The locus coeruleus and norepinephrine release appear to be one important mediator of withdrawal symptoms. Opioids should be gradually tapered to avoid withdrawal symptoms (Ballantyne and LaForge 2007). Dose reductions of 10–25 tend to be safe. Preclinical data suggest that flavonol glycosides may ameliorate opioid withdrawal syndrome (Capasso 2007).

Addiction

Neuronal circuits that induce opioid rewarding effects involve mesocorticolimbic dopamine neurotransmission (Ballantyne and LaForge 2007). This pleasure/reward circuitry consists of an in-series sequence of synaptic circuitry between the ventral limbic diencephalon and forebrain (Wise and Bozarth 1984). The first stage neuron circuitry originates from a group of ventral limbic forebrain nuclei located rostral to the anterior hypothalamus, which is loosely termed by neuroanatomists as the anterior bed nuclei of the medial forebrain bundle (MFB) (Gardner 2008). The second stage neurons ascend rostrally within the MFB to synapse in the Acb of the ventral limbic forebrain, upon the cell bodies/ dendrites of the third stage reward neurons (Gardner 2008). These third stage neurons are GABAergic medium spiny neurons that appear to co-localize an endogenous opioid neurotransmitter. The third stage neurons project from the Acb to synapse in the ventral pallidum (Gardner 2000, 2005). Addiction medicine specialists call drug addiction the "disease of the 5 Cs": chronic disease with impaired control, compulsive use, continued use despite harm, and drug craving (Gardner 2008). Importantly, addictive behaviours appear to be habit based (Di Chiara 1998, 1999; Everitt et al. 2001; Robbins and Everitt 2002). Thus, drugs with addictive potential are also described as habit-forming, a useful term so as to distinguish them from many medications that produce physical dependence which are nonhabit-forming and nonaddictive (Gardner 2008).

Addiction should not be mistaken for pseudoaddiction, which is opioid-seeking behaviour because of gross under treatment of pain. Opioid diversion can be behaviour of nonaddicted individuals in an attempt to financially profit from opioids by diverting prescription opioids from the intended recipient (Ballantyne and LaForge 2007).

Conclusion

Opioid pharmacology provides a basis for understanding variability in opioid responses. Opioid pharmacodynamics are complex and unique. The recent discovery of receptor splice variants, receptor dimers, and the process of bias agonism explains in part analgesic noncross tolerance between opioids. Individuals are also obviously unique, and therefore treatment must be individualized. Molecular medicine has unravelled many of the mysteries behind individual variability in the art and science of optimizing opioid responses; analgesia while minimizing side effects is a continual clinical challenge.

Acknowledgment

The author would like to thank Michele Wells and Pamela Gamier for lending their technical skills to the preparation of this manuscript.

References

Ballantyne JC, LaForge KS. Opioid dependence and addiction during opioid treatment of chronic pain. *Pain.* 2007;129(3):235–255.

Bozarth MA, Wise RA. Intracranial self-administration of morphine into the ventral stegmental area in rats. *Life Sci.* 1981;28(5):551–555.

Bozarth MA, Wise RA. Localization of the reward-relevant opiate receptors. *NIDA Res Monogr.* 1982;41:158–164.

Bullingham RE, Moore RA, Symonds HW, et al. A novel form of dependency of hepatic extraction ratio of opioids in vivo upon the portal vein concentration of drug: comparison of morphine, diamorphine, fentanyl, methadone and buprenorphine in the chronically cannulated cow. *Life Sci.* 1984;34(21):2047–2056.

Callaghan R, Desmond PV, Paull P, et al. Hepatic enzyme activity is the major factor determining elimination rate of high clearance drugs in cirrhosis. *Hepatology.* 1993;18(1):54–60.

Capasso A. The effect of flavonol glycosides on opiate withdrawal. *Med Chem.* 2007;3(4):327–331.

Chang G, Chen L, Mao J. Opioid tolerance and hyperalgesia. *Med Clin N Am.* 2007;91(2):199–211.

Chauvin M, Bonnet F, Montembault C, et al. The influence of hepatic plasma flow on alfentanil plasma concentration plateaus achieved with an infusion model in humans: measurement of alfentanil hepatic extraction coefficient. *Anesth Analg.* 1986;65(10):999–1003.

Davis MP. Methadone. In Davis M, Glare P, Hardy J, eds. *Opioids in Cancer Pain.* New York: Oxford University Press; 2005;173–198.

Davis M, Pasternak GW. Opioid receptors and opioid pharmacodynamics. In Davis M, Glare P, Hardy J, eds. *Opioids in Cancer Pain.* New York: Oxford University Press; 2005;11-41.

Di Chara G. A motivational learning hypothesis of the role of mesolimbic dopamine in compulsive drug use. *J Psychopharmacol.* 1998;12(1):54–67.

Di Chiara G, Tanda G, Bassereo V, et al. Drug addiction as a disorder of associate learning. Role of nucleus accumbens shell/extended amygdale dopamine. *Ann N Y Acad Sci.* 1999;877:461–485.

Everitt BJ, Dickinson A, Robbins TW. The neuropsychological basis of addictive behaviour. *Brain Res Rev.* 2001;36(2-3):129–138.

Finnegan TF, Li DP, Chen SR, et al. Activation of mu-opioid receptors inhibits synaptic inputs to spinally projecting rostral ventromedial medulla neurons. *J Pharmacol Exp Ther.* 2004;309(2):476–483.

Gardner EL. What we have learned about addiction from animal models of drug self-administration. *Am J Addict.* 2000;9(4):285–313.

Gardner EL. Brain-reward mechanisms. In Lowinson JH, Ruiz P, Millman RB, et al., eds. *Substance Abuse: A Comprehensive Textbook.* 4th ed. Philadelphia: Lippincott Williams and Wilkins, 2005; 48–97.

Gardner EL. Pain management and the so-called "risk" of addiction: a neurobiological perspective. In Smith HS, Passik SD, eds. *Pain and Chemical Dependency.* New York: Oxford University Press, 2008;427–435.

Garzón J, Rodr'guez-Muñoz M, de la Torre-Madrid E, et al. Effector antagonism by the regulators of G protein signalling (RGS) proteins causes desensitization of mu-opioid receptors in the CNS. *Psychopharmacology.* 2005;180(1):1–11.

Hall T, Hardy JR. The lipophilic opioids: fentanyl, alfentanil, sufentanil and remifentanil. In Davis M, Glare P, Hardy J, eds. *Opioids in Cancer Pain.* New York: Oxford University Press; 2005;155–171.

Ingelman-Sundberg M. Pharmacogenetics of cytochrome P450 and its applications in drug therapy: the past, present and future. *Trends Pharmacol Sci.* 2004;25(4):193–200.

Inturrisi CE. Clinical pharmacology of opioids for pain. *Clin J Pain.* 2002; 18(4 Suppl):S3–S13.

Kenakin T. Collateral efficacy in the drug discovery: taking advantage of the goo (allosteric) nature of 7TM receptors. *Trends in Pharmacol Sci* 2007a;28(8):407–15.

Kenakin T. Functional selectivity through protean and biased agonism: who steers the ship? *Molecular Pharmacol* 2007b;72(6):1393–1401.

Kenakin T. Functional sensitivity and biased receptor signalling. *JPET* 2011; 336(2):296–302.

Kiang TK, Ensom MH, Chang TK. UDP-glucuronosyltransferases and clinical drug-drug interactions. *Pharmacol Ther*. 2005;106(1):97–132.

Lamba J, Lin YS, Schuetz EG, et al. Genetic contribution to variable human CYP3A mediated metabolism. *Adv Drug Deliv Rev*. 2002;54(10):1271–1294.

Laugsand EA, Kaasa S, Klepstad P. Management of opioid-induced nausea and vomiting in cancer patients: systematic review and evidence based recommendations. *Palliat Med* 2011;25(5):442–53.

Law PY, Erickson LJ, El-Kouhen R, et al. Receptor density and recycling affect the rate of agonist-induced desensitization of mu-opioid receptor. *Mol Pharmacol*. 2000;58(2):388–398.

Lehmann KA. Opioids: overview on action, interaction and toxicity. *Support Care Cancer*. 1997;5(6):439–444.

Leppert W. CYP2D6 in the metabolism of opioids for mild to moderate pain. *Pharmacology* 2011;87(5–6):274285.

Lin J, Lu AY. Inhibition and induction of cytochrome P450 and the clinical implications. *Clin Pharmacokinetics*. 1998;35(5):361–390.

McNicol E, Horowicz-Mehler N, Fisk RA, et al. Management of opioid side effects in cancer related and chronic noncancer pain: a systematic review. *J Pain*. 2003;4(5):231–256.

O'Brien JA, Nation RL, Evans AM. The disposition of morphine and morphine-3-glucuronide in the isolated perfused rat liver: effects of altered perfusate flow rate. *J Pharm Pharmacol*. 1996;48(5):498–504.

Olds ME. Hypothalamic substrate for the positive reinforcing properties of morphine in the rat. *Brain Res*. 1979;168(2):351–360.

Olds ME. Reinforcing effects of morphine in the nucleus accumbens. *Brain Res*. 1982;237(2):429–440.

Ossipov MH, Lai J, King T, et al. Underlying mechanisms of pronociceptive consequences of prolonged morphine exposure. *Biopolymers*. 2005;80(2–3):319–324.

Pasternak GW. Molecular biology of opioid analgesia. *J Pain Symptom Manage*. 2005;29(5 Suppl):S2–S9.

Peng PW, Sandler AN. A review of the use of fentanyl analgesia in the management of acute pain in adults. *Anesthesiology*. 1999;90(2):576–599.

Robbins TW, Everitt BJ. Limbic-striatal memory systems and drug addiction. *Neurobiol Learn Mem*. 2002;78(3):625–636.

Ross J, Rutter D, Welsh D, et al. Clinical response to morphine in cancer patients and genetic variation in candidate genes. *Pharmacogenomics J*. 2005;5(5):324–336.

Shand DG, Kornhauser DM, Wilkinson GR. Effects of route of administration and blood flow on hepatic drug elimination. *J Pharmacol Exp Ther*. 1975;195(3):424–432.

Scholz J, Steinfath M, Schulz M. Clinical pharmacokinetics of alfentanil, fentanyl and sufentanil. An Update. *Clin Pharmacokinet*. 1996;31(4):275–292.

Smith HS. The metabolism of opioid agents and the clinical impact of the active metabolites. *Clin J Pain.* 2011;—27(9):824–838.

Stein EA, Olds J. Direct intracerebral self-administration of opiates in the rat. *Soc Neurosci Abstr.* 1977;3:302.

Stone P, Minton O. European Palliative Care Research collaborative pain guidelines. Central side-effects management: what is the evidence to support best practice in the management of sedation, cognitive impairment and myoclonus? *Palliat Med* 2011; 25(5):431–41.

Surratt C, Adams WR. G protein-coupled receptor structural motifs: relevance to the opioid receptors. *Curr Top Med Chem.* 2005;5(3):315–324.

Tegeder I, Lotsch J, Geisslinger G. Pharmacokinetics of opioids in liver disease. *Clin Pharmacokinet.* 1999;37(1):17–40.

Tukey RH, Strassburg CP. Human UDP-glucuronosyltransferases: metabolism, expression, and disease. *Annu Rev Pharmacol Toxicol.* 2000;40:581–616.

Volles DF, McGory R. Pharmacokinetic considerations. *Crit Care Clin.* 1999;15(1):55–75.

Wilkinson G. Drug metabolism and variability among patients in drug response. *N Engl J Med.* 2005;352(21):2211–2221.

Wise RA, Bozarth MA. Brain reward circuitry: four circuit elements "wired" in apparent series. *Brain Res Bull.* 1984;12(2):203–208.

Zhang Y, Benet LZ. The gut as a barrier to drug absorption. *Clin Pharmacokinetics.* 2001;40(3):159–168.

Chapter 5a

Optimizing Pharmacologic Outcomes: Drug Selection

Kenneth C. Jackson II and Howard S. Smith

Selecting an opioid analgesic requires clinicians to consider a multitude of patient specific dynamics. There is significant individual variation in the analgesic response to different opioids; therefore, a previous response to an earlier trial of opioid therapy (according to both patient report and medical records) should be reviewed when selecting a new opioid. The severity, duration, and pattern of the pain should be considered along with individual opioid-specific differences. The patient's age, metabolic considerations, medical comorbidities, mental status, history of compliance with medical regimens, and history of substance misuse are all factors to consider.

Individual Opioid Analgesics

Opioid analgesics have traditionally been classified into three pharmacological classes—the full agonists, partial agonists, and mixed agonist-antagonists (Table 5a.1). The opioids most commonly used in chronic opioid therapy (COT) are the pure agonists because they have no clinically relevant ceiling effect to analgesia. As the dose is increased, analgesia increases until either full analgesia is achieved or dose-limiting side effects occur. The partial agonists have a low intrinsic activity, so that a ceiling effect occurs at less than the maximum effect produced by an agonist. A mixed agonist–antagonist produces agonist effects at one receptor and antagonist effects at another. Agonist-antagonists (e.g., butorphanol, nalbuphine, pentazocine) do not have a significant place among agents used for COT.

For drugs acting at the Mu-opioid receptor (MOR), published measurements of binding affinity ($K(i)$) are incomplete and inconsistent due to differences in methodology and assay system, leading to a wide range of values for the same drug thus precluding a simple and meaningful relative ranking of drug potency (Volpe et al. 2011). Experiments were conducted to obtain $K(i)$'s for 19 approved opioid drugs using a single binding assay in a cell membrane preparation expressing recombinant human MOR. The $K(i)$ values obtained ranged from 0.1380 nM (sufentanil) to 12.486 µM (tramadol). The drugs were separated into three categories based upon their $K(i)$ values: $K(i) > 100$ nM (tramadol, codeine, meperidine, propoxyphene, and pentazocine), $K(i)=1$-100 nM (hydrocodone, oxycodone, diphenoxylate, alfentanil, methadone, nalbuphine, fentanyl, and morphine) and $K(i) < 1$ nM (butorphanol, levorphanol,

Table 5a.1 Opioid Analgesics Classified by Mechanism of Activity

Full (Pure) Agonists	Partial Agonists	Mixed Agonist-Antagonists
Codeine	Buprenorphine	Butorphanol
Fentanyl		Nalbuphine
Hydromorphone		Pentazocine
Levorphanol		
Meperidine		
Methadone		
Morphine		
Oxycodone		
Oxymorphone		
Propoxyphene		

Table 5a.2 Long-Acting Oral Opioids

Pharmacologically Long-Acting	Pharmaceutically Long-Acting
Levorphanol (Levo-Dromoran)	Hydromorphone (Exalgo)
Methadone (Dolophine)	Morphine sulfate (Kadian, AVINZA, MS Contin, Oramorph SR)
	Oxycodone (Oxycontin)
	Oxymorphone (Opana ER)
	Transdermal fentanyl (3 day patch) (Duragesic)
	Transdermal Buprenorphine (7 day patch) (Butrans)
	Tramadol ER (Ultram ER, Ryzolt)
	Tapentadol ER (Nucynta)

oxymorphone, hydromorphone, buprenorphine, and sufentanil) (Volpe et al. 2011).

There are two main groups of oral long-acting opioid analgesics (Table 5a.2). The most commonly utilized are the pharmaceutically enhanced opioid analgesics. A second group comprises methadone and levorphanol, two agents with inherently long-acting pharmacokinetic profiles. In general, the pharmaceutically modified agents are much easier to dose and titrate and typically can be managed in most primary care settings with little special training. Methadone and levorphanol are more difficult to use, as discussed below. Clinicians who prescribe opioid analgesics should be familiar with their metabolism (Smith 2009a; Smith 2011a).

Opioids for Dyspnea/Air Hunger in Palliative Medicine

Opioids may also be used for alleviation of other symptoms besides pain, such as for anti-tussive effects and diminishing the perception of dyspnea in the palliative care population. Unpleasant dyspneic sensations may include the sense of excessive work of breathing, air hunger ("starved for air"), and perhaps the sensation of chest tightness or constriction. Air hunger has been proposed to be due to a mismatch or dissociation between central respiratory drive (which in part may be stimulated be sensory receptors [mechanoreceptors and chemical receptors] in the lung and respiratory muscles/chest wall) versus actual ventilation. Exogenous opioids (morphine and other opioids) (Jennings et al. 2002) and endogenous opioids (Gifford et al. 2011) may modulate the intensity and unpleasantness of breathlessness in certain patients/medical conditions (e.g., chronic obstructive lung disease [COPD]) but may not be all that effective in others (e.g., congestive heart failures [CHF]) (Oxberry et al. 2011).

Banzett et al. found that for each given level of PET_{CO2}, infused morphine, as compared with the same-day baseline, induced a similar and substantial decrease in induced air hunger for both its sensory and primary affective dimension (intensity and discomfort, respectively) (Banzett et al. 2011). Additionally, over a similar range of PET_{CO2}, morphine induced a significant decrease in the spontaneous ventilatory response to hypercapnia (hypercapnic ventilatory response [HCVR]). Banzett and colleagues also showed a further significant impact of morphine, namely, a decrease in dyspnea-related anxiety that was independent of its effect on immediate discomfort (Banzett et al. 2011). There is no robust evidence supporting dramatic advantages of one opioid versus another opioid with respect to their effects on dyspnea.

Morphine

Morphine is the prototype exogenous mu opioid receptor (MOR) agonist. It is relatively hydrophilic, and 90% of its molecules are ionized at normal oral pH. The onset of analgesia with oral morphine is approximately 20 to 30 minutes, with a time to peak analgesia of 60 to 90 minutes. The oral bioavailability of morphine is roughly 25% to 35%, but demonstrates marked interindividual variability. Its plasma half-life of two to three hours is somewhat shorter than its duration of analgesia of three to six hours. The duration of analgesia with modified-release formulations (e.g., MS Contin, Oramorph, Kadian, AVINZA) ranges from eight to 24 hours, depending on the specific drug and individual variation.

With recognition of its active metabolites, the role of morphine in the management of chronic pain has evolved (Sjogren 1997). Morphine-6-glucuronide, an active metabolite that may contribute to the analgesia and side effects observed during morphine therapy, can accumulate in patients with renal insufficiency and has been associated with toxicity in some renally impaired patients. Morphine-3-glucuronide also may cause toxicity, possibly leading to myoclonus and worsening pain. Patients who develop morphine toxicity, particularly in the setting of renal insufficiency, should be offered an alternative opioid in the hope that lesser metabolite accumulation may contribute to a better response.

Morphine sulphate and naltrexone hydrochloride extended release capsule (MS-sNT) [Embeda®] are safe and effective for the management of chronic, moderate-to-severe pain, and are designed to reduce morphine-induced subjective effects (e.g., drug liking and euphoria) upon tampering by crushing (Smith 2011b). Embeda® was voluntarily recalled from US wholesalers and retailers because a pre-specified stability requirement was not met during routine testing (the intent is to resolve the stability issue and make Embeda available again).

Fentanyl

Fentanyl is a synthetic phenylpiperidine MOR agonist that is roughly 80 times more potent than morphine. It is highly lipophilic and binds avidly to plasma proteins. After intramuscular administration of fentanyl citrate, the time to onset of analgesia is roughly seven to 15 minutes. The time to peak analgesia can be extremely variable but may be estimated as 15 to 45 minutes; the duration of analgesia is about one to two hours. Fentanyl is largely metabolized by piperidine N-dealkylation to norfentanyl via hepatic microsomal CYP3A4 (Janicki and Parris 2003).

Oral transmucosal fentanyl citrate (OTFC) is a candy matrix formulation administered orally as a lozenge on a stick. It is applied against the buccal mucosa, with roughly 25% of the total dose of OTFC being rapidly absorbed via the buccal mucosa, making it systemically available almost immediately. The remaining 75% of the total dose is swallowed with saliva and slowly absorbed from the gastrointestinal (GI) tract. About one-third of this (25% of the total dose) escapes hepatic and intestinal first-pass elimination and becomes systemically available. The apparent 50% bioavailability represents 25% from rapid transmucosal absorption and 25% from slower GI absorption. OTFC appears to be particularly well suited for breakthrough pain (which is present in roughly two-thirds of cancer patients with pain), owing to its rapid onset. Meaningful analgesia occurs faster than with comparable doses of immediate-release oral opioids. Peak plasma concentrations are achieved at 20 minutes, and the duration of analgesia is roughly two hours (Lichtor et al. 1999). The fentanyl buccal tablet, or FBT (Fentora), is another oral transmucosal formulation of fentanyl available in the United States. This formulation enhances buccal delivery of fentanyl by utilizing an effervescent drug delivery system and achieves an absolute bioavailability of 65%. The onset of pain relief occurs within 15 minutes in some patients, with the duration of analgesia ranging up to 60 minutes (Pather et al. 2001; Durfee et al. 2006). The rate and extent of fentanyl absorption is greater following administration of FBT compared to OTFC (largely due to dynamic shifts in pH within the different microenvironments [dissolving tablet versus buccal mucosa]), making FBT well suited for breakthrough pain (Darwish et al. 2006; Darwish et al. 2007).

Oxycodone

Oxycodone (14-hydroxydihydrocodeinone) is a potent MOR agonist, and it appears to have effects at the κ opioid receptor as well. It is available as a controlled-release formulation and as a short-acting analgesic in various strengths, both alone and in combination with acetaminophen or aspirin. The opioid effects of oxycodone are related to the parent drug and not to its metabolites (Lalovic et al. 2006).

OXECTA® (oxycodone HCl) Tablets which utilizes Acura's AVERSION® Technology, is available in 5 mg and 7.5 mg dosage strengths and was approved by the FDA in June 2011.

Watson and colleagues (2003) studied patients with painful diabetic neuropathy who were treated for four weeks with controlled-release oxycodone or placebo. The only side effects that occurred on a statistically more significant basis in the oxycodone-treated group were dry mouth and constipation (Watson et al. 2003). The number needed to treat with oxycodone for the relief of neuropathic pain is 2.5. This means that one in every 2.5 (or 4 out of 10) patients with neuropathic pain treated with oxycodone will achieve around a 50% reduction in pain.

Marshall and colleagues (2006) have assessed the cost of producing pain relief in patients with osteoarthritis of the hip or knee when controlled-release oxycodone or a combination of acetaminophen and oxycodone is used. They found that 62% of patients using controlled-release oxycodone alone had pain relief, compared to 46% taking the combination of that drug and acetaminophen. Consequently, from an economic perspective, use of controlled-release oxycodone alone was more cost effective than use of the combination product (Marshall et al. 2006).

Oxymorphone

Oxymorphone, a 3-0-demethylation metabolite of oxycodone, is a potent opioid that has a MOR affinity three to five times higher than that of morphine (Gimbel and Ahdieh 2004). Oxymorphone has been studied for postsurgical pain in an oral immediate-release formulation (Gimbel and Ahdieh 2004) and also as an oral extended-release (ER) formulation for moderate to severe pain secondary to osteoarthritis (Matsumoto et al. 2005). In June 2006, the FDA approved oxymorphone hydrochloride (Opana) tablets (5mg and 10mg) and ER tablets (5mg, 10mg, 20mg, and 40mg). Oxymorphone ER uses the TIMERx (Penwest Pharmaceuticals Co., Danbury, CT) delivery system (Pharmaceuticals P., 2005) to provide pharmacokinetic characteristics consistent with 12-hour dosing (Adams and Ahdieh 2004; Smith 2009b). The major metabolites of oxymorphone include 6-OH-oxymorphone-3-glucuronide. It appears that oxymorphone ER does not affect the CYP2C9 or CYP3A4 metabolic pathways (Adams and Ahdieh 2005). Noroxymorphone demonstrated a 3- and 10-fold higher affinity for the MOR than did oxycodone and noroxycodone, respectively (Lalovic et al. 2004).

In a randomized, double-blind, placebo-controlled, 12-week study, oxymorphone ER twice daily was shown to be effective and safe for opioid-experienced patients with chronic moderate to severe low back pain (Hale et al. 2007). Over half of opioid-experienced patients were successfully converted and titrated to twice-daily oxymorphone ER, and efficacy and tolerability were maintained during 12 weeks of treatment (Hale et al. 2007). Oxymorphone ER was also effective and well tolerated in opioid-naïve patients with chronic low back pain; after titration to stabilized dose, patients were randomized to continue oxymorphone ER or to receive placebo for 12 weeks, with immediate-release oxymorphone available for rescue. After randomization, 68% of oxymorphone ER and 47% of placebo patients completed 12 weeks of doubling treatment, with pain intensity increasing significantly more in the placebo group than the oxymorphone ER group (Katz et al. 2007). The safety, tolerability, and effectiveness of oxymorphone ER for patients with moderate to severe osteoarthritis pain was also demonstrated in a 52-week, multicenter, open-label extension study (40% of patients—61 of 153—completed the study). Average daily dosing remained stable throughout the study (median: 40mg/day). At each assessment (weeks one, two, six, and 10, and every six weeks thereafter), at least 80% of patients rated their global satisfaction with oxymorphone ER as "excellent," "very good," or "good" (McIlwain and Ahdieh 2005).

Methadone

Methadone is a unique opioid of the class that has been termed the diphenylheptanes. The chemical name for methadone is d1(SR) 4,4-diphenyl-6-dimethylamine-3-heptanone. It is structurally dissimilar to the standard alkaloid-type ringed-type structures (Bruera and Sweeney 2002). It is distinguished as being an openchain (linear-type) molecule. In this sense it is most similar to propoxyphene. Methadone contains a single chiral carbon atom and so exists as two enantiomers. The l(R)-enantiomer is primarily responsible for analgesia (Kristensen et al. 1996), with a 10-fold higher affinity for MORs and up to 50 times the analgesic activity of the d(S)-enantiomer (Scott et al. 1948).

The l(R)-isomer is a potent pure, full MOR agonist with low affinity for delta and kappa receptors (Kristensen et al. 1995). Multiple studies with cloned human receptors and with mu knockout mice show full delta receptors show no significant effective methadone agonist action at δ opioid receptors (Bot et al. 1997). The d(S)-enantiomer, although relatively inactive at the MOR, functions as a modest noncompetitive N-methyl-D-aspartate (NMDA) antagonist and also prevents the reuptake of 5-hydroxytryptamine and norepinephrine (Codd et al. 1995).

In the United States, methadone is available in racemic form, as a 50:50 mixture of two enantiomers (l[R]-enantiomer and d[S]-enantiomer). Germany has access to the pure l(R)-enantiomer, which exhibits twice the potency of the racemic product (Kristensen et al. 1996; Bruera and Sweeney 2002).

Methadone is a relatively lipophilic basic drug with a pK_a of about 9.1; it is available as a hydrochloride salt. Methadone is extremely versatile in terms of potential routes of administration and has been given via oral (tablet, solution), rectal (using tablets to compound a suppository), parenteral (subcutaneous, intramuscular, intravenous) (Mathew and Storey 1999), and spinal (epidural [Shir et al. 2001] and intrathecal [Jacobson et al. 1990]) routes.

Methadone can be detected in the blood 15 to 45 minutes after oral administration (Eap 2002). The onset of action of methadone is roughly 0.5 to 1.5 hours after oral administration and about 10 to 20 minutes after parenteral administration (Wolff et al. 1997; Davis and Walsh 2001). The peak analgesic effect occurs 1 to 2 hours after parenteral administration and 2 to 4 hours after oral administration (Wolff et al. 1997; Kreek 2000; Davis and Walsh 2001). The duration of action of methadone for the purpose of suppressing opioid withdrawal is substantially longer (24 to 48 hours) (Gutstein and Akil 2001; Fishman et al. 2002).

Methadone undergoes hepatic biotransformation, primarily via N-demethylation, and is cleared via both urine and feces (Kreek et al. 1976). The major enzyme for N-demethylation is CYP3A4, with minor roles for CYP1A2, CYP2D6, and possibly CYP2B6 (Davis and Walsh 2001; Crettol et al. 2005). The primary N-demethylation metabolite, 2-ethylidene-1,5-dimethyl-3,3-diphenylpyrrolidine, is further N-demethylated to 2-ethyl-5-methyl-3,3-diphenylpyrroline.

The clinically significant major drug interactions of methadone include rifampin, phenytoin, barbiturates, and carbamazepine. The antiepileptic drugs phenytoin, phenobarbital, and carbamazepine are inducers of CYP3A4 and therefore may diminish the concentration of methadone in the blood.

Methadone has a uniquely long and highly variable half-life, irrespective of the patient population; this presents additional issues in drug selection. Its half-life can vary from 12 hours to more than 150 hours (Plummer et al. 1988). Therefore, the time to approach steady state after treatment begins or is changed can be as brief as several days or as long as two weeks. If the dose is rapidly increased to an effective level, the plasma concentration can continue to rise toward steady-state levels, and late toxicity can occur. For this reason, prescibers should carefully monitor patients for a prolonged period after methadone dosing is initiated or increased. This issue has become even more salient in recent years, as the death rate associated with methadone use has risen exponentially (Webster 2011a). Prescribers should exercise extreme caution when initiating or modifying a methadone based analgesic regimen.

The use of methadone for the treatment of pain is increasing as evidence mounts that the drug has a unique pharmacology which, in some cases, leads to a much greater potency than anticipated (Bruera and Neumann 1999; Scholes et al. 1999). Based on this growing experience, a trial of methadone should especially be considered for patients whose opioid requirements are increasing and whose side effects—such as sedation, confusion, and myoclonus—are compromising therapy. Methadone may also be useful if the cost of therapy is an important consideration, as it is substantially less expensive than other opioids typically used for chronic therapy.

When converting patients to methadone from another opioid, the clinician must consider several issues. First, the equianalgesic conversion ratios may not be bidirectional (i.e., the morphine-to-methadone conversion ratio may not be the same as the methadone-to-morphine ratio). Second, in converting from a specific opioid to methadone, the higher the opioid dose, the higher the conversion ratio. At morphine equivalence of less than 90mg, a conversion of 5:1 (morphine: methadone) is recommended, but at morphine doses over 300mg a rotation of 8:1 is recommended (Bruera and Sweeney 2002). Third, its unpredictable half-life may make methadone a challenging medication to use unless the prescriber is experienced in its use. In general there does not appear to be good evidence to support the superiority of any specific method for methadone dose conversions (Weschules 2008).

It has recently been suggested that using methadone as a co-analgesic might be useful as an alternative to attempting a dose conversion when switching to methadone (McKenna 2011). This approach uses the addition of low doses of methadone to the opioids already being utilized by the patient. This interesting approach appears worthy of further investigation.

Given its long and variable half-life and a potency that can be far greater than indicated on standard relative potency tables, the safe use of methadone requires more careful dosing and monitoring at the start of therapy than is typical for other drugs. Clinicians who offer this therapy must be aware of the need for caution.

Some early data also indicate that methadone can prolong the QTc interval (Kornick et al. 2003; Cruciani et al. 2005). Although the risk of cardiac toxicity appears very low, and while there is no consensus concerning electrocardiograph (ECG) monitoring, it is reasonable to obtain a baseline ECG in patients with heart disease, who are undergoing concurrent treatment with cardioactive drugs, who may be predisposed to a prolonged QT interval, or whose methadone dose reaches relatively high levels (e.g., above 200mg/day).

Clinicians who prescribe methadone as an analgesic must also be clear about the differences between this use and its administration for opioid addiction. In the United States, any clinician may prescribe methadone for pain, but a special license is required to use the drug in maintenance therapy for addiction. In contrast to the once-daily administration that is adequate for treating addiction, the use of methadone as an analgesic requires multiple daily doses in most patients.

Hydrocodone

Hydrocodone is a codeine derivative, and because of its high bioavailability (50%) it is available in oral formulations, mostly in combination with nonopioid analgesics (e.g., acetaminophen, ibuprofen). The FDA has recommended limiting the dose of acetaminophen to 325 mg per pill for combined prescription products. Hydrocodone in similar doses is equivalent to morphine in effectiveness after oral administration. It possesses analgesic and antitussive activity, and its half-life is similar to that of codeine. Hydrocodone undergoes extensive hepatic conjugation and oxidative degradation to a variety of metabolites, which are excreted mainly in urine (Janicki and Parris 2003) (Figure 5a.1).

The major metabolites of hydrocodone excreted into urine are dihydrocodeine and nordihydrocodeine (both conjugated to approximately 65%). The O-demethylation to dihydromorphine (DHM) conversion is mediated by the polymorphically expressed cytochrome P-450 CYP2D6 enzyme; however, DHM is produced in minor amounts, and 85% is conjugated further. Traces

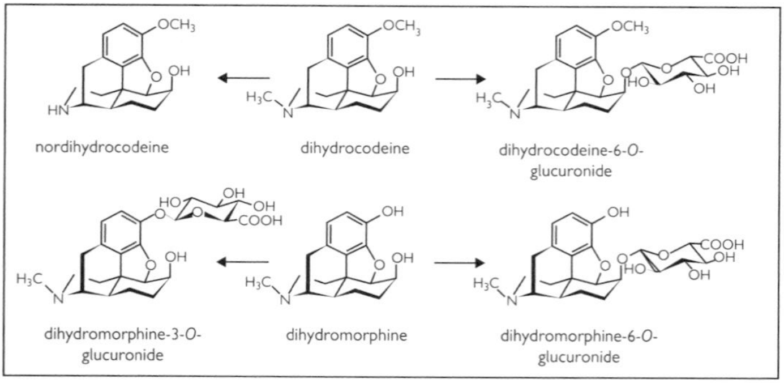

Figure 5a.1 Chemical structure of dihydrocodeine and its essential metabolic steps.

of nordihydromorphine and hydrocodone have been confirmed, and other metabolites of dihydrocodeine can be detected. Some of the hydrocodone metabolites (DHM, hydromorphone, dihydrocodeine) are pharmacologically active at the opioid receptors and may contribute in various degrees to the analgesic activity of hydrocodone or produce unexpected side effects when their excretion is impaired (e.g., renal dysfunction) (Janicki and Parris 2003). An ER hydrocodone/acetaminophen formulation (Vicodin CR) has been undergoing trials, but the FDA did not approve it.

Also there is a novel formulation of hydrocodone bitartrate that does not contain acetaminophen pending FDA approval. Preliminary results of a Phase II trial suggest that this single-entity hydrocodone therapy (Zohydro®) is effective for the treatment of moderate to severe chronic pain. In a 12-week multicenter study, 300 opioid-experienced patients with moderate to severe chronic low back pain and inadequate analgesia from their current medical regimen were administered hydrocodone bitartrate (10-, 20-, 30-, 40- and 50-mag capsules) every 12 hours or placebo. The study met its primary efficacy end point, which was a mean change in average 24-hour pain intensity ratings based on the Numerical Rating Scale.

Codeine

Codeine is the prototype of the opioid analgesics for mild pain. It has weak affinity to the MOR and about 15% of the analgesic potency of morphine. The half-life of codeine is 2.5 to three hours. Codeine is metabolized predominantly by glucuronidation to codeine-6-glucuronide (C6G). Minor metabolic pathways include N-demethylation to norcodeine and O-demethylation to morphine (Yue et al. 1991). The latter is catalyzed by the polymorphically expressed CYP2D6 (Yu et al. 1989). There is increasing evidence that the analgesic effect of codeine is mediated by morphine, its O-demethylated metabolite (Eckhardt et al. 1998), and the glucuronidated morphine metabolite M6G. In humans, the analgesic activity of C6G has not been reported; however, antinociceptive responses after intracerebroventricular administration have been reported in rats (Srinivasan et al. 1996). Constipation and nausea are the major side effects of codeine. Doses of codeine greater than 65mg may not be appropriate, especially in older persons, because of the increasing side effects (particularly constipation) (Janicki and Parris 2003).

Levorphanol

Levorphanol is a MOR agonist that represents a useful alternative for patients unable to tolerate morphine and methadone. It is similar to methadone in that (1) it is long-acting, with a plasma half-life longer than that of most opioids (roughly 12 to 16 hours); (2) caution must be used to avoid accumulation; and (3) it appears to have functional activity as an NMDA receptor antagonist (McNulty 2007). Levorphanol (Levo-Dromoran) is the enantiomer of dextromethorphan. The starting oral dose is generally 2 to 4mg, and 2mg of parenteral levorphanol may be roughly equipotent to 10mg of parenteral morphine sulfate. The oral-to-parenteral potency ratio of levorphanol is 1:2.

Meperidine

Meperidine should not have a significant place among agents used for LTOT. It is a relatively weak MOR agonist (with 10% the efficacy of morphine) having significant anticholinergic and local anesthetic properties. The oral-to-parenteral ratio is 1:4. The anticholinergic properties of meperidine might be responsible for associated tachycardia, mydriasis, and clinically uncertain spasmolytic effects (e.g., decreased pressure in the biliary and urinary tracts). The half-life of meperidine is three hours. It is demethylated in the liver to normeperidine (with a half-life of 15 to 30 hours), which has significant neurotoxic properties. Normeperidine is accumulated after long-term meperidine administration, particularly in patients with renal dysfunction, and may cause CNS excitatory effects (dysphoria, tremulousness, hyperreflexia); it may also produce naloxone-irreversible multifocal myoclonus and grand mal seizures. Short-term administration of meperidine has been associated with mild dysphoria. Meperidine must not be given to patients being treated with monoamine oxidase inhibitors, because this combination can produce severe respiratory depression, hyperpyrexia, CNS excitation, delirium, seizures, and death. In postanesthesia care units, meperidine is often used to treat postanesthetic shivering (Janicki and Parris 2003). Meperidine should not be used for the treatment of chronic pain.

Dihydrocodeine

Dihydrocodeine (Synalgos-DC) is similar in many respects to codeine and has a pharmacokinetic pattern similar to that of codeine. It was previously unclear whether the analgesic effect of dihydrocodeine, similar to that of codeine, was attributable to the drug itself or to its metabolite, DHM. Most of the dihydrocodeine is conjugated to inactive dihydrocodeine-6-glucuronide. Less than 10% of dihydrocodeine is metabolized by N-demethylation to nordihydrocodeine and via O-demethylation to DHM; this latter conversion is mediated by the cytochrome P-450 CYP2D6 enzyme. However, the CYP2D6 phenotype appears not to dramatically affect opioid-receptor-mediated effects of a single 60mg dihydrocodeine dose (Schmidt et al. 2003a,b). DHM, which has a stronger affinity to the MOR than morphine itself, is conjugated further to the next active metabolite, DHM-6-glucuronide, and inactive DHM-3-glucuronide (Aderjan and Skopp 1998). Studies of the relative contributions of dihydrocodeine and DHM to analgesia after dihydrocodeine administration (Webb et al. 2001) indicate that polymorphic differences in dihydrocodeine metabolism to DHM have little or no impact on the analgesic effect (Janicki et al. 2003) (Figure 5a.1).

Propoxyphene

Propoxyphene, a commonly used opioid, is most often combined with acetaminophen (Darvocet) or aspirin (Darvon) and is no longer available in the United States; having been taken off the market due to safety concerns. The analgesic activity is confined to its d-stereoisomer (dextropropoxyphene). In addition to being a MOR agonist, propoxyphene is a weak and noncompetitive NMDA receptor antagonist. Propoxyphene is an odorless, white, crystalline powder with a bitter taste and a molecular weight of 375.94. Chemically, it is (2S,3R)-(+)-4-(dimethylamino)-3-methyl-1,2-diphenyl-2-butanol propionate (ester), and structurally it is somewhat related to methadone. Both are somewhat linear, as opposed to the ringed opioids (5 rings distinguish the phenanthrenes [e.g., morphine], and 2 rings distinguish the phenylpiperidines [e.g., fentanyl]). Peak plasma concentrations of propoxyphene are reached in about two to 2.5 hours after oral administration (its half-life is about 30 to 36 hours). Norpropoxyphene has significantly fewer CNS-depressant effects than propoxyphene but a greater local anesthetic effect, which may lead to prolonged intracardiac conduction times (e.g., increased PR and QRS intervals) (Nicklander et al. 1977). Propoxyphene itself can produce seizures (naloxone-reversible) after overdose (Smith 2003).

Propoxyphene has a *Physician's Desk Reference* black box warning that includes the following instructions:

- Do not prescribe propoxyphene for patients who are suicidal or addiction-prone.
- Prescribe propoxyphene with caution for patients taking tranquilizers or anti-depressant drugs and patients who use alcohol in excess.
- Tell your patients not to exceed the recommended dose and to limit their intake of alcohol.

In a 1975 survey of deaths due to propoxyphene overdosage, roughly 20% of the deaths occurred within the first hour following ingestion (5% occurred in 15 minutes).

Propoxyphene comes in two forms, propoxyphene hydrochloride (Darvon compound-65, with 65mg of propoxyphene hydrochloride) and propoxyphene napsylate (Darvocet-N 50 or Darvocet-N 100, with 50 or 100mg of propoxyphene napsylate). Following administration of 65, 130, or 195mg of propoxyphene hydrochloride, the bioavailability of propoxyphene is equivalent to that of 100, 200, or 300mg, respectively, of propoxyphene napsylate. The napsylate salt tends to be absorbed more slowly than the hydrochloride. The maximum recommended daily dose of propoxyphene hydrochloride is 390mg, and the maximum recommended daily dose of propoxyphene napsylate is 600mg (Smith 2003).

Smith (1971) reported that the analgesic activity of propoxyphene was less than that of aspirin. Propoxyphene may exhibit potent local anesthetic properties at clinical doses. As a result, it may lead to depression of the cardiac conduction system in cases of overdose (Holland and Steinberg 1979). Propoxyphene toxicity is a real concern in patients with liver disease because of significant first-pass metabolism to norpropoxyphene (propoxyphene may facilitate hepatic insult). Rare instances of jaundice have occurred in patients without known preexisting liver disease (Giacomini et al. 1980). In patients with renal failure, high blood levels of both propoxyphene and norpropoxyphene can accumulate, which, owing to secondary high protein binding, tend not to be removed well by hemodialysis (Mather 1992). Propoxyphene should be avoided for patients with renal insufficiency. Subacute painful myopathy has occurred following chronic propoxyphene overdosage (Mather 1992; Smith 2003).

Furthermore, propoxyphene remains a potentially inappropriate medication for use in older adults, according to the updated Beers criteria (Fick et al. 2003), and it appears to be associated with an increased risk for hip fractures in older adults (Kamal-Bahl et al. 2006). Despite these concerns, it seems that there was a continuing high prevalence of propoxyphene use in the community-dwelling older Medicare population from 1993 through 1999, with more than 2 million beneficiaries receiving the drug in 1999 (Kamal-Bahl et al. 2005).

Hydromorphone

Hydromorphone is a semi-synthetic opioid agonist and a hydrogenated ketone of morphine (Quigley 2002). It was first synthesized in Germany in 1921 and was introduced into clinical practice by 1926 (Murray and Hagen 2005). Hydromorphone is structurally very similar to morphine; it differs from morphine by the presence of a 6-keto group and the hydrogenation of the double bond at the 7-8 position of the molecule (Babul et al. 1995). Hydromorphone-3-glucuronide is the major hydromorphone metabolite (Zheng et al. 2002). Hydromorphone is available in the following oral preparations: powder, solution, immediate release tablet, and modified-release tablet. It is absorbed in the upper small intestine, is extensively metabolized by the liver, and has a variety of renally excreted, water-soluble metabolites. Approximately 62% of the oral dose is eliminated by the liver on first pass, partly accounting for oral bioavailability in the range of 1:2 to 1:8 (Vallner et al. 1981). For orally-administered, immediate release preparations, the onset of action is approximately 30 minutes with a duration of action of about 4 hours (Benedetti and Butler 1990). Hydromorphone can be administered parenterally by intravenous, intramuscular, and subcutaneous routes. The oral to parenteral equianalgesic ratio has been estimated as 5:1, although a range has been described and clearly there is a great deal of interindividual variablility (Benedetti and Butler 1990). Subcutaneous administration has been found to have 78% of the bioavailability of intravenous dosing (Moulin et al. 1991). Onset of action of hydromorphone after intravenous dosing is approximately five minutes, although maximum effect is not achieved for as long as 20 minutes (Murray and Hagen 2005). The equianalgesic ratio for parenteral morphine to parenteral hydromorphone is roughly 5:1 (Houde 1986; Bruera et al. 1996; Dunbar et al. 1996; Rapp et al. 1996).

The bioavailability of hydromorphone from OROS hydromorphone is minimally affected by food or alcohol (ethanol) (Lussier et al. 2010). Hydromorphone is mainly metabolized in the liver and is excreted in the urine. Unlike morphine, hydromorphone does not have an active 6-glucuronide metabolite. This metabolite of morphine can accumulate in the presence of renal failure; therefore, the lack of an active 6-glucuronide metabolite may make hydromorphone a useful alternative to morphine in elderly patients with renal failure. However, hydromorphone is similar to morphine in that it is metabolized to hydromorphone-3-glucuronide, which may be neuroexcitatory (Lussier et al. 2010).

Snarr and colleagues attributed prolonged sinus pauses (up to 7.12 seconds with no escape rhythm) to hydromorphone administration in a patients without known cardiac conduction disease or cardiac history (Snarr et al. 2011).

Although this is certainly not typical for hydromorphone or any opioid/opioid-like analgesic agent, all opioids with the exception of meperidine may lead to bradycardia.

A Cochrane review found that hydromorphone is a potent analgesic that the clinical effects of hydromorphone for acute and chronic pain appear to be dose-related, and that the adverse effect profile of hydromorphone is similar to that of other mu opioid receptor agonists (Quigley 2002).

Felden and colleagues performed a meta-analysis which suggested some advantage of hydromorphone over morphine for analgesia (Felden et al. 2011). Side-effects were similar, for example, nausea (P=0.383, nine studies, 456 patients receiving hydromorphone and 460 morphine); vomiting (P=0.306, six studies, 246 patients receiving hydromorphone and 239 morphine); or itching (P=0.249, eight studies, 405 patients receiving hydromorphone, 410 morphine) Additional potential clinical pharmacological advantages with regard to side-effects, such as safety in renal failure or during acute analgesia titration, are based on limited evidence and require substantiation by further studies.

The FDA has approved the opioid agonist hydromorphone in a once-daily extended-release (ER) oral tablet formulation (Exalgo®) for the management of moderate to severe pain in opioid-tolerant patients requiring continuous, long-term therapy. A twice-daily hydromorphone ER formulation (Palladone®) was available previously, but was withdrawn from the market because taking it with alcohol could interfere with the extended-release mechanism and lead to rapid release of potentially lethal amounts of the drug ("dose-dumping") (Palladone 2005). Hydromorphone Extended-Release (ER) (Exalgo®) is a formulation delivers hydromorphone at a controlled rate for up to 24 hours (Wallace et al. 2007). Steady-state concentrations are reached after three to four days, and are within the same range as those with immediate-release (IR) hydromorphone administered four times daily, but with less fluctuation in peaks and troughs. In a double-blind, placebo-controlled withdrawal study of 268 opioid-tolerant patients with moderate to severe low back pain, hydromorphone ER significantly reduced pain intensity compared to placebo (Hale et al. 2010).

Buprenorphine

Buprenorphine is classified as a partial mu opioid agonist. It has been available in the United States in parenteral formulation for pain and in sublingual tablets for opioid dependence (Subutel® [buprenorphine] sublingual and Suboxone® [buprenorphine and naloxone] sublingual). In 2011 the food and drug administration (FDA) has approved a transdermal formulation of buprenorphine, the Buprenorphine Transdermal System (BTS) (Butrans®) for treatment of moderate to severe chronic pain. Buprenorphine binds to the MOR with high affinity and slow dissociates from it (exhibiting prolonged receptor occupancy). In high doses it can act as a mu opioid antagonists. It is highly lipophilic and thus has a large volume of distribution. It tends to have a slow onset in the transdermal formulation (steady state achieved in about three days after initial application). Buprenorphine is hepatically metabolized (slowly cleared by liver via CYP2A4 and conjugases) to an active metabolite, norbuprenorphine, and excreted in the bile and urine. CYP3A4 accounts for about 65% of norbuprenorphine production and CYP2C8 for about 30% (Picard et al. 2005). Minor metabolites include hydroxybuprenorphine and hydroxyl-norbuprenorphine (Picard et al. 2005). Its terminal half-life is roughly 26 hours. Although its predominant mechanisms of action are from being a mu-opioid receptor agonist, it may also exhibit actions as a partial/full agonist at the nociceptin opioid peptide (NOP) receptor (formerly called orphan-related ligand-1 receptor) and as a kappa opioid receptor agonist. It is conceivable that its action as a NOP agonist may be partially useful in certain neuropathic pain states where NOP receptors may be upregulated.

Transdermal buprenorphine is available in three strengths delivering 5 mcg/h, 10 mcg/h, or 20 mcg/h. Patients who are opioid-naïve or taking an opioid equivalent of less than 30 mg/day of oral morphine should start with the 5 mcg/h strength. The maximum dose is 20 mcg/h since higher doses may lead to QTc prolongation. It is worn for seven days and then changed and it should not be cut. It should be applied to hairless skin at one of the eight possible sites: upper outer arm, upper back, upper chest, or the side of the chest (on the right or left sides of the body). After seven days, a new transdermal system should be applied to a new site thereby rotating sites. It is recommended to wait 21 days before reusing the same site. Heat from a heating pad or from a fever can increase absorption and serum concentration of the drug.

Kouya and colleagues studied and compared the antinociceptive and anti-hyperalgesic effect of the partial opioid receptor agonist buprenorphine in normal and neuropathic rats (Kouya et al. 2002). In normal rats, systemic buprenorphine produced dose-dependent antinociception on the hot plate test. In rats with peripheral nerve or spinal cord injury, buprenorphine markedly alleviated neuropathic pain-related behaviors, including mechanical and cold allodynia/hyperalgesia at doses comparable to that producing antinociception. They suggested that buprenorphine may be a useful analgesic for treating neuropathic pain (Kouya et al. 2002).

Opioid-Like Analgesic Agents

Opioid-like analgesic agents (OLAs) are agents that bind to or interact with an opioid receptor and produce analgesia at least in part due to this binding/interaction. They may include so-called atypical opioids or dial mechanism agents as well as other agents in the future.

Tramadol

Tramadol, a centrally acting analgesic available as both immediate release (IR) and extended release (ER) formulations, is structurally related to codeine and morphine, consists of two enantiomers, both of which contribute to analgesic activity via different mechanisms (Grond and Sablotzki 2004). (+)-Tramadol and the metabolite (+)-O-desmethyl-tramadol (M1) are agonists of the mu opioid receptor. (+)-Tramadol inhibits serotonin reuptake and (-)-tramadol inhibits norepinephrine reuptake, enhancing inhibitory effects on pain transmission in the spinal cord (Grond and Sablotzki 2004).

Tramadol has a better potency ratio relative to morphine in neuropathic than in nociceptive pain models (Christoph et al. 2007). The doses of drug that were calculated to result in 50% pain inhibition (ED[50]) for tramadol and morphine were 2.1 and 0.9 mg/kg, respectively, in CCI rats and 4.3 and 3.7 mg/kg, respectively, in SNL rats (Christoph et al. 2007). In the tail-flick assay of acute nociception, the potency of the two drugs differed markedly, as seen by ED(50) values of 5.5 and 0.7 mg/kg intravenously for tramadol and morphine, respectively. Accordingly, the analgesic potency ratio (ED[50] tramadol/ED[50] morphine) of both compounds differed in neuropathic (potency ratio 2.3 in CCI and 1.2 in SNL) and nociceptive pain models (potency ratio 7.8), suggesting a relative increase in potency of tramadol in neuropathic pain compared with nociceptive pain (Christoph et al. 2007).

Harati and colleagues conducted a placebo-controlled, double-blind trial that showed tramadol was effective and safe in treating the pain of diabetic neuropathy (Harati et al. 1998). Harati et al. also evaluated the efficacy and safety of tramadol in a six-month open extension (Harati et al. 2000), following a six-week double-blind randomized trial (Harati et al. 1998). They concluded that tramadol safely provides long-term relief of the pain of diabetic neuropathy. Freeman and colleagues conducted a randomized study of tramadol/acetaminophen versus placebo in painful diabetic peripheral neuropathy. Tramadol/acetaminophen was more effective than placebo and was well tolerated in the management of painful DPN (Freeman et al. 2007). They identified six eligible trials, four comparing tramadol with placebo, one comparing tramadol with clomipramine, and one comparing tramadol with morphine. In 2006, Hollingshead and colleagues performed a Cochrane review on tramadol for neuropathic pain (Hollingshead et al. 2006). All four trials comparing tramadol with placebo showed a significant reduction in neuropathic pain with tramadol. Three of the trials that compared tramadol to placebo (total 269 participants) were combined in a meta-analysis. The number needed to treat with tramadol compared to placebo to reach at least 50% pain relief was 3.8 (95% confidence interval 2.8 to 6.3). There were insufficient data to draw conclusions about the effectiveness of tramadol compared to either clomipramine or morphine. One trial considered subcategories of neuropathic pain. It found a significant therapeutic effect of tramadol on paraesthesiae, allodynia, and touch evoked pain. Numbers needed to harm were calculated for side effects resulting in withdrawal from the placebo-controlled trials. Three trials provided these data, and the combined number needed to harm was 8.3 (95% confidence interval 5.6 to 17) (Hollingshead et al. 2006). Hollingshead et al. concluded that tramadol is an effective treatment for neuropathic pain (Hollingshead et al. 2006). Tramadol was also found to provide effective analgesia in the treatment of neuropathic cancer pain from a 2007 randomized, double-blind, placebo-controlled study (Arbaiza and Vidal 2007) as well as in the treatment of neuropathic pain after spinal cord injury from a 2009 randomized, double-blind, placebo-controlled trial (Norrbrink and Lundeberg 2009).

Tapentadol

Tapentadol is a novel centrally acting analgesic, initially formulated as an imme-diate-release preparation. It is a potent Schedule II analgesic approved for use by the US Food and Drug Administration (FDA) in 2009. In 2011, the FDA approved the extended-release formulation. Tapentadol extended release is available as 50, 100, 150, 200, and 250 mg tablets with a recommended interval between dosing of about 12 hours. Tapentadol immediate-release is avail-able as 50, 75, and 100 mg tablets and provides four to six hours of analgesia. Tapentadol immediate-release was shown to provide analgesia comparable with that of 10–15 mg of immediate-release oxycodone in patients recovering from dental extraction pain3 and pain following bunionectomy. The controlled release formulation provides a 12-hour duration of activity, as well as the con-venience and analgesic uniformity associated with twice per day dosing. It was also as effective as oxycodone in patients presenting with chronic osteoarthritis pain and chronic low back pain (Vadovelu et al. 2011). Of importance in the comparator trials was the finding that patients treated with tapentadol had a lower incidence of adverse gastrointestinal events, including nausea, vomiting, and constipation than those treated with oxycodone.

Tapentadol produces potent analgesic effects via its dual mechanism of action, that is, mu opioid receptor agonism and norepinephrine reuptake inhi-bition. In animal models, tapentadol behaves as a weak opioid agonist, with 50 times less affinity than morphine for the mu receptor (Vadovelu et al. 2011). Tapentadol exists as a single active enantiomer and is metabolized mainly by O-glucuronidation. Its principal metabolite is inactive, having no affinity for the mu opioid receptor or the norepinephrine transporter. Because the anal-gesic activity of tapentadol is limited to the primary molecule, no enzymes are needed to convert it to an active metabolite, as is the case for tramadol and codeine (Vadovelu et al. 2011).

Tapentadol, but not morphine, selectively inhibits disease-related thermal hyperalgesia in a mouse model of diabetic neuropathic pain (Christoph et al. 2010). Tapentadol was more potent than morphine against heat hyperalgesia, with ED(50) (minimal effective dose) values of 0.32 (0.316) and 0.65 (1)mg/kg, respectively. Christoph and colleagues hypothesized that this superior efficacy profile of tapentadol for neuropathic pain is due to simultaneous activation of MOR and inhibition of NA reuptake (Christoph et al. 2010).

Schröder and colleagues analyzed the contribution of opioid and monoamin-ergic mechanisms to the activity of tapentadol in rat models of nociceptive and neuropathic pain (Schröder et al. 2010). Antinociceptive efficacy was inferred from tail withdrawal latencies of experimentally naive rats using a tail flick test. Antihypersensitive efficacy was inferred from ipsilateral paw withdrawal thresh-olds toward an electronic von Frey filament in a spinal nerve ligation model of mononeuropathic pain. Tapentadol showed clear antinociceptive and antihyper-sensitive effects (>90% efficacy) with median effective dose (ED[50]) values of 3.3 and 1.9 mg/kg, respectively. While the antinociceptive ED(50) value of tap-entadol was shifted to the right 6.4-fold by naloxone (21.2mg/kg) and only 1.7-

fold by yohimbine (5.6 mg/kg), the antihypersensitive ED(50) value was shifted to the right 4.7-fold by yohimbine (8.9 mg/kg) and only 2.7-fold by naloxone (5.2mg/kg) (Schröder et al. 2010). Activation of both mu-opioid receptors and alpha2-adrenoceptors contribute to the analgesic effects of tapentadol. The relative contribution is, however, dependent on the particular type of pain, as mu-opioid receptor agonism predominantly mediates tapentadol's antinociceptive effects, whereas noradrenaline reuptake inhibition predominantly mediates its antihypersensitive effects (Schröder et al. 2010).

Further support of the inhibition of norepinephrine reuptake being a major factor in tapentadol's effects on neuropathic pain was seen in a rat model (Bee et al. 2011). Bee and colleagues performed a series of in vivo electrophysiological tests in spinal nerve ligated and sham-operated rats to show that systemic tapentadol (1 and 5mg/kg) dose-dependently reduced evoked responses of spinal dorsal horn neurones to a range of peripheral stimuli, including brush, punctate mechanical and thermal stimuli (Bee et al. 2011). They also showed that spinal application of the selective (2)-adrenoceptor antagonist atipamezole, or alternatively the mu-opioid receptor antagonist naloxone, produced near complete reversal of tapentadol's inhibitory effects, which suggested not only that the spinal cord is the key site of tapentadol's actions, but in addition that no pharmacology other than mu-opioid receptor agonism norepinephrine reuptake inhibition (MOR-NRI) is involved in its analgesia. Moreover, according to the extent that the antagonists reversed tapentadol's inhibitions in sham and SNL rats, they suggested that there may be a shift from predominant opioid inhibitory mechanisms in control animals, to predominant noradrenergic inhibition in neuropathic animals (Bee et al. 2011).

Tapentadol IR (Hale et al. 2009) as well as tapentadol ER has been shown to be safe and efficacious for the short term (Afilalo et al. 2010; Buynak et al. 2010) and long term (Wild et al. 2010) management of chronic osteoarthritis (knee or hip) and low back pain.

Selection of One Opioid Over Another

One major question that continues to be of relevance is whether individual opioids have distinct advantages over other members of this class. For example, some investigators favor methadone for the treatment of neuropathic pain. Staahl and colleagues (2006) have compared the effects of morphine and oxycodone in healthy human volunteers. They utilized a crossover study design, so each subject received morphine and an equianalgesic dose of oxycodone. They have shown that both oxycodone and morphine are equipotent in modulating induced skin and muscle pain. In contrast, when used for mechanically and thermally induced visceral pain of the esophagus, oxycodone produced significantly superior analgesia (Staahl et al. 2006). On the other hand, the ACTION study—a randomized, open-label, multicenter trial comparing once-a-day ER morphine sulfate (AVINZA) to twice-a-day controlled-release oxycodone hydrochloride (OxyContin) for the treatment of chronic, moderate to severe low back pain—and its extension phase suggested that ER morphine was significantly better than controlled-release oxycodone for reducing pain as well as improving sleep and physical functioning at a lower daily opioid dose (Rauck et al. 2006). No conclusions should be drawn from the selected findings in these studies, which are not of the highest quality. There are still no well-designed large, multicenter studies that reveal any significant distinct analgesic benefits for any particular opioid over another for certain painful conditions. The general principle is that, all other things being equal, there is no clear analgesic advantage to using a particular opioid for a specific diagnosis. However, it is conceivable that certain opioids may have particular characteristics that make them well-suited to treat neuropathic pain (Methadone, buprenorphine, oxycodone, tramadol, tapentadol (Smith 2012).

Opioids and Renal Insufficiency

In the terminal phase of end-of-life care, end-organ insufficiency is not uncommon. In renal failure, morphine, codeine, dihydrocodeine, meperidine, and propoxyphene should be avoided. Commercial morphine preparations may contain bisulfite, which can contribute to somnolence if very large doses are used (Gregory et al. 1992). Morphine is metabolized to morphine-3-glucuronide (M3G) and M6G. M3G is inactive at opioid receptors, and M3G and/or normorphine may contribute to hyperexcitability with the accumulation of large amounts (Mcquay et al. 1990; Glare et al. 1990).

In patients with renal insufficiency, hydromorphone may be used with caution; however, there is only limited evidence for a need for this (Dean 2004; Murtagh et al. 2006). Hydromorphone is mainly metabolized to hydromorphone-3-glucuronide, which is a reasonable opioid metabolite relative to others, although it may contribute to hyperexcitability if it accumulates in large amounts (Babul and Darke 1992). Additionally, based on their relative lack of active metabolites, fentanyl and methadone have been recommended for use in patients with renal insufficiency (Dean 2004). This recommendation is tempered, however, by the challenges inherent in the use of drugs with long half-lives in patients with poor renal function.

Opioids and Substance Misuse

The clinical use of opioids in LTOT is often complicated by a host of issues that include patient, family and societal perceptions of the potential for medication misuse. A significant concern is the potential for addiction in patients exposed to opioids. This concern has evolved and may be better explained by the concept of aberrant drug-related behaviors (Portenoy 2004). Aberrant behaviors may include issues such as pseudo-addiction, which has wide ranging implications that include issues ranging from poor pain control to the potential for medication diversion. In recent years the stigma related to opioid use has increased with the marked increase in death rates associated with opioid prescriptions (Webster 2011a). There appear to be many factors associated with opioid overdose deaths, including poor prescriber knowledge, unanticipated or poorly evaluated mental health issues (e.g., prior history of substance abuse) and nonadherence to their opioid regimen. This nonadherence could also include the nonmedical use of an opioid, either by the patient or another individual (i.e., diversion).

As a reaction to the changing environment associated with opioid analgesics the pharmaceutical industry has responded with a new class of opioids, the abuse-deterrent and abuse-resistant opioids. In reality this approach is not a new concept and can be traced back to combination opioid formulations that contained an active antagonist agent such as naloxone (e.g., Talwin NX). Currently there is only one FDA approved long-acting opioid using the agonist/antagonist approach with morphine and naltrexone to provide deterrence (e.g., Embeda). Other agents are in various stages of research and development and it is likely other combinations will be available in the US. Another variation on this approach is the use of an additive agent (e.g., niacin) that can be used to produce unpleasant effects when the dosage form is manipulated (e.g., snorted or used IV) or when used in excessive oral doses. In this approach the additive agent would not cause any untoward event with appropriate medical use.

Similar to deterrence, abuse-resistance offers an avenue to decrease the potential for unintended use of opioids. Abuse-resistance opioids provide a variety of mechanisms that prevent the crushing and extraction of the active opioid ingredient from the dosage form. There are currently formulations with this technology for oxycodone (OxyContin tamper-resistant), hydromorphone (Exalgo) and tramadol (Ultram ER).

At this time it is difficult to determine the role for abuse-deterrent and resistant opioids. There are multiple questions as to how to best integrate these medications into an effective approach to COT. Chief among these questions is whether these agents should become the standard approach for all patients. At this time this does not appear to be an acceptable approach, if for no other reason than the limited number of agents available and the limitation this places on options for prescribers (Webster 2011b). Other key questions exist about the role of these agents. These include the need for a more established evidence base and the profound impact related to health care professional education. Last, but certainly not least, is to consider that even with these approaches there is no guarantee that individuals will not continue to misuse these substances (excessive dosing) or find ways to promote nonmedical opioid use by supplanting the deterrence or resistance mechanism (Webster 2011b).

While addiction and diversion are issues worthy of significant evaluation in any candidate for COT, recent data suggest a wider paradigm of opioid related concerns (Sullivan 2010). Sullivan and colleagues have begun an exploration of patient perspectives that appear to be more encompassing than only the concern of addiction. These concerns include issues that do not necessarily reflect an active substance abuse issue. These issues include the desire to stop or cut down opioid use, and concerns of dependence or the impression of family and friends related to appearance of dependence. Sullivan and colleagues present compelling evidence of these and other patient-centered concerns that do not appear to be strongly associated with objective measures of substance abuse or aberrant opioid use (Sullivan 2010). This data would appear to indicate the importance of an interdisciplinary approach to patient care, involving a priori discussions about patient beliefs and concerns related to opioid therapy.

References

Adams MP, Ahdieh H. Pharmacokinetics and dose-proportionality of oxymorphone extended release and its metabolites: results of a randomized crossover study. *Pharmacotherapy.* 2004;24(4):468–476.

Adams MP, Ahdieh H. Single- and multiple-dose pharmacokinetic and dose-proportionality study of oxymorphone immediate-release tablets. *Drugs RD.* 2005;6(2):91–99.

Aderjan RE, Skopp G. Formation and clearance of active and inactive metabolites of opiates in humans. *Ther Drug Monit.* 1998;20(5):561–569.

Afilalo M, Etropolski MS, Kuperwasswer B, et al. Efficacy and safety of Tapentadol extended release compared with oxycodone controlled release for the management of moderate to severe chronic pain related to osteoarthritis of the knee: a randomized, double-blind, placebo- and active-controlled phase III study. *Clin Drug Investig.* 2010;30(8):489–505.

Arbaiza D, Vidal O. Tramadol in the treatment of neuropathic cancer pain: a double-blind, placebo-controlled study. *Clin Drug Invest.* 2007;27(1):75–83.

Babul N, Darke AC, Hagen N. Hydromorphone metabolite accumulation in renal failure. *J Pain Symptom Manage.* 1995;10(3):184–186.

Babul N, Darke AC. Putative role of hydromorphone metabolites in myoclonus. *Pain.* 1992;51(2):260–261.

Banzett RB, Adams L, O'Donnell CR, Gilman SA, Lansing RW, Schwartzstein RM. Using laboratory models to test treatment: morphine reduces dyspnea and hypercapnic ventilatory response. *Am J Respir Crit Care Med.* 2011;184(8):920–927.

Bee LA, Bannister K, Rahman W, et al. Mu-opioid and noradrenergic A(2)-adrenoceptor contributions to the effects of tapentadol on spinal electrophysiological measures of nociception in nerve-injured rats. *Pain.* 2011;152(1):131–139.

Benedetti CB, Butler SH. Systemic analgesics. In Bonica JJ, ed. *The Management of Pain.* Philadelphia: Lea & Febiger, 1990; 1640–1658.

Bolan EA, Tallarida RJ, Pasternak GW. Synergy between µ opioid receptor subtypes. *JPET.* 2002;303(2):557–562.

Bot G, Blake AD, Li S, et al. Opioid regulation of the mouse opioid receptor expressed in human embryonic kidney 293 cells. *Mol Pharmacol.* 1997;53(2):272–281.

Bruera E, Sweeney C. Methadone use in cancer patients with pain. *J Palliat Med.* 2002;5(1):127–137.

Bruera E, Neumann CM. Role of methadone in the management of pain in cancer patients. *Oncology.* 1999;13(9):1275–1284.

Bruera E, Pereira J, Watanabe S, et al. Opioid rotation in patients with cancer pain. A retrospective comparison of dose ratios between methadone, hydromorphone, and morphine. *Cancer.* 1996;78(4):852–857.

Buynak R, Shapiro DY, Okamoto A, et al. Efficacy and safety of tapentadol extended release for the management of chronic low back pain: results of a prospective, randomized, double-blind, placebo- and active-controlled Phase III study. *Expert Opion Pharmacother.* 2010;11(11):1787–1804.

Christoph T, De Vry J, Tzschentke TM. Tapentadol, but not morphine, selectively inhibits disease-related thermal hyperalgesia in a mouse model of diabetic neuropathic pain. *Neurosci Lett.* 2010;470(2):91–94.

Christoph T, Kögel B, Strassburger W, et al. Tramadol has a better potency ratio relative to morphine in neuropathic than in nociceptive pain models. *Drugs RD.* 2007;8(1):51–57.

Codd EE, Shank RP, Schupsky JJ, et al. Serotonin and norepinephrine uptake inhibiting activity of centrally acting analgesics: structural determinants and role in antinociception. *J Pharmacol Exp Ther.* 1995;274(3):1263–1270.

Crettol S, Deglon JJ, Besson J, et al. Methadone enantiomer plasma levels, CYP2B6, CYP2C19, and CYP2C9 genotypes, and response to treatment. *Clin Pharmacol Ther.* 2005;78(6):593–604.

Cruciani RA, Homel P, Yap Y, et al. QTc measurements in patients on methadone. *J Pain Symptom Manage.* 2005;29(4):385–391.

Darwish M, Kirby M, Robertson P Jr, et al. Absolute and relative bioavailability of fentanyl buccal tablet and oral transmucosal fentanyl citrate. *J Clin Pharmacol.* 2007;47(3):343–350.

Darwish M, Tempero K, Kirby M, et al. Relative bioavailability of the fentanyl effervescent buccal tablet (FEBT) 1,080 pg versus oral transmucosal fentanyl citrate 1,600 pg and dose proportionality of FEBT 270 to 1,300 microg: a single-dose, randomized, open-label, three-period study in healthy adult volunteers. *Clin Ther.* 2006;28(5):715–724.

Davis M, Walsh D. Methadone for the relief of cancer pain: a review of pharmacokinetics, pharmacodynamics, drug interactions and protocols of administration. *Support Care Cancer.* 2001;9(2):73–83.

Dean M. Opioids in renal failure and dialysis patients. *J Pain Symptom Manage.* 2004;28(5):497–504.

Dunbar PJ, Chapman CR, Buckley FP, et al. Clinical analgesic equivalence for morphine and hydromorphone with prolonged PCA. *Pain.* 1996;68(2–3):265–270.

Durfee S, Messina J, Khankari R. Fentanyl effervescent buccal tablets: enhanced buccal absorption. *Am J Drug Deliv.* 2006;4(1):1–5.

Eap CB, Buclin T, Baumann P. Interindividual variability of the clinical pharmacokinetics of methadone: implications for the treatment of opioid dependence. *Clin Pharmacokinet.* 2002;41(14):1153–1193.

Eckhardt K, Li S, Ammon S, et al. Same incidence of adverse drug events after codeine administration irrespective of the genetically determined differences in morphine formation. *Pain.* 1998;76(1–2):27–33.

Felden L, Walter C, Harder S, et al. Comparative clinical effects of hydromorphone and morphine: a meta-analysis. *Br J Anaesth.* 2011;107(3):319–328.

Fick DM, Cooper JW, Wade WE, et al. Updating the Beers criteria for potentially inappropriate medication use in older adults. *Arch Intern Med.* 2003;163(22):2716–2724.

Fishman S, Wilsey B, Mahajan G, et al. Methadone reincarnated: novel clinical applications with related concerns. *Pain Med.* 2002;3(4):339–348.

Freeman R, Raskin P, Hewitt DJ, et al. CAPSS-237 Study Group. Randomized study of tramadol/acetaminophen versus placebo in painful diabetic peripheral neuropathy. *Curr Med Res Opi.* 2007;23(1):147–161

Giacomini K, Giacomini JC, Gibson TP, et al. Propoxyphene and norpropoxyphene plasma concentrations after oral propoxyphene in cirrhotic patients with and without surgically constructed porta caval shunt. *Clin Pharmacol Ther.* 1980;28(3):417–424.

Gifford AH, Mahler DA, Waterman LA, et al. Neuromodulatory effect of endogenous opioids on the intensity and unpleasantness of breathlessness during resistive load breathering in COPD. *COPD.* 2011;8(3):160–166.

Gimbel J, Ahdieh H. The efficacy and safety of oral immediate release oxymorphone for postsurgical pain. *Anesth Analg.* 2004;99(5):1472–1477.

Glare PA, Walsh TD, Pippenger CE. Normorphine, a neurotoxic metabolite. *Lancet.* 1990;335(8691):725–726.

Gregory RE, Grossman S, Sheidler VR. Grand mal seizures associated with high dose intravenous morphine infusions: incidence and possible etiology. *Pain.* 1992;51(2):255-258.

Grond S, Sablotzki A. Clinical pharmacology of tramadol. *Clin Pharmacokinet.* 2004;43(13):879–923.

Gutstein H, Akil H. Opioid analgesics. In Hardman J, Goodman Gilman A, Limbird L, eds. *The Pharmacological Basis of Therapeutics.* 10th ed. New York: McGraw-Hill, 2001; 569–620.

Hale M, Khan A, Kutch M, et al. Once-daily OROS hydromorphone ER compared with placebo in opioid-tolerant patients with chronic low back pain. *Curr Med Res Opin.* 2010;26(6):1505–1508.

Hale M, Upmalis D, Okamotoa A, et al. Tolerability of tapentadol immediate release in patients with lower back pain or osteoarthritis of the hip or knee over 90 days: a randomized, double-blind study. *Curr Med Res Opin.* 2009;25(5):1095–1104.

Hale ME, Ahdieh H, Ma T, et al. Efficacy and safety of OPANA ER (oxymorphone extended release) for relief of moderate to severe chronic low back pain in opioid-experienced patients: a 12-week, randomized, double-blind, placebo-controlled study. *J Pain.* 2007;8(2):175–184.

Harati Y, Gooch C, Swenson M, et al. Maintenance of the long-term effectiveness of tramadol in treatment of the pain of diabetic neuropathy. *J Diabetes Complications.* 2000;14(2):65–70.

Harati Y, Gooch C, Swenson M, et al. Double-blind randomized trial of tramadol for the treatment of the pain of diabetic neuropathy. *Neurology.* 1998;50(6):1842–1846.

Holland D, Steinberg M. Electrophysiological properties of propoxyphene or norpropoxyphene in canine cardiac conducting tissues in vitro and in vivo. *Toxicol Appl Pharmacol.* 1979;47(1):123–133.

Hollingshead J, Dühmke RM, Cornblath DR. Tramadol for neuropathic pain. *Cochrane Database Syst Rev.* 2006;3: DOI: 10.1002/14651858.CD003726.

Houde R. Clinical analgesic studies of hydromorphone. In Foley K, ed. *Advances in Pain Research and Therapy.* Vol. 8. New York: Raven Press, 1986; 129–135.

Jacobson L, Chabal C, Brody MC, et al. Intrathecal methadone: a dose-response study and comparison with intrathecal morphine 0.5mg. *Pain.* 1990;43(2):141–148.

Janicki PK, Parris WC. Clinical pharmacology of opioids. In Smith HS, ed. *Drugs for Pain.* Philadelphia: Hanley & Belfus, 2003; 97–118.

Jennings AL, Davies AN, Higgins JP, Gibbs JS, Broadley KE. A systematic review of the use of opioids in the management of dyspnoea. *Thorax*. 2002;57(11):939–944.

Kamal-Bahl S, Stuart BC, Beers MH. National trends in and predictors of propoxyphene use in community-dwelling older adults. *Am J Geriatr Pharmacother*. 2005;3(3):186–195.

Kamal-Bahl SJ, Stuart BC, Beers MH. Propoxyphene use and risk for hip fractures in older adults. *Am J Geriatr Pharmacother*. 2006;4(3):219–226.

Katz N, Rauck R, Ahdieh H, et al. A 12-week, randomized, placebo-controlled trial assessing the safety and efficacy of oxymorphone extended release for opioid-naïve patients with chronic low back pain. *Curr Med Res Opin*. 2007;23(1):117–128.

Kornick CA, Kilborn MJ, Santiago-Palma J, et al. QTc interval prolongation associated with intravenous methadone. *Pain*. 2003;105(3):499–506.

Kouya PF, Hao JX, Xu XJ. Buprenorphine alleviates neuropathic pain-like behaviors in rats after spinal cord and peripheral nerve injury. *Eur J Pharmacol*. 2002;450(1):49–53.

Kreek MJ, Gutjahr CL, Garfield JW, et al. Drug interactions with methadone. *Ann N Y Acad Sci*. 1976;281:350–371.

Kreek MJ. Methadone-related opioid agonist pharmacotherapy for heroin addiction: history, recent molecular and neurochemical research and future in mainstream medicine. *Ann N Y Acad Sci*. 2000;909:186–216.

Kristensen K, Christensen CB, Christup LL. The mu1, mu2, delta, kappa opioid receptor binding profiles of methadone stereoisomers and morphine. *Life Sci*. 1995;56(2):PL45–PL50.

Kristensen K, Blemmer T, Angelo HR, et al. Stereoselective pharmacokinetics of methadone in chronic pain patients. *Ther Drug Monit*. 1996;18(3):221–227.

Lalovic B, Phillips B, Risler LL, et al. Quantitative contribution of CYP2D6 and CYP3A to oxycodone metabolism in human liver and intestinal microsomes. *Drug Metab Dispos*. 2004;32(4):447–454.

Lalovic B, Kharasch E, Hoffer C, et al. Pharmacokinetics and pharmacodynamics of oral oxycodone in healthy human subjects: role of circulating active metabolites. *Clin Pharmacol Ther*. 2006;79(5):461–479.

Lichtor JL, Sevarino FB, Joshi GP, et al. The relative potency of oral transmucosal fentanyl citrate compared with intravenous morphine in the treatment of moderate to severe post-operative pain. *Anesth Analg*. 1999;89(3):732–738.

Lussier D, Richarz U, Finco G. Use of hydromorphone, with particular reference to the OROS formulation, in the elderly. *Drugs Aging*. 2010;27(4):327–335.

Marshall DA, Strauss ME, Pericak D, et al. Economic evaluation of controlled-release oxycodone vs. oxycodone-acetaminophen for osteoarthritis pain of the hip or knee. *Am J Manag Care*. 2006;12(4):205–214.

Mather L. Clinical pharmacokinetics of analgesic drugs. In Ray PP, ed. *Practical Management of Pain*. 2nd ed. St. Louis: Mosby, 1992; 620–635.

Mathew P, Storey P. Subcutaneous methadone in terminally ill patients: manageable local toxicity. *J Pain Symptom Manage*. 1999;18(1):49–52.

Matsumoto AK, Babul N, Ahdieh H. Oxymorphone ER tablets relieve moderate to severe pain and improve physical function in osteoarthritis: results of a randomized double-blind, placebo- and active-controlled Phase III trial. *Pain Med*. 2005;6(5):357–366.

McKenna M, Nicholson AB. Use of methadone as a coanalgesic. *J Pain Symptom Manage* 2011;42(6):e4–e6.

McIlwain H, Ahdieh H. Safety, tolerability, and effectiveness of oxymorphone extended release for moderate to severe osteoarthritis pain: a one-year study. *Am J Ther.* 2005;12(2):106–112.

McNulty JP. Can levorphanol be used like methadone for intractable refractory pain? *J Palliat Med.* 2007;10(2):293–296.

Mcquay HF, Carrol D, Foura CC, et al. Oral morphine in cancer pain: influences on morphine and metabolite concentration. *Clin Pharmacol Ther.* 1990;48(3):236–244.

Moulin DE, Kreeft JH, Murray-Parsons N, et al. Comparison of continuous subcutaneous and intravenous hydromorphone infusions for management of cancer pain. *Lancet.* 1991;337(8739):465–468.

Murray A, Hagen NA. Hydromorphone. *J Pain Symptom Manage.* 2005;29(5 Suppl):S57–66.

Murtagh FE, Addinton-Hall JM, Donohoe P, et al. Symptom management in patients with established renal failure managed without dialysis. *EDTNA ERCA J.* 2006;32(2):93–98.

Nicklander R, Smits S, Steinberg M. Propoxyphene and norpropoxyphene: pharmacology and toxic effects in animals. *JPET.* 1977;200(1):245–253.

Norrbrink C, Lundeberg T. Tramadol in neuropathic pain after spinal cord injury: a randomized, double-blind, placebo-controlled trial. *Clin J Pain.* 2009;25(3): 177–184.

Oxberry SG, Torgerson DJ, Bland JM, et al. Short-term opioids for breathlessness in stable chronic heart failure: a randomized controlled trial. *Eur J Heart Fail.* 2011;13(9):1006–1012.

Palladone for chronic pain. *Med Lett Drugs Ther.* 2005;47(1204):21–23.

Pather SI, Siebert JM, Hontz J, et al. Enhanced buccal delivery of fentanyl using the OraVescent drug delivery system. *Drug Deliv Tech.* 2001;1:54–57.

Pharmaceuticals P. TIMERx control release delivery systems. *Penwest Pharmaceuticals Web site.* www.penwest.com/timerx.html. Accessed January 10, 2005.

Plummer JL, Gourlay GK, Cherry DA, et al. Estimation of methadone clearance: application in the management of cancer pain. *Pain.* 1988;33(3):313–322.

Picard N, Cresteil T, Djebli N, et al. In vitro metabolism study of buprenorphine: evidence for new metabolic pathways. *Drug Metab Dispos.* 2005;33(5):689–695.

Portenoy RK. Appropriate use of opioids for persistent non-cancer pain. Lancet 2004;364(9436):739–40.

Quigley C. Hydromorphone for acute and chronic pain. *Cochrane Database Syst Rev.* 2002(1): DOI: 10.1002/14651858. CD003447.

Rapp SE, Egan KJ, Ross BK, et al. A multidimensional comparison of morphine and hydromorphone patient-controlled analgesia. *Anesth Analg.* 1996;82(5):1043–1048.

Rauck RL, Bookbinder SA, Bunker TR, et al. The ACTION study: a randomized, open-label, multicenter trial comparing once-a-day ER morphine sulfate capsules (AVINZA) to twice-a-day controlled-release oxycodone hydrochloride tables (OxyContin) for the treatment of chronic, moderate to severe low back pain. *J Opioid Manag.* 2006;2(3):155–166.

Schmidt H, Vormfelde SV, Walchner-Bonjean M, et al. The role of metabolites in dihydrocodeine effects. *Int J Clin Pharmacol Ther.* 2003a;41(3):95–106.

Schmidt H, Vormfelde SV, Klinder K, et al. Affinities of dihydrocodeine and its metabolites to opioid receptors. *Pharm Tox.* 2003b;91(2):57–63.

Scholes CF, Gonty N, Trotman IF. Methadone titration in opioid-resistant cancer pain. *Eur J Cancer Care*. 1999;8(1):26–29.

Schröder W, Vry JD, Tzschentke TM, et al. Differential contribution of opioid and noradrenergic mechanisms of tapentadol in rat models of nociceptive and neuropathic pain. *Eur J Pain*. 2010;14(8):814–821.

Scott CC, Robbins EB, Chen KK. Pharmacologic comparison of the optical isomers of methadone. *J Pharmacol Exp Ther*. 1948;93(3):282–286.

Shir Y, Rosen G, Zeldin A, et al. Methadone is safe for treating hospitalized patients with severe pain. *Can J Anaesth*. 2001;48(11):1109–1113.

Sjogren P. Clinical implications of morphine metabolites. In Portenoy RK, Bruera EB, eds. *Topics in Palliative Care*. Vol. 1. New York: Oxford University Press, 1997; 163–177.

Smith R. Federal government faces painful decision on Darvon. *Science*. 1971;203(4383):857–858.

Smith HS. The metabolism of opioid agents and the clinical impact of their active metabolites. *Clin J Pain*. 2011a;27(9):824–838.

Smith HS. Morphine sulphate and naltrexine hydrochloride extended release capsules for the management of chronic, moderate-to-severe pain, while reducing morphine-induced subjective effects upon tampering by crushing. *Expert Opin Pharmacother*. 2011b;12(7):1111–1125.

Smith HS. Opioids and Neuropathic Pain. *Pain Physician*. 2012; 2012; 15(3S): ES93–ES110.

Smith HS. Opioid metabolism. *Mayo Clin Proc*. 2009a;84(7):613–624.

Smith HS. Clinical Pharmacology of Oxymorphone. *Pain Med*. 2009b;10(Suppl 1):S3–S10.

Smith HS. Potential analgesic interactions. In Smith HS, ed. *Drugs for Pain*. Philadelphia: Hanley & Belfus, 2003; 453–463.

Snarr BS, Rowley CP, Phan SV, et al. Prolonger Sinus Pauses with Hydromorphone in the Absence of Cardiac Conduction Disease. *South Med J*. 2011;104(3):239–240.

Srinivasan V, Wielbo D, Simpkins J, et al. Analgesic and immunomodulatory effects of codeine and codeine 6-glucuronide. *Pharm Res*. 1996;13(2):296–300.

Staahl C, Christrup LL, Andersen SD, et al. A comparative study of oxycodone and morphine in a multi-modal tissue-differentiated experimental pain model. *Pain*. 2006;123(1-2):28–36.

Sullivan MD, Von Korff M, Banta-Green C, et al. Problems and concerns of patients recieving chronic opioid therapy for chronic non-cancer pain. *Pain* 2010;149(2):345–353.

Vadovelu N, Timchenko A, Huang Y, et al. Tapentadol extended-release for treatment of chronic pain: a review. *J Pain Res*. 2011;4:211–218

Vallner JJ, Stewart JT, Kotzan JA, et al. Pharmacokinetics and bioavailability of hydromorphone following intravenous and oral administration to human subjects. *J Clin Pharmacol*. 1981;21(4):152–156.

Volpe DA, McMahon Tobin GA, Mellon RD, et al. Uniform assessment and ranking of opioid Mu receptor binding constants for selected opioid drugs. *Regul Toxicol Pharmacol*. 2011;59(3):385–390.

Wallace M, Rauck RL, Moulin D, et al. Once-daily OROS hydromorphone for the management of chronic nonmalignant pain: a dose-conversion and titration study. *Int J Clin Pract*. 2007;61(10):1671–1676.

Watson CP, Moulin D, Watt-Watson J, et al. Controlled-release oxycodone relieves neuropathic pain: a randomized controlled trial in painful diabetic neuropathy. *Pain.* 2003;105(1-2):71–78.

Webb JA, Rostami-Hodjegan A, Abdul-Manap R, et al. Contribution of dihydrocodeine and dihydromorphine to analgesia following dihydrocodeine administration in man: a PK-PD modeling analysis. *Br J Clin Pharm.* 2001;52(1):35–43.

Webster LR, Butera PG, Moran LV, et al. Oxytrex minimizes physical dependence while providing effective analgesia: a randomized controlled trial in low back pain. *J Pain.* 2006;7(12):937–946.

Webster LR, Cochella S, Dasgupta N, et al. An analysis of the root causes for opioid-related overdose deaths in the United States. *Pain Medicine* 2011a;12(Suppl 2): S26–35.

Webster L, St. Marie B, McCarberg B, et al. Current status and evolving role of abuse-deterrent opioids in managing patients with chronic pain. J of Opioid Manage 2011b; 7(3):235–45.

Weschules DJ, Bain KT. A systematic review of opioid conversion ratios used with methadone for the treatment of pain. Pain Medicine 2008;9(5):595–611.

Wild JE, Grond S, Kuperwasser B, et al. Long-term safety and tolerability of tapentadol extended release for the management of chronic low back pain or osteoarthritis pain. *Pain Pract.* 2010;10(5):416–427.

Wolff K, Rostami-Hodjegan A, Shires S, et al. The pharmacokinetics of methadone in healthy subjects and opiate users. *Br J Clin Pharmacol.* 1997;44(4):325–334.

Yue QY, Hasselstrom J, Svennson JO, et al. Pharmacokinetics of codeine and its metabolites in Caucasian healthy volunteers: comparisons between extensive and poor hydroxylators of debrisoquine. *Br J Clin Pharmacol.* 1991;31(6):635–642.

Yue QY, Svensson JO, Alm C, et al. Codeine O-demethylation co-segregates with polymorphic debrisoquine hydroxylation. *Br J Clin Pharmacol.* 1989;28(6):639–645.

Zheng M, McErlane KM, Ong MC. LC-MS-MS analysis of hydromorphone and hydromorphone metabolites with application to a pharmacokinetic study in the male Sprague-Dawley rat. *Xenobiotica.* 2002;32(2):141–151.

Chapter 5b

Optimizing Pharmacologic Outcomes: Route Selection

Howard S. Smith

For chronic therapy, the oral route of opioid delivery is usually attempted first, and the transdermal route for fentanyl is a widely accepted alternative (Donner et al. 1996; Ahmedzai and Brooks 1997). The availability of controlled-release oral formulations allows convenient dosing, either once or twice daily. Some patients require doses three times per day to optimize therapy, but this, too, is usually accommodated well. The transdermal route offers a 48- to 72-hour dosing interval and is very useful for patients who are unable to swallow or absorb an orally administered opioid, as well as for those who perceive nonoral administration as a convenience. It allows a trial of fentanyl during opioid rotation and appears to improve adherence to therapy in some cases. The observation that transdermal fentanyl produces less constipation than oral morphine (Ahmedzai and Brooks 1997; Staats et al. 2004a; Allan et al. 2005) suggests that the presence of severe constipation may be a trigger to consider an opioid switch from morphine to fentanyl.

The use of the transdermal system is limited by the difficulties involved in delivering high doses and the need for an alternative route to provide supplemental doses for breakthrough pain. It is also not preferred when rapid dose titration is needed for severe pain. Because drug delivery is influenced by the patient's temperature, frequent fever spikes could lead to unstable absorption from the transdermal system and thus complicate the use of this approach.

Patients who are unable to swallow or absorb oral opioid drugs and who do not experience intolerable side effects from systemic administration are also candidates for other approaches to long-term parenteral dosing. Repetitive injections are painful and should be avoided. Continuous infusion techniques are generally preferred because they reduce the need for nursing support, eliminate the potential for bolus effects (side effects at peak concentration or pain breakthrough at the end of the dosing interval), and can be implemented in the home with relative ease. Any opioid available in an injectable formulation can be used for continuous infusion. Long-term intravenous administration is possible if the patient has an indwelling venous access device. If subcutaneous infusion is chosen, a 25-gauge butterfly needle is conventionally used. This indwelling needle, which can be placed at any convenient site, is usually changed weekly.

Rapid Onset Opioids

Rapid-onset opioids FDA approved in the United States include: oral transmucosal fentanyl citrate (OTFC) (Actiq®), fentanyl buccal tablet (FBT) (Fentora®), fentanyl buccal soluble film (FBSF) (Onsolis®), sublingual fentanyl (SLF) (Abstral®), and fentanyl pectin nasal spray (FPNS) (Lazanda®) and fentanyl sublingual spray (FSS) [Subsys®] (Smith 2012a). Potential future rapid-onset opioids may include: intranasal fentanyl spray (INFS) (Instanyl®) and fentanyl dry powder intrapulmonary inhaler (TAIFUN®). Clinicians should initiate therapy with the lowest dose available (100 mcg if possible), and should attempt to only use a maximum of two doses per breakthrough pain episode and preferably no more than four breakthrough pain episodes per day.

Oral Transmucosal Fentanyl Citrate (OTFC)

OTFC (Actiq®) is a sweetened lozenge containing fentanyl citrate that is attached to a stick to help the patient sweep the medication across the buccal mucosa (lining of the cheek). Administration of the lozenge takes approximately 15 min (Actiq®, 2009). OTFC was approved in the United States in 1998 for breakthrough pain (BTP) in adults with cancer who are receiving, and are tolerant of, opioid analgesics for underlying chronic cancer pain. OTFC was approved in Europe for the same indication in 2002. OTFC is available in six dose strengths: 200, 400, 600, 800, 1200, and 1600 µg lozenges. The oral mucosal route of delivery offers some advantages. The oral mucosa is highly permeable, 20 times more than skin, and highly vascularized.

When the OTFC lozenge is administered as directed, 25% of the total dose of fentanyl is absorbed by the buccal mucosa and becomes systemically available. Approximately 75% of the OTFC dose is swallowed and is then absorbed from the gastrointestinal tract where two-thirds is eliminated via first-pass metabolism (Streisand et al. 1991). The bioavailability of OTFC is therefore approximately 50% of the total dose, split evenly between transmucosal and (slower) gastrointestinal absorption (Streisand et al. 1991).

Fentanyl Buccal Tablet (FBT)

The FBT Fentora® was approved in the United States in 2006 for BTP in adults with cancer pain who are receiving and are tolerant of opioid analgesics for underlying chronic cancer pain. FBT is available in doses of 100, 200, 400, 600, and 800 µg buccal tabs. FBT uses OraVescent® delivery technology to alter the pH of the oral environment in order to assist with dissolution and maximize absorption of fentanyl. Dissolution takes 14–25 min with FBT and does not require active participation from the patient (Fentora®, 2011). The OraVescent® system produces an effervescence reaction that releases carbon dioxide to produce carbonic acid in the buccal cavity. The resultant decrease in pH optimizes tablet dissolution. FBT then releases carbon dioxide which is subsequently lost from solution with a resultant increase in the pH in order to increase permeation of fentanyl through the buccal mucosa (Durfee et al. 2006; Pather et al. 2001). The buccal pH changes orchestrated by this effervescence reaction result in a greater proportion of fentanyl being absorbed transmucosally instead of being swallowed and absorbed by the slower gastrointestinal route. Furthermore, because about 50% of the fentanyl in FBT is absorbed transmucosally (Darwish et al. 2007), cytochrome P450 metabolism is bypassed to a greater extent than with traditional short-acting opioids and OTFC, so a greater proportion of fentanyl enters the systemic circulation (Darwish et al. 2006). (Absolute bioavailablity for FBT=65%, which is 48% buccal absorption plus 17% GI absorption versus OTFC where absolute bioavailability is 47% buccal absorption is 22% plus GI absorption is 25%.)

Fentanyl Buccal Soluble Film (FBSF)

The fentanyl buccal soluble film (FBSF) Onsolis™ utilizes BioErodible MucoAdhesive (BEMA™) technology (BioDelivery Sciences International). It was approved in the USA in 2009 for BTP in adults with cancer who are receiving and who are tolerant of opioid analgesics for chronic cancer pain. FBSF is available in doses of 200, 400, 600, 800, and 1200 μg per film.

FBSF presents fentanyl in a layer that adheres to the inside of the patient's cheek; an outer layer isolates the fentanyl-containing layer from saliva. In this way, the FBSF minimizes the quantity of fentanyl that is swallowed in the saliva and which is consequently lost during first-pass metabolism (Vasisht et al. 2010). The absolute bioavailability of fentanyl from FBSF was reported to be 71%, with approximately 51% of the administered dose being absorbed through the buccal mucosa (Vasisht et al. 2010).

Sublingual Fentanyl (SLF)

SLF (Abstral®) was approved in the USA for opioid-tolerant adults with cancer in 2011. The sublingual mucosa is highly vascularized and has good permeability, allowing rapid absorption of fentanyl (Lennernas et al. 2010). SLF is a tablet comprising water-soluble carrier particles that are coated with fentanyl and a mucoadhesive agent to hold the tablet under the tongue. SLF is available in doses of 100 μg, 200, 300, 400, 600, and to 800 μg sublingual tabs.

Fentanyl Pectin Nasal Spray (FPNS)

The fentanyl pectin nasal spray (FPNS), Lazanda® (US trade name), was approved in the United States in 2011 for BTP in adults with cancer who are receiving and who are tolerant of opioid analgesics for chronic cancer pain T_{max} ~ 20 min.). The addition of pectin in FPNS promotes the formation of a gel on contact with calcium cations on the nasal mucosa, prolonging the residence time of fentanyl at the mucosa and giving a rounded pharmacokinetic profile compared with the sharp profile of nongelling sprays (Fisher et al. 2010; Watts et al. 2009). This pectin-based drug delivery system is referred to as PecSys (Watts et al. 2009).

Fentanyl Sublingual Spray (FSS)

SUBSYS®, a fentanyl sublingual spray (FSS), is a sublingually administered formulation of fentanyl in a novel delivery device that was approved by the USFDA in January of 2012. This spray formulation differs from the sublingual fentanyl tablet (Abstral®). Inactive ingredients include: dehydrated alcohol 63.6% purified water, propylene glycol, xylitol, and L-menthol. The initial dose is 100 mcg but it comes in units of 100 mcg, 200 mcg, 400 mcg, 800 mcg, 1200 mcg, and 1600 mcg. For each BTP episode that is unrelieved after 30 minutes, patients may take only one additional dose of the same strength. Patients must wait 4 hours before treating another BTP episode.

Risk Evaluation and Mitigation Strategy (REMS) for Transmucosal Immediate-Release Fentanyl (TIRF) Medicines

On December 28, 2011, the FDA approved a single, shared system Risk Evaluation and Mitigation Strategy (REMS) for the entire class of transmucosal immediate-relaes fentanyl (TIRF) prescription medicines. This REMS, called the TIRF REMS Access program, consists of a restricted distribution program to reduce the risk of misuse, abuse, addiction, and overdose with TIRF medicines. The TIRF REMS Access program is the first approved class REMS for drugs in the opioid class. However, TIRF may be a suboptimal term to use instead of rapid onset opioid (ROO) since (in the minds of some clinicians) these agents may be grouped with other immediate-release formulations (oxycodone [oxyIR} morphine [MSIR]) (Smith 2012b).

A Useful Clinical Niche for Rapid Onset Opioids

A particularly useful clinical niche for rapid onset opioids is for the treatment of rapid-onset breakthrough pain in advanced painful osseous metastases. In painful osseous metastases (POM), there are generally two types of break-through pain: gradual onset breakthrough pain (GOBTP) (usually coming on in a predictable fashion in 15 to 30 minutes and fading within an hour) and ROBTP (often unpredictable in nature may be paroxysmal and/or lacinating coming on and reaching a peak severe intensity within five minutes and fading within 15 minutes). These ROBTP episodes are extremely challenging to address and require treatment with rapid onset opioids.

A triple opioid therapy (TOT) approach to using opioid analgesics may be optimal to treat painful osseous metastases (Smith 2012c). A triple opioid therapy approach utilizes three different opioid formulations: a controlled release opioid (CRO), an immediate release opioid (IRO), and a rapid onset opioid (ROO). Enteral or transdermal extended release (ER) or controlled release (CR) opioids are employed for "maintenance" therapy to control the baseline or background constant pain. The patient receiving TOT then evaluates BTP episodes: (a) if a BTP episode seems relatively predictable and gradually intensifies over a half-hour or more gradual onset breakthrough pain (GOBTP), then it may be treated early with an immediate release (IR) opioid formulation; however, (b) if a BTP episode is unpredictable and/or the intensity suddenly increases rapidly (ROBTP), then it should be treated with a rapid onset opioid (Figure 5b.1).

An iontophoretic fentanyl HCl–activated transdermal system has been developed for the management of postoperative pain. The self-contained needle-free system is roughly the size of a credit card (5cm by 7.5cm); it attaches to the upper arm or chest and delivers a set amount of fentanyl (40µg) when an imperceptible, low-intensity electric current is initiated by quickly double-clicking the dose-activation button (Viscusi et al. 2006a).

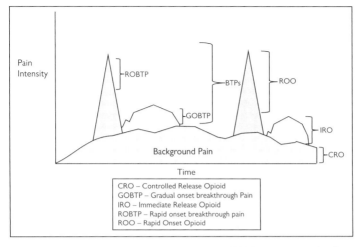

Figure 5b.1 Two different types of breakthrough pains (BTPs) and their "matching" opioid treatment

The rectal route is occasionally used for prolonged therapy, particularly at the end of life. Rectal administration of a controlled-release oral morphine preparation and specially compounded methadone suppositories have been effective.

Spinal Opioids

Extended-release epidural morphine (DepoDur) is available for treating postoperative pain and may reduce the need for other supplemental analgesia (Viscusi et al. 2006b).

Chronic intrathecal analgesic therapy

A variety of techniques for intraspinal opioid delivery have been adapted to long-term treatment, and properly selected patients can benefit greatly (Du Pen and Du Pen 2000). The clearest indication is intolerable somnolence or confusion in a patient who is not experiencing adequate analgesia during systemic opioid treatment of a pain syndrome located below the level of the mid-chest. Continuous epidural infusion or patient-controlled epidural analgesia can be accomplished through either a percutaneous or implanted epidural catheter. These approaches are generally preferred if life expectancy is measured in a few months. Intrathecal infusion or patient-controlled intrathecal analgesia using a totally implanted pump should be considered for patients with longer life expectancies. Epidural or intrathecal administered opioids may vary significantly with respect to their retention time in the epidural or intrathecal space as well as their spread, with lipiphilic opioids having short retention time, little or segmental spread, rapid onset, and short duration (Figure 5b.2). Hydrophilic opioids have longer retention times, large spread, delayed onset, longer duration, and may lead to delayed respiratory depression.

Intraspinal drug infusions via implantable intrathecal drug delivery systems (IDDS) are a viable therapeutic option that may be used for the treatment of intractable, persistent pain that is unresponsive to less invasive approaches (Smith et al. 2008; Hayek et al. 2011). Efforts to review the current literature, revise the algorithm for drug selection developed in 2000, and develop current guidelines (among other goals) led to the organization of the 2003, 2007, and 2011 Polyanalgesic Consensus conferences. Opioids have been and continue to be a mainstay agent for intraspinal therapy. Guidelines developed at the 2007 Polyanalgesic Consensus Conference suggest that the first-line intraspinal agent should be an opioid, either preservative-free, sterile morphine sulphate or hydromorphone, or a nonopioid (ziconotide) (Deer et al. 2008). It also suggested switching from one agent to another (e.g., hydromorphone) or adding agents (e.g., ziconotide) if the suggested maximum dose is reached (e.g., 15mg/day of morphine) or if side effects occur (Hassenbusch et al. 2004). The three potential first-line intrathecal analgesics that were suggested in the 2007 guidelines were morphine, hydromorphone, and ziconotide (Deer et al. 2008; Smith et al. 2008) (Figure 5b.3).

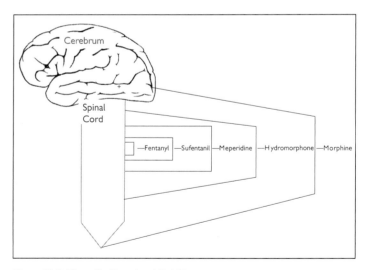

Figure 5b.2 "Spread" of Intrathecal Opioids

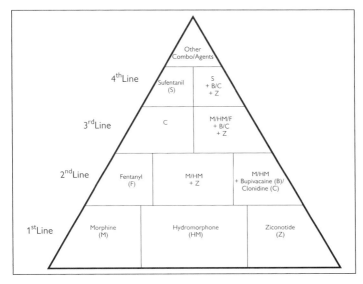

Figure 5b.3 Intrathecal Analgesic Therapies

With further evidence of favorable outcomes in the oncology population, the use of intraspinal infusion in the management of cancer pain is likely to increase. Smith et al. (2002) conducted a controlled trial comparing neuraxial infusion and comprehensive medical management, and they found that the spinal opioid treatment improved pain, side effects, quality of life, and even survival. The potential for intraspinal infusion has increased further with the use of drug combinations. The long-term spinal administration of combinations of analgesic agents (e.g., opioid, local anesthetic, and clonidine) may be utilized for a wide variety of populations but has not been rigorously studied. Ziconotide (Prialt), an N-type calcium-channel blocker, has been shown to be effective for cancer pain (Staats et al. 2004b) and may be combined with opioids (Smith and Deer 2009; Alicino et al. 2012), although strong evidence-based data are limited (Wallace et al. 2010). Suggestions for selection of patients for chronic intrathecal analgesic therapy (CIAT) have been advanced for noncancer pain (Deer et al. 2010) as well as for cancer pain (Deer et al. 2011). The results of the 2011 Polyanalgesic Consensus Conference were presented during the North American Neuromodulation Society Annual Meeting, December 8–11, in Las Vegas, Nevada, and included treatment suggestions as well as recommendations on trialing (Deer et al 2012a) and issues surrounding catheter-tip granulomas (Deer et al. 2012b). Among other recommendations, ziconotide was again suggested as a first-line intrathecal treatment for nociceptive and neuropathic chronic pain and as the preferred option for intrathecal administration compared to opioids when there was a concern for recurrent granuloma. As new drugs are tested for intraspinal therapy, the indications for this approach are likely to increase.

References

Ahmedzai S, Brooks D. Transdermal fentanyl versus sustained-release oral morphine in cancer pain: preference, efficacy, and quality of life. The TTS-Fentanyl Comparative Trial Group. *J Pain Symptom Manage.* 1997;13(5):254–261.

Allan L, Richarz U, Simpson K, et al. Transdermal fentanyl sustained release oral morphine in strong-opioid naïve patients with chronic back pain. *Spine.* 2005;30(22):2484–2490.

Actiq® Package Insert. Actiq® (oral transmucosal fentanyl citrate) Package Insert. Salt Lake City, UT: Cephalon, Inc. 2009.

Alicino I, Giglio M, Manca F, et al. Intrathecal combination of ziconotide and m orphine for refractory cancer pain: A rapidly acting and effective choice. *Pain.* 2012;153(1):245–259.

Darwish M, Kirby M, Robertson P, Jr., Tracewell W, Jiang JG. Absolute and relative bioavailability of fentanyl buccal tablet and oral transmucosal fentanyl citrate. *J Clin Pharmacol.* 2007;47(3):343–350.

Darwish M, Tempero K, Kirby M, Thompson J. Relative bioavailability of the fentanyl effervescent buccal tablet (FEBT) 1,080 pg versus oral transmucosal fentanyl citrate 1,600 pg and dose proportionality of FEBT 270 to 1,300 microg: a single-dose, randomized, open-label, three-period study in healthy adult volunteers. *Clin Ther.* 2006;28(5):715–724.

Deer TR, Smith HS, Burton AW, et al. Comprehensive consensus based guidelines on intrathecal drug delivery systems in the treatment of pain caused by cancer pain. *Pain Physician.* 2011;14(3):E283–312.

Deer TR, Smith HS, Cousins M, et al. Consensus guidelines for the selection and implantation of patients with noncancer pain for intrathecal drug delivery. *Pain Physician.* 2010;13(3):E175–213.

Deer T, Krames ES, Hassenbusch S, et al. Future Directions for Intrathecal Pain Management: A Review and Update From the Interdisciplinary Polyanalgesic Consensis Conference 2007. *Neuromodulation.* 2008;11(2):92–97.

Deer TR, Prager J, Levy R, et al. Polyanalgesic Consensus Conference-2012: Recommendations on Trialing for Intrathecal (Intraspinal) Drug Delivery: Report of an Interdisciplinary Expert Panel. *Neuromodulation.* 2012a;In press.

Deer TR, Prager J, Levy R, et al. Polyanalgesic Consensus Conference-2012: Consensus on Diagnosis, Detection, and Treatment of Catheter-Tip Granulomas (Inflammatory Masses). *Neuromodulation.* 2012b;In press.

Donner B, Zenz M, Tryba M, et al. Direct conversion from oral morphine to transdermal fentanyl: a multicenter study in patients with cancer pain. *Pain.* 1996;64(3):527–534.

Du Pen SL, Du Pen AR. Intraspinal analgesic therapy in palliative care: evolving perspective. In Portenoy RK, Bruera EB, eds. *Topics in Palliative Care.* Vol. 4. New York: Oxford University Press, 2000; 217–235.

Durfee S, Messina J, Khankari R. Fentanyl effervescent buccal tablets. *Am J Drug Deliv.* 2006;4(1):1–5.

Fentora® Package Insert. Fentora® (fentanyl buccal tablet) Package Insert; Salt Lake City, UT: Cephalon, Inc. 2011.

Fisher A, Watling M, Smith A, Knight A. Pharmacokinetics and relative bioavailability of fentanyl pectin nasal spray 100–800 microg in healthy volunteers. *Int J Clin Pharmacol Ther.* 2010;48(12):860–867.

Hassenbusch SJ, Portenoy RK, Cousins M, et al. Polyanalgesic Consensus Conference 2003: an update on the management of pain by intraspinal drug delivery—report of an expert panel. *J Pain Symptom Manage.* 2004;27(6):540–563.

Hayek SM, Deer TR, Pope JE, et al. Intrathecal therapy for cancer and non-cancer pain. *Pain Physician.* 2011;14(3):219–48.

Lennernas B, Frank-Lissbrant I, Lennernas H, Kalkner KM, Derrick R, Howell J. Sublingual administration of fentanyl to cancer patients is an effective treatment for breakthrough pain: results from a randomized phase II study. *Palliat Med.* 2010;24:286–293.

Pather SI, Siebert JM, Hontz J, Khankari RK, Gupte SV, Kumbale R. Enhanced buccal delivery of fentanyl using the oravescent drug delivery system. *Drug Deliv Technol.* 2001;1(1): 54–57.

Smith HS. A Comprehensive Review of Rapid-Onset Opioids for Breakthrough Pain. *CNS Drugs.* 2012a;26(6):509–535.

Smith HS. Painful bone metastases – Can we do better? *Ann Palliat Med.* 2012b;1(1):81–82.

Smith HS. Rapid onset opioids in palliative medicine. *Ann Palliat Med.* 2012c;1(1):45–52.

Smith HS, Deer TR. Safety and efficacy of intrathecal ziconotide in the management of severe chronic pain. *Ther Clin Risk Manag.* 2009;5(3):521–534.

Smith HS, Deer TR, Staats PS, et al. Intrathecal drug delivery. *Pain Physician.* 2008;11(2 Suppl):S89–S104.

Smith TJ, Staats PS, Deer T, et al. Implantable Drug Delivery Systems Study Group. Randomized clinical trial of an implantable drug delivery system compared with comprehensive medical management for refractory cancer pain: impact on pain, drug-related toxicity, and survival. *J Clin Oncol.* 2002;20(10):4040–4049.

Staats PS, Markowita J, Schein J. Incidence of constipation associated with long-acting opioid therapy: a comparative study. *South Med J.* 2004a;97(2):129–134.

Staats PS, Yearwood T, Charapata SG, et al. Intrathecal ziconotide in the treatment of refractory pain in patients with cancer or AIDS: a randomized controlled trial. *JAMA.* 2004b;291(1):63–70.

Streisand JB, Varvel JR, Stanski DR, et al. Absorption and bioavailability of oral transmucosal fentanyl citrate. *Anesthesiology.* 1991;75(2):223–239.

Vasisht N, Gever LN, Tagarro I, Finn AL. Single-dose pharmacokinetics of fentanyl buccal soluble film. *Pain Med.* 2010;11(7):1017–1023.

Viscusi ER, Reynolds L, Tait S, et al. An iontophoretic fentanyl patient-activated analgesic delivery system for postoperative pain: a double-blind, placebo-controlled trial. *Anesth Analg.* 2006a;102(1):188–194.

Viscusi ER, Kopacz D, Hartrick C, et al. Single-dose extended-release epidural morphine for pain following hip arthroplasty. *Am J Ther.* 2006b;13(5):423–431.

Wallace MS, Rauck RL, Deer T. Ziconotide combination intrathecal therapy: rationale and evidence. *Xlin J Pain.* 2010;26(7):635–644.

Watts P, Smith A. PecSys: in situ gelling system for optimised nasal drug delivery. *Expert Opin Drug Deliv.* 2009;6(5):543–552.

Chapter 5c

Optimizing Pharmacologic Outcomes: Assessing and Managing Opioid Side Effects

Howard S. Smith, Gary McCleane, and Gary Thompson

Better known opioid side effects may include constipation, nausea and vomiting, sedation, and pruritus. Other adverse effects may include cognitive disturbances, perceptual distortions, delirium, myoclonus, urinary retention, headache and dizziness, fatigue, anorexia, dry mouth, sweating, decreased sexual desire (libido), hormonal disturbance, abdominal discomfort, cramping, and bloating, and infrequent respiratory depression. In addition, the potential euphoriant effects of opioids may encourage drug abuse. In the long term paradoxical pain may also occur where the use of opioid induces, rather than alleviates pain. Opioid toxicity will be different between individuals. Individuals do not develop

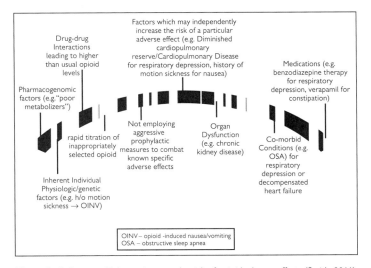

Figure 5c.1 Factors which may increase the risk of opioid adverse effects (Smith, 2011)

every potential adverse effect or toxicity and differ greatly as to the magnitude of various effects and how much distress is experienced. In general, tolerance develops to most side effects. There remains a dearth of high-quality evidence for the treatment of opioid side effects in populations both with and without cancer pain (McNicol et al. 2003) A number of factors that may affect the risk of opioid adverse effects (Smith 2011) (Figure 5c.1).

Opioid-Induced Bowel Dysfunction

Opioid-induced bowel dysfunction (OIBD) is a symptom characterized by retention of bowel content leading to gastro-oesophageal reflux, nausea, bloating, constipation, and incomplete evacuation (Kurz and Sessler 2003; Pappagallo 2001). Approximately 30% of patients reduce or terminate treatment with opioids as a result of OIBD (Bell et al. 2009). Therefore, alleviation of constipation (which is the most frequently reported symptoms of OIBD) in patients with cancer may help to optimize pain management with opioids (Candrilli et al. 2009; Olesen and Drewes 2011).

Opioids may affect the entire gastro intestinal (GI) tract including: upper GI tract (decreased gastric motility, increased pyloric tone, delayed gastric emptying), small intestine (inhibition of small bowel propulsion, increased nonpropulsive smooth muscle segmental contractions, decreased intestinal secretions), and large intestine (increased fluid absorption, inhibition of large bowel propulsion, increased nonpropulsive contractions, increased anal sphincter tone, increased water absorption from bowel).

Opioid-Induced Constipation

Functional constipation has been defined by Rome III criteria (Table 5c.1) (Longstreth et al. 2006). Opioid bowel syndrome occurs as a result of activation of opioid receptors within the myenteric and submucosal plexuses. The

Table 5c.1 Rome III Diagnostic Criteria for Functional Constipation
1. Must include two or more of the following:
a. Straining during at least 25% of defecations
b. Lumpy or hard stools in at least 25% of defecations
c. Sensation of incomplete evacuation for at least 25% of defecations
d. Sensation of anorectal obstruction/blockage for at least 25% of defecations
e. Manual maneuvers to facilitate at least 25% of defecations (e.g., digital evacuation, support of the pelvic floor)
f. Fewer than three defecations per week
2. Loose stools are rarely present without the use of laxatives
3. There are insufficient criteria for irritable bowel syndrome
Criteria fulfilled for the last 3 months with symptom onset at least 6 months prior to diagnosis
(Longstreth et al. 2006)

result is inhibition of peristalsis due to inhibition of longitudinal muscle and disinhibition of circular muscle, leading to segmental contraction; colic; and dry, desiccated stool due to reduced secretion and increased absorption from submucosal plexus binding (Kurz and Sessler 2003; Davis 2005).

Opioid-induced constipation (OIC) is a component of overall opioid bowel dysfunction. Opioids may lead to constipation via multiple mechanisms (Sykes 1998), including the following:

1. Increased ileocecal and anal sphincter tone;
2. Decreased defecation reflexes;
3. Decreased peristalsis/increased intestinal tone (opioids bind to mu opioid receptors [MORs] in the gastrointestinal tract [GI] [myenteric plexus], thereby inhibiting the release of acetylcholine, with resultant increased intestinal tone and increased resting contractile tone in the small and large intestinal circular muscle with subsequent reduced peristalsis leading to decreased intestinal motility; opioids also act in the spinal cord and brain to suppress intestinal transit); and
4. Decreased enterocyte secretion/increased liquid and electrolyte absorption from the intestinal lumen (opioids bind to GI MORs, leading to release of serotonin predominantly from neurons in the submucosal plexus, with resultant activation of $5\text{-}HT_4$ receptors and subsequent release of norepinephrine, which activates a_2 adrenergic receptors in the GI tract, thereby inhibiting enterocyte secretion [Pappagallo et al. 1999]).

Constipation is a common side effect of opioid therapy (especially in patients with advanced cancer), and this often impairs quality of life. Constipation may be present in over half of all opioid-treated cancer patients (Vanegas et al. 1998). Wirz and Klaschik (2005) reported an OIC occurrence of 42.7%. In noncancer pain patients the incidence is somewhat lower (15% to 40%); this may be partly due to a lower prevalence of comorbidities and the higher activity level in this population (Kalso et al. 2004). Risk factors for constipation (other than opioid therapy and advanced malignancy) include inadequate food intake, low-fiber diet, dehydration, weakness, inactivity, confusion, electrolyte disturbances (hypercalcemia), neurologic disorders, depression, and unfamiliar or difficult toilet arrangements. Inadequate analgesia may occur if patients discontinue opioid therapy because they feel that their constipation is more distressing than their pain.

History taking should include questions regarding frequency of evacuation, description of evacuation (color, shape), previous baseline frequency and description of bowel movements, medications that may be exacerbating bowel dysfunction, diet, history of ingestion of liquids, and comorbidities. An evaluation for fecal impaction should be included in the physical examination, during which the physician should look for palpable masses and assess anal sphincter tone. If impaction is found, manual digital evacuation may be required before any other therapeutic strategies can be initiated.

Assessment of OIC May Be Challenging

In 2010 a consensus document was developed by a multidisciplinary group of leading Canadian palliative care specialists that supported the inclusion of a portion of the Victoria Hospice Society Bowel Performance Scale, only including the part about constipation (Librach et al. 2010). The use of images to describe stool consistency has been shown to be meaningful to patients (Librach et al. 2010). Instruments that may be helpful in addition to the history and physical examination include: the Bristol Stool Form Scale (Lewis and Heaton 1997), the PAC-SYM (Frank et al. 1999), the PAC-QOL (Marquis et al. 2005), the Cleveland Clinic Constipation Score (CCS) (Agachan et al. 1996), the Constipation Severity Instrument (CSI) (Varma et al. 2008), the Constipation Assessment Scale (CAS) (McMillan and Williams 1989), and the Victoria Bowel Performance Scale (BPS) (Downing et al. 2007).

Opioids appear to differ to a certain extent in terms of the incidence and frequency of side effects associated with their use. Although no well-designed, large-scale prospective studies have attempted to compare commonly used opioids to one another with respect to constipating effects, codeine appears to be associated with a relatively high incidence of constipation. Staats and colleagues (2004) retrospectively studied 1836 patients receiving treatment with transdermal fentanyl, sustained-release oxycodone, and sustained-release morphine. Patients receiving transdermal fentanyl had a lower risk of developing constipation than those taking either of the other two strong opioids. The claim of a lower incidence of constipation with transdermal fentanyl is supported by other studies (van Seventer et al. 2003; Allan et al. 2005).

General measures to combat constipation include increasing physical activity (e.g., walking); increasing food, fiber, or liquid intake; treating confusion or depression; addressing other contributory comorbidities and electrolyte abnormalities; and providing easy and familiar toileting arrangements. Nonpharmacologic strategies for OIC may include physical therapy (Harrington and Haskvitz 2006).

A number of strategies exist to counteract OIC. Two categories of laxatives are commonly used:

1. Stool softeners, which increase liquid in the intestinal lumen via osmosis or secretion and/or decrease the absorption of fluids and electrolytes out of the intestinal lumen. There are three categories of stool softeners:
   a. bulk-forming agents (methylcellulose, psyllium), which also stimulate transit via increased volume, leading to intestinal stretching;
   b. osmotic agents (magnesium citrate, lactulose)—salts that may partially inhibit Na^+/K^+ ATPase activity; and
   c. surfactants (docusate sodium).
2. Stimulating agents ("contact cathartics"), which increase intestinal motility. The two types of stimulating agents are:
   a. anthraquinones (senna); and
   b. diphenylmethanes (bisacodyl), which can be used intermittently.

Other pharmacologic strategies for dealing with OIC include lubricants (paraffin, mineral oil), prokinetic agents (metoclopramide, bethanecol), rectal agents (suppositories such as glycerol, which produce anal/rectal stimulation leading to defecation), enemas (phosphate, high-volume saline), and miscellaneous agents that lead to diarrhea as a side effect (e.g., colchicine, misoprostol). Also, erythromycin may promote colonic transit by stimulating motilin receptors (Hasler et al. 1992).

Alvimopan is an orally administered, systemically available peripherally acting mu-opioid receptor antagonist approved in the United States for short-term, in hospital management of postoperative ileus in patients undergoing bowel resection. Jansen and colleagues (2011) examined its use in patients taking opioids for chronic noncancer pain and found that it reduced OIC without antagonizing opioid analgesia.

Oral naloxone for refractory OIC has been used with slow, careful titration from 1mg twice a day to doses above 20mg/day if required. Although the bioavailability of naloxone is roughly 3%, opioid withdrawal syndrome has been noted infrequently. The Cochrane Review Group (Candy et al. 2011) have examined available evidence for the use of methylnaltrexone (and laxatives) for the management of constipation in palliative care patients. They included seven studies (of 616 patients in their examination) and concluded that subcutaneous methylnaltrexone was effective in reducing OIC. Currently an oxycodone/naloxone combination product is available in the United Kingdom. In Scotland, the Scottish Medicines Consortium (a body that decides on the use of medicinal compounds in the Scottish health care system) has not approved this combination on the basis that comparative studies between the combination and conventional therapy of opioid and regular laxative treatment have not been undertaken and so evidence of superiority is lacking.

The neutral opioid antagonist 6β-naltrexol acts as a potent, peripherally selective opioid antagonist (Yancey-Wrona et al. 2011). Oral-cecal transit time was measured using the lactulose-hydrogen breath test in ten healthy opioid-naïve male volunteers. 6β-Naltrexol potently blocked morphine-induced slowing of gastrointestinal transit, with a median effective dose (ED(50)) of ~3 mg. In contrast, no effect was observed with 6β-naltrexol doses up to 20 mg on morphine-induced analgesia or pupil constriction. Intravenous 6β-naltrexol infusion over 30 minutes was well-tolerated up to the highest dose tested (Yancey-Wrona et al. 2011).

Another novel potential alternative for OIC treatment is lubiprostone, a locally acting type 2 chlorine channel activator, approved for the treatment of chronic idiopathic constipation and irritable bowel syndrome with constipation may be effective in OIC.

Opioid-Induced Nausea/Vomiting

Nausea and vomiting tend to resolve several days after opioids are started. These symptoms occur in about one-third of those started on morphine, and the severity is about the same for all opioids (Lehmann 1997). However, patients who have experienced these symptoms from a phenanthrene opioid with a hydroxyl group at position 6 (6-OH) (e.g., morphine), may be able to tolerate a dehydroxylated phenanthrene opioid (lacking a 6-OH) (e.g., hydromorphone) with less nausea (Wirz et al. 2008). Tapentadol, a dual acting opioid agent (a mu opioid receptor agonist and inhibitor of norepinephrine reuptake) may also be useful as far as having somewhat less opioid-induced nausea/vomiting than some other opioids. Approximately 60% of patients with advanced cancer report nausea and 30% report vomiting (Davis 2005). Nausea is highly distressing with or without vomiting and can affect overall outcome, medication compliance/enteral absorption, and quality of life.

The experience of nausea/vomiting may involve multiple receptors (Smith 2005). Opioid-induced nausea/vomiting (OINV) may be difficult to tease apart from chemotherapy-induced nausea/vomiting (CINV), radiation-induced nausea or vomiting, or postoperative nausea/vomiting (PONV); thus it has not been studied alone extensively. Opioid-induced emesis/OINV may be due to multiple opioid effects, including (a) direct effects on the chemoreceptor trigger zone, (b) enhanced vestibular sensitivity (symptoms may include vertigo and worsening with motion), and (c) delayed gastric emptying (symptoms of early satiety and bloating, worsening postprandially).

The emetic effects of some opioids seem most likely to occur secondary to activation of the d opioid receptor (DOR). In clinical settings, multiple receptors may play a role in contributing to nausea/vomiting. Some of the emetogenic receptors that have been proposed are dopamine-2 (D_2), histamine-1 (H_1), DOR, 5-hydroxy tryptamine (serotonin) (5-HT_3), acetylcholine (ACh), neurokinin-1 (NK-1), and cannabinoid receptor-1 (CB_1). Antimemetics that antagonize these receptors include the following:

- D_2—haloperidol
- H_1—promethazine
- DOR—naloxone
- 5-HT_3—ondansetron, tropisetron, dolasetron, granisetron
- ACh—scopolamine
- NK-1—aprepitant
- CB_1—dronabinol

The substituted benzamide metoclopramide (at high doses) blocks both dopamine and 5-HT3 receptors and also increases lower esophageal sphincter tone; it exhibits prokinetic activity (facilitating gastric emptying) but may lead to extrapyramidal side effects (Mehendale and Yuan 2006) and can, like other D_2 antagonists, have a negative impact on hedonic tone (Smith 2006).

Based largely on data from perioperative studies, transdermal scopolamine appears to help ameliorate OINV (Kotelko et al. 1989; Loper et al. 1989; Ferris et al. 1991; Harris et al. 1991; Tarkkila et al. 1995). Although aprepitant has not been studied for alleviating "pure" OINV, it seems, intuitively, that it could be a promising agent for this purpose. The acute administration of morphine may cause an increase in central nervous system (CNS) expression of substance P (Cantarella and Chahl 1996). Furthermore, morphine upregulates functional expression of the NK-1 receptor (NK-1R) in cortical neurons (as evidenced by mRNA levels, as well as immunofluorescence and Western blot assays using specific antibody to NK-1R protein), possibly via MOR-induced changes in cyclic adenosine monophosphate, leading to activation of the p38 MAPK signaling pathway (via phosphorylation) and activation of the NK-1R promoter (Wan et al. 2006). Therefore, it does not seem unreasonable to study aprepitant—an NK-1R antagonist used for the treatment of PONV and CINV—for its efficacy in treating OINV.

Although the use of drug combinations for OINV has not been studied, it is not uncommon for clinicians to empirically combine multiple antiemetic agents in attempts to optimize outcomes. Corticosteroids, despite their uncertain mechanism of action, have been utilized as antiemetic adjuvants in combination with other antiemetic agents (Münstedt et al. 1999).

Preliminary preclinical data suggest that LNS5662 (Flavonol-PgP Modulator)—a flavonol thought to activate PgP efflux of pump ligands at the blood–brain barrier—may ameliorate opioid adverse effects in OINV, thereby improving tolerability without interfering with analgesic efficacy. This agent may therefore deserve further study (Gordon et al. 2007).

Opioid-Induced Sedation

Opioid-induced sedation (OIS) has been defined as a unique, disordered level of consciousness in which both arousal mechanisms and content processing are functional but attenuated because of the action of opioids at receptors within the CNS. Attenuated arousal manifests as decreased wakefulness, and attenuated content processing manifests as a slowed interpretation of the environment (Young-McCaughan and Miaskowski 2001a). Various strategies have been proposed to measure OIS (Young-McCaughan and Miaskowski 2001b), which is most likely largely mediated via the MOR. It appears that activation of the MOR with opioid binding inhibits rapid eye movement (REM) sleep, thus disrupting normal sleep–wake cycles; this may contribute to OIS.

Patients with OIS often report symptoms such as feeling drowsy, sleepy, groggy, dizzy, dreamy, cloudy, mentally foggy, or lethargic. Signs of OIS may include cognitive impairment, lack of coordination, slowed reaction time, and performance deficits. Patients with OIS may be able to perform motor and/or cognitive tasks during evaluation; however, once they are no longer actively engaged in performing a specific task, they may drift back into a sedated state (Young-McCaughan and Miaskowski 2001a). Before assuming that observed/reported sedation is due to opioids, clinicians should consider other possible causes of sedation, including interactions with other drugs/substances, sleep disturbances/sleep-disordered breathing (e.g., sleep apnea), and so on.

OIS is usually most intense upon initiation or escalation of opioids. Although most patients develop tolerance to OIS within days to weeks (O'Mahony et al. 2001), some patients may never develop significant tolerance to sedation. OIS may limit dose titration, contribute to noncompliance, diminish quality of life, and put the sedated patient at risk. General measures to combat OIS may include opioid dose reduction, opioid rotation, elimination of other sedating medications (when possible), and appropriate diet, activity, and sleep hygiene.

Pharmacologic treatment of OIS may be useful in certain patients/settings. The following three agents appear to be particularly beneficial:

1. Methylphenidate (an amphetamine) at a dose of 10 to 15mg/day (Bruera et al. 1989; Bruera et al. 1992; Wilwerding et al. 1995);
2. Donepezil (an acetylcholinesterase inhibitor) at a dose of 2.5 to 15mg/day (Slatkin 2001; Bruera et al. 2003); and
3. Modafinil (a CNS stimulant) at a dose of 100 to 600mg/day (Webster et al. 2003).

Opioid-Induced Pruritus

More than 340 years ago, Samuel Hafenreffer, a German physician, defined itch as an "unpleasant sensation that elicits the desire or reflex to scratch." At the level of the skin, neuronal or immune-cell-derived cannabinoids can lead to the release of b-endorphin from keratinocytes (via CB_2 activation), which conceivably could play a role in modulating certain pruritic states. At least some opioid-induced pruritis (OIP), from topically or systemically administered opioids, may be due in part from the opioid binding to peripheral mu opioid receptors (peripheral OIP) (Yamamoto and Sugimoto 2010). Therefore, it is possible in the future that agents like the peripherally restricted opioid antagonist naloxone methiodide (Yamamoto and Sugimoto 2010), may be a useful treatment at least for peripheral OIP. At the spinal level, it appears that mu opioids are pruritic in certain settings (Andrew et al. 2003) and k opioids are antipruritic (Wakasa et al. 2004; Wikström et al. 2005). Furthermore, the MOR appears to play an important role in certain pruritic states (especially chronic cholestatic pruritus). Administered systemically, naltrexone, an opioid antagonist, can treat some pruritic conditions (Wolfhagen et al. 1997; Terg et al. 2002); it has also been administered topically in a 1% Excipial-type cream (Bigliardi et al. 2007). In the future, specially designed MOR antagonist agents, which may peripherally antagonize opioid-induced pruritus (OIP) while maintaining adequate analgesia, may be useful for patients on long-term opioid therapy (LTOT) who are suffering from significant OIP.

Intense pruritus is not a very common side effect of systemic opioids, but it is a common side effect with epidural or intrathecal morphine administered for postoperative pain or refractory cancer pain. In the perioperative period, naloxone or mixed agonist-antagonists (e.g., butorphanol) may reverse pruritus, indicating that activation of the opioid receptor is needed for OIP to develop (Lehmann 1997); however, these agents can not be advocated to treat pruritus associated with LTOT. Antihistamines/anticholinergics (e.g., diphenhydramine) or serotonin-receptor blockers (e.g., cyproheptadine) may relieve pruritus to varying degrees in some individuals. Opioid switch or opioid dose reduction plus the addition of an adjuvant analgesic should be attempted if pruritus is distressful (Lehmann 1997; Cherny et al. 2001; McNicol et al. 2003).

Opioid-Induced Respiratory Depression

There have been parallel increases in both opioid use and the incidence of reportable adverse events such as respiratory depression. According to the Adverse Event Reporting System (AERS) used by the Food and Drug Administration (FDA) to track adverse effects as reported by health care professionals, oxycodone and fentanyl were the two most frequently reported drugs associated with fatal or serious nonfatal outcomes from 1998 to 2005 (Moore et al. 2007). Webster et al. concluded that causes of opioid-related deaths are multifactorial, so solutions must address prescribed behaviours, patient contributory factors, nonmedical use patterns, and systemic failures (Webster et al. 2011). Clinical strategies to reduce opioid-related mortality should be empirically tested, should not reduce access to needed therapies, should address risk from methadone as well as other opioids, and should be incorporated into any risk evaluation and mitigation strategies enacted by regulators (Webster et al. 2011).

Hospital inpatients may be at significant risk of opioid-induced respiratory depression (OIRD) as well. Patients with severe acute pain may be given large doses of opioids rapidly in efforts to ameliorate pain. OIRD associated with the treatment of postoperative pain may occur from multiple causes. (Patients may be particularly susceptible to OIRD, organ function may be diminished, hypovolemia, altered pharmacokinetics/pharmodynamics, or errors in prescribing opioids.) One of the most common errors in prescribing opioids in the hospital is changing from 2 mg of intravenous morphine to 2 mg of intravenous hydromorphone without taking into account that hydromorphone is about five times as potent as morphine. Cronrath and colleagues utilized the Healthcare Failure Mode Effect Analysis (HFMEA) model with multidisciplinary team to look at processes, diagramming the steps involved to identify potential failure points in efforts to prevent PCA oversedation (Cronrath et al. 2011). The changes implemented identified 16 failure points with a hazard score of 16 or greater. One year later, the established systems HFMEA goal was met: oversedation events were reduced by 50% (Cronrath et al. 2011).

Mechanisms of OIRD

The precise mechanisms responsible for opioid-induced respiratory depression (OIRD) are uncertain. Initially, it was thought that the pre-Bötzinger complex, a small area in the ventrolateral medulla in the rat, but not found as of yet in humans, was the pacemaker for respiratory rhythm. It is becoming appreciated that control of respiratory rhythm/drive is extremely complex and likely involves neural circuitry communicating with multiple cortical regions (e.g., insula, frontal operculum, secondary somatosensory cortex), brainstem, and periphery.

Central chemoreceptors provide tonic drive to the respiratory motor output by sensing changes in pH (Pattison 2008). The retrotrapezoid nucleus and midline raphe nuclei contain brainstem carbon dioxide-sensitive neurons (central chemoreceptors) that activate premotor neurons of the ventral respiratory group (VRG) that includes the pre-Bötzinger complex, an area with respiratory rhythm-generating neurons (Dahan et al. 2010). The retrotrapezoid nucleus (RTN) is thought to be an important site of chemoreception; select neurons (i.e., chemoreceptors) in this region sense changes in $CO(2)/H(+)$ and send excitatory glutamatergic drive to respiratory centers to modulate the depth and frequency of breathing (Mulkey and Wenker 2011). Purinergic signaling may also contribute to chemoreception. $CO(2)/H(+)$ facilliates ATP release within the RTN to stimulate breathing, and $CO(2)/H(+)$- sensitive astrocytes are the source of this purinergic drive to breath (Mulkey and Wenker 2011).

Chemoreceptive areas that modulate respiration include the nucleus tractus solitaries (NTS), midline medullary raphe, pre-Bötzinger complex, and the RTN.pFRG in the medulla (Feldman et al. 2003), the locus coreuleus (Oyamada et al. 1998) in the pons, and the fastigial nucleus in the cerebellum (Martino et al. 2007). Afferent sensory input from the peripheral chemoreceptors of the carotid bodies activates the nucleus tractus solitaries, which also projects to the VRG (Dahan et al. 2010) (Figure 5c.2).

LC noradrenergic neurons play an important role in the ventilator response to CO_2 acting on tidal volume (Blandina et al. 1991). Serotonin (5-HT) modulates the LC role in the hypercapnia-induced hypernea. Hypercapnia induces an increase in the release of 5-HT in the LC, which acts on postsynaptic 5-HT$_{2A}$ receptors to inhibit noradrenergic (NA) neurons (with resultant altered tidal volumes) and may act on presynaptic 5-HT$_{1A}$ receptors to regulate its own release and have opposite effects from 5-HT$_{2A}$ (de Souza Moreno et al. 2010). Thus, it is possible that 5-HT released from the dorsal raphe (DR) nucleus during hypercapnia acts on 5-HT$_2$ receptors in the LC. As a consequence, neuronal firing rate and therefore NA release in LC projection sites would be decreased, reducing the ventilator response to 7% CO_2 (de Souza Moreno et al. 2010).

The mechanisms contributing to OIRD are likely multifactorial in nature. With regard to respiration, opioid receptors are abundant in respiratory control centers (Wamsley 1983) that include the brainstem (Akil et al. 1984), but also include higher centers such as insula, thalamus, and anterior cingulated cortex (Banzett et al. 2000; Baumgartner et al. 2006; McKay et al. 2003). Opioid receptors are also located in the carotid bodies (Lundberg et al. 1979a; Wharton et al. 1980) and in the vagi (Lundberg et al. 1979b). Mechanosensory receptors located in the epithelial, submucosal, and muscular layers of the airways (Kubin et al. 2006; Yu 2005) relay mechanical and sensory information from the lungs and express opioid receptors (Zebraski et al. 2000; Pattison 2008).

Opioids profoundly depress the hypoxic ventilatory response (HVR) and hypercapnic ventilatory response (HCVR) (Weil et al. 1975) through depression of central and peripheral chemoreception, described above. The degree of respiratory depression varies between drugs, but there are currently no opioids available that are devoid of respiratory side effects (Pattison 2008). However, perhaps the predominant contribution to OIRD is due to recent MOR agonists inhibiting activity in the dorsolateral and medial parts of the NTS

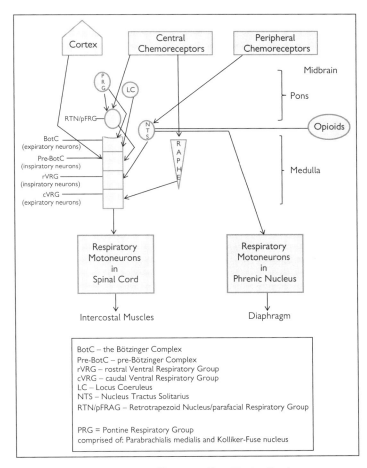

Figure 5c.2 Simplified Schematic of Respiratory Drive/Rhythm Circuitry

(Poole et al. 2007), an area which contains chemoreceptive neurones (Paton et al. 2001) and is the location of the afferent inputs from the carotid body (Finley and Katz 1992), thus, Pattison hypothesized that opioids affect the peripheral chemoreflex pathway by interrupting it where impulses synapse in the brainstem (Pattison 2008).

Opioids have profound effects on the cortical centers that control breathing, which potentiates their actions in the brainstem. Using functional magnetic resonance imaging, Pattison and colleagues found that awareness of respiration, reflected by an urge-to-breathe score, was profoundly reduced with remifentanil (Pattison et al. 2009). Urge to breathe was associated with activity in the bilateral unsula, frontal operculum, and secondary somatosensory cortex. Localized remifentanil-induced decreases in breath hold-related activity were observed in the left anterior insula and operculum. Pattison and colleagues also observed remifentanil-induced decreases in the **b**lood **o**xygenation **l**evel-**d**e-pendent (BOLD) response to breath holding in the left dorsolateral prefrontal cortex, anterior cingulated, the cerebellum, and peraqueductal gray, brain areas that mediate task performance (Pattison et al. 2009).

It is clinically important to recognize that acute pain may antagonize OIRD. Opioid-induced respiratory depression is also less severe in patients with chronic pain likely due to chronic pain (particularly chronic neuropathic pain), enhancing 5-HT$_{4A}$ receptor systems in the brainstem (Kamei et al. 2011). However, with acute pain, once the acute pain has resolved, caution must be utilized to make sure that the patient does not all of a sudden develop severe OIRD, since post-resolution of pain, there will be no pain to antagonize the OIRD.

In the future, it appears that a number of nonopioid agents may be useful to reverse OIRD without diminishing opioid-induced analgesia. Respiratory drive may be restored via modulation of neuronal transmitter systems in the regions contributing to respiratory drive, especially boosting serotonergic systems which tend to increase levels of cyclic adenosine monophosphate (cAMP) in the region which correlates with the pre-Bötzinger complex, opposing the decrease in cAMP. Agents which may contribute to reversing OIRD include 5HT$_{1A}$ ago-nists [8-hydroxy-2-(di-n-propylamino)tetralin (8-OH-DPAT), the partial agonist busprione], 5HT$_{4A}$ agonists [BIMU8 zacopride, mosapride], ampakines, [CX546, CXH7], and microglial inhibitors [minocycline] (Dahan et al. 2010).

Additionally, it is conceivable that reversal of OIRD stimulation of respira-tory drive may occur due to: enhancement of dopaminergic neurotransmis-sion (Lalley 2008), methylxanthine administration (Ruangkittisakul and Ballanyi 2010), and modulation of neurokinin receptors (Shvarev et al. 2010).

Respiratory depression remains one of the most feared effects of opioids; however, this effect is unusual if opioids are appropriately titrated to pain re-lief (Davis et al. 2004). Parenteral opioid titration for relief of cancer pain has not been associated with respiratory depression, as demonstrated by the ab-sence of significant changes in end-tidal carbon dioxide or oxygen saturation in nonoxygen-dependent cancer patients (Estfan 2007). Experienced palliative care clinicians are generally adamant that, as long as escalations in opioids are carefully titrated on the basis of appropriate control of symptoms (usually pain, dyspnea, or cough), and signs (mental status, respiratory rate), concerns that death will be hastened by opioids are unwarranted (Forrow and Smith 2004). Twycross (1982) argues that "the use of morphine in the relief of cancer pain carries no greater risk than the use of aspirin *when used correctly*," and, far from being the cause of death, "the correct use of morphine is more likely to prolong a patient's life because he is more rested and pain-free." Portenoy and Coyle (1990) report that "the development of new respiratory symptoms is virtually never a primary drug effect in patients who have been receiving stable doses or who are undergoing dose increases following substantial prior opioid intake."

Foley (1991) maintains that "respiratory depression is not a significant limiting factor in the management of patients with pain because with repeated doses, tolerance develops to this effect." Respiratory depression may occur if large doses are used in an opioid-naïve patient, if doses are titrated without regard to opioid half-life, if drug-drug interactions occur that prevent opioid clearance, or if sedative medications (e.g., benzodiazepines) are started in conjunction with an opioid (particularly methadone) (McNicol 2003).

Dahan et al. (2001) studied MOR knockout mice (i.e., mice lacking the MOR) and concluded that opioid activation of MORs (and not d, k, or opioid-receptor-like 1 receptors) is almost solely responsible for the respiratory effects of opioids, independent of their analgesic behavior. Opioid-induced respiratory depression (OIRD) is most pronounced during sleep (Dahan 2007). Buprenorphine, a partial MOR agonist, displays ceiling effects with respect to respiratory depression, and morphine-6-glucuronide has only limited effects on hypoxemic breathing response. However, with acute pain (especially postoperative pain), opioid-naïve patients may receive significant doses or increases in doses in efforts to combat severe pain. In acute/perioperative pain OIRD may occur < 1% of the time; although this number is likely significantly higher when selecting out specific patient subtypes who may be more susceptible to OIRD than average. One example of this patient subtype is the group of morbidly obese (MO) patients with obstructive sleep apnea (OSA). A simple eight-item questionnaire attempting to identify patients at risk for OSA is the STOP-BANG tool (Table 5c.2) (Chung et al. 2008). When administrating significant doses of opioids to these MO patients with OSA, capnography trends may be

Table 5c.2 STOPBANG screening tool for Obstructive Sleep Apnea (OSA)	
STOPBANG	
Yes = 1, No = 0	
S (Snore) Have you been told that you snore?	_____
T (Tired) Are you often tired during the day?	_____
O (Obstruction) Has anyone observed you stopping breathing during your sleep?	_____
P (Pressure) Do you have or are you being treated for high blood pressure?	_____
B (BMI) Is your body mass index greater than 35 kg/m^2?	_____
A (Age) Are you 50 years old or older?	_____
N (Neck) Is your neck circumference > 40 cm? [Are you a male with a neck circumference > 17 inches or a female with a neck circumference > 16 inches?]	_____
G (Gender) Are you a male?	_____
Total score: add all eight questions	_____
High Risk of OSA $\geq$ 3	
Low Risk of OSA < 3	

useful in efforts to identify early respiratory depression by increasing end tidal carbon dioxide levels.

If the clinician is faced with serious respiratory depression, the agent of choice to antagonize OIRD is naloxone. Naloxone is a short-acting medication; therefore, once OIRD is reversed by intravenous naloxone boluses, it appears best to follow up with a continuous infusion. Alternatively, it may sometimes be better for the patient to be transiently intubated and mechanically ventilated (e.g., in a patient with severe coronary artery disease, as the use of naloxone in such a patient may result in pulmonary edema, hypertension, tachycardia, and severe pain).

Although appropriate opioid titration will not necessarily lead to respiratory depression in patients with severe pain, if a patient whose severe pain is partially controlled by large doses of opioids has all of the pain acutely alleviated (e.g., by nerve block), it would be prudent to monitor him or her closely and proactively and to cut the opioid dose in half immediately after the procedure.

Opioid-Induced Androgen Deficiency (OPIAD)

Morphine may induce a dramatic long-lasting decrease in testosterone, which persists during opioid therapy even if the treatment lasts for months or years, in both males and females (Aloisi et al. 2005). The effect can occur after a few hours, with testosterone concentrations reaching castration levels (< 1ng/ml) (Aloisi et al. 2005), although typically it is not generally appreciated in clinical practice until after a week of intrathecal opioid or a month of oral opioid therapy with doses exceeding 100 mg of oral morphine equivalents daily (Smith and Elliott 2011). Aloisi and colleagues have also shown that once opioid treatment is interrupted, testosterone levels recover in a few hours or days (Aloisi et al. 2009; Ceccarelli et al. 2006).

The occurrence of significantly reduced testosterone levels during morphine administration has largely been attributed to the inhibitory action of morphine on gonadotropin-releasing hormone secretion in the hypothalamus (Kalyani et al. 2007; Daniell et al. 2006). This inhibition causes decreased gonadotropin production, and, consequently, gonadal hormone secretion.

Patients who chronically consume opioids should be asked about symptoms such as reduced libido, erectile dysfunction, depression, fatigue, hot flashes or night sweats, and irregular menses (Elliott et al. 2011). Laboratory testing to assess for the presence of opioid-induced hypogonadism may include TT, FT, SHBG, LH, FSH, DHEAS, and estradiol (E2) (Katz and Mazer 2009).

Acute administration of opioids increases levels of prolactin, growth hormone, thyroid-stimulating hormone, and adrenocorticotropic hormone while inhibiting the release of luteinizing hormone (LH) (Grossman 1983; Su et al. 1987; Paice et al. 1994). When opioids are administered on a long-term basis, different endocrine results are observed. Hypogonadotropic hypogonadism may occur with opioids, particularly at high doses. Levels of follicle-stimulating hormone (FSH) and LH will be low, and testosterone or estrogen levels will be below normal. Hot flashes, irritability, and loss of libido may occur due to lowered hormone levels. A significant decrease in testosterone levels (hypogonadism) may be linked to osteoporosis, lowered pain threshold, and impaired wound healing. Testosterone injections or administration via patches or gels (for male hormone replacement) and co administration of testosterone and estrogen (e.g., Estratest, an esterified estrogen/methyltestosterone used for female hormone replacement) may be utilized in attempts to address this issue, as hormone replacement may improve symptoms (Rajagopal et al. 2003; Strasser et al. 2006).

Abs and colleagues (2000) extensively investigated 73 patients receiving intrathecal opioids for chronic nonmalignant pain for an average duration of 26 months. Decreased libido and impotence were present in 23 of the 24 men studied. Nine of the men had a significantly reduced testosterone level, and most had a decreased LH level. All of the premenopausal women had either amenorrhea or an irregular cycle, with ovulation in only one patient, as well as decreased LH and FSH levels compared to controls. The 24-hour urinary cortisol excretion was significantly lower in 14 of the 73 patients than in controls. Most of these men and all of the women developed hypogonadotrophic hypogonadism, 15% of all patients developed central hypocorticism, and about 15% developed growth hormone deficiency (Abs et al. 2000).

Sleep-Disordered Breathing and Chronic Opioid Therapy

The use of opioids has been associated with development of sleep-disordered breathing, including central apneas, nocturnal oxygen desaturations, and abnormal breathing patterns (Guilleminault et al. 2010). It appears that opioids may promote sleep-disordered breathing phenomena (Zutler and Holty 2011). Studies looking at the effects of chronic opioid use on breathing and sleep have found that repetitive central apneas during nonrapid eye movement (NREM) sleep are common (Walker et al. 2007; Wang et al. 2005; Farney et al. 2003). Walker et al. (2007) showed the development of ataxic breathing and central apneas during NREM sleep in 70% of patients chronically using opioids compared to 5% of controls. Furthermore, this appeared to be a dose-dependent relationship. Farney et al. (2003) reported on three patients who developed sleep-disordered breathing associated with long-term opioid therapy.

Hajiha et al. (2009) concluded that mu-opioid receptor stimulation suppresses motor output from a central respiratory motoneuronal pool that activates genioglossus muscle, and this suppression does not involve muscarinic receptor-mediated inhibition (Hajika et al. 2009). This mu-opioid receptor-induced suppression of tongue muscle activity by effects at the hypoglossal motor pool may underlie the clinical concern regarding adverse upper airway function with mu-opioid analgesics. The inhibitory effects of mu- and delta-opioid receptors at the hypoglossal motor nucleus (HMN) also indicate an influence of endogenous enkephalins and endorphins in respiratory motor control (Hajiha et al. 2009).

Webster and colleagues performed an observational study of chronic pain patients on opioid therapy who received overnight polysomnographies (Webster et al. 2008). They found a direct relation between the central apnea index and the daily dosage of methadone (P = 0.008) and also with benzodiazepines calls for increased vigilance (Webster et al. 2008).

Other Opioid Adverse Effects

A recurrent concern associated with the chronic administration of an opioid is for severe pain the drug's effect on cognition and motor tasks such as driving. Schindler and colleagues (2004) examined this issue in opioid addicts (without chronic pain) using an Austrian standard test battery, the Act and React Test (ART) system, to measure performance related to driving. Subjects were taking either methadone or buprenorphine and were compared to healthy controls. It was found that the performance of those taking opioids for severe pain did not differ significantly from that of the healthy controls in the majority of standard ART tests (Schindler et al. 2004).

Similarly, Sabatowski and colleagues (2003) measured attention, reaction, visual orientation, motor coordination, and vigilance in 30 subjects using a stable dose of transdermal fentanyl for noncancer pain and compared the results to those of 90 healthy volunteers. None of the results differed significantly between the fentanyl-treated and volunteer subjects. The investigators concluded that in patients treated with stable doses of transdermal fentanyl, the threshold for fitness to drive did not differ significantly from that of control subjects.

The psychotomimetic adverse effects of opioids (myoclonus, visual hallucinations, and confusion) occur in a minority of patients, usually only at high doses (Lehmann 1997; Inturrisi 2002). Dysphoria, feelings of unreality, depersonalization, vivid daydreams, nightmares, twilight visual hallucinations, and paradoxical pain (opioid-induced hyperalgesia) have been reported. Patients usually do not report hallucinations voluntarily. These side effects can appear in individuals taking antipsychotic medications and are dose-limiting to opioid titration. Anecdotally, baclofen, diazepam, clonazepam, midazolam, valproic acid, and dantrolene sodium have been used to treat myoclonus (Cherny et al. 2001). It is possible that hyperexcitability/confusion secondary to high-dose opioids (especially in renal failure) may be mediated via spinal antiglycinergic effects and therefore are not responsive to, and perhaps even worsened by, naloxone administration (Hagen and Swanson 1997). Dose reduction (with the addition of an adjuvant analgesic) or opioid switch will be necessary in most patients who have symptomatic psychotomimetic opioid effects.

It appears that opioids may modulate the immune system and also may affect cancer in the human body. Morphine when administered in large enough doses may suppress complement receptor expression, phagocytosis, and respiratory burst in neutrophils (Welters et al. 2000) and natural killer cell activity (Saurer et al. 2006a; Saurer et al. 2006b); however, when it is administered for the treatment of acute inflammatory pain, which also reduces NK cell activity, morphine may suppress the reduction caused by acute inflammatory pain (Sakaue et al. 2011). Moreover, buprenorphine and methadone may exhibit less potential immunosuppresion. Morphine also has dual effects on tumor cell proliferation and survival either by activation of different opioid receptors on the cell surface or via opioid receptor-independent pathways. Both pro- and anti-migratory effects have been reported for morphine (Afsharimani et al. 2011a). At the moment evidence does not draw a clear picture of morphine as a tumor-promoting or inhibiting agent (Afsharimani et al. 2011b).

A variety of possible adverse effects may have clinical significance in certain circumstances, including issues of analgesic tolerance and opioid-induced hyperalgesia. It appears that sleep-disordered breathing may be associated with LTOT (Farney et al. 2003; Wang et al. 2005). A single case report highlights a different possible side effect of fentanyl use. Kokko and colleagues (2002) reported apparent inappropriate antidiuretic hormone (ADH) release in a patient with a known lung tumor who was being treated with fentanyl. Withdrawal of fentanyl terminated the ADH release, while reinstitution of fentanyl at a later date triggered further inappropriate ADH release.

Opioid Abuse Deterrence Medication

With the increased use of opioids and particularly opioids for severe pain in the treatment of chronic noncancer pain, along with the increasing prevalence of substance abuse; the issue of opioid misuse is more important than ever. While careful patient screening prior to prescription is a fundamental prerequisite of strong opioid use, measures that may counteract the tendency for abuse may have merit. One strategy is to provide the strong opioid with sequestered naltrexone. If the extended release opioid is chewed or crushed in an attempt to get a quick "hit" from the opioid, the release of the naltrexone counteracts the normal "high" from the opioid. Katz and colleagues (2010) studied patients given morphine with sequestered naltrexone for chronic osteoarthritis pain. In their enriched enrolment study of 547 patients they were able to show that the combination of morphine and naltrexone provided the same degree of relief as an equal dose of morphine. As Smith (2011) has stated, only longer-term epidemiology studies will prove whether this has an impact on drug misuse. Brushwood and colleagues (2010) raise the interesting question as to whether the health care provider has a legal liability when a product without abuse-deterrence qualities is used and a person suffers harm that would not have occurred had an abuse-deterrent formulation been given in its place.

Conclusion

Opioid side effects are generally mediated through opioid receptors; certain side effects (myoclonus, hallucinations, and opioid-induced hyperalgesia) will not respond to MOR antagonists. Tolerance develops to most side effects (e.g., sedation, nausea). Opioid dose reduction with the addition of an adjuvant analgesic, route conversion (usually to spinal opioids), or opioid rotation will reduce or relieve most opioid side effects.

References

Abs R, Verhelst J, Maeyaert J, et al. Endocrine consequences of long term intrathecal administration of opioids. *J Clin Endocrinol Metab.* 2000;85(6):2215–2222.

Afsharimani B, Cabot P, Parat MO. Morphine and tumor growth and metastasis. *Cancer Metastasis Rev.* 2011a;30(2):225–238.

Afsharimani B, Cabot PJ, Parat MO. Morphine use in cancer surgery. *Front Pharmacol.* 2011b;2:46.

Agachan F, Chen T, Pfeifer J, et al. A constipation scoring system to simplify evaluation and management of constipated patients. *Dis Colon Rectum.* 1996;39(6):681–685.

Akil H, Watson SJ, Young E, et al. Endogenous opioids: biology and function. *Annu Rev Neurosci.* 1984;7:223–255.

Allan L, Richarz U, Simpson K, et al. Transdermal fentanyl sustained release oral morphine in strong-opioid naive patients with chronic back pain. *Spine.* 2005;30(22):2484–2490.

Aloisi AM, Pari G, Ceccarelli I, et al. Gender related effects of chronic non-malignant pain and opioid therapy on plasma levels of macrophage migration inhibitory factor (MIF). *Pain.* 2005;115(1-2):142–151.

Aloisi AM, Aurilio C, Bachiocco V, et al. Endocrine consequences of opioid therapy. *Psychoneuroendocrinology.* 2009;34(Suppl 1):S162–168.

Andrew D, Schmeiz M, Ballantyne JC. Itch—mechanisms and mediators. In Dostrovsky JO, Carr DB, Koltzenburg M, eds. *Progress in Pain Research and Management.* Seattle: IASP Press, 2003; 213–226.

Banzett RB, Mulnier HE, Murphy K, et al. Breathlessness in humans activates insular cortex. *Neuroreport.* 2000;11(10):2117–2120.

Baumgartner U, Buchholz HG, Bellosevich A, et al. High opiate receptor binding potential in the human lateral pain system. *Neuroimage.* 2006;30(3):692–699.

Bell TJ, Panchal SJ, Miaskowski C, et al. The prevalence, severity, and impact of opioid-induced bowel dysfunction: results of a US and European Patient Survey (PROBE 1). *Pain Med.* 2009;10(1):35–42.

Bigliardi PL, Stammer H, Jost G, et al. Treatment of pruritus with topically applied opiate receptor anatagonist. *J Am Acad Dermatol.* 2007;56(6):979–988.

Blandina P, Goldfarb J, Walcott J, et al. Serotonergic modulation of the release of endogenous norepinephrine from rat hypothalamic slices. *J Pharamcol Exp Ther.* 1991;256(1):341–347.

Bruera E, Brenneis C, Paterson A, et al. Use of methylphenidate as an adjuvant to narcotic analgesics in patients with advanced cancer. *J Pain Symptom Manage.* 1989;4(1):3–6.

Bruera E, Strasser F, Shen L, et al. The effects of donepezil on sedation and other symptoms in patients receiving opioids for cancer pain: a pilot study. *J Pain Symptom Manage.* 2003;26(5):1049–1054.

Bruera E, Fainsinger R, MacEachern T, et al. The use of methylphenidate in patients with incident cancer pain receiving regular opiates. A preliminary report. *Pain.* 1992;50(1):75–77.

Brushwood DB, Rich BA, Coleman JJ, Bolen J, Wong W. Legal liability perspectives on abuse-deterrent opioids in the treatment of chronic pain. *J Pain Palliat Care Pharmacother* 2010;24(4):333–48.

Candrilli SD, Davis KL, Iyer S. Impact of constipation on opioid use patterns, health care resource utilization, and costs in cancer patients on opioid therapy. *J Pain Palliat Care Pharmacother.* 2009;23(3):231–241.

Candy B, Jones L, Goodman ML, Drake R, Tookman A. Laxatives or methylnaltrexone for the management of constipation in palliative care patients. *Cochrane Database Syst Rev.* 2011 DOI: 10.1002/14651858. CD003448.

Cantarella PA, Chahl LA. Acute effects of morphine on substance P concentrations in microdissected regions of guinea-pig brain. *Behav Pharmacol.* 1996;7(5):470–476.

Ceccarelli I, De Padova AM, Fiorenzani P, et al. Single opioid administration modifies gonadal steroids in both the CNS and plasma of male rats. *Neurosci* 2006;140(3):929–937.

Cherny N, Ripamonti C, Pereira J, et al. Strategies to manage the adverse effects of oral morphine: an evidence-based report. *J Clin Oncol.* 2001;19(9):2542–2554.

Chung F, Yegneswaran B, Liao P, et al. STOP questionnaire: a tool to screen patients for obstructive sleep apnea. *Anesthesiology.* 2008;108(5):812–821.

Cronrath P, Lynch TW, Gilson LJ, et al. PCA oversedation: application of Healthcare Failure Mode Effect (HFMEA) Analysis. *Nurs Econ.* 2011;29(2):79–87.

Dahan A, Aarts L, Smith TW. Incidence, Reversal, and Prevention of Opioid-induced Respiratory Depression. *Anesthesiology.* 2010;112(1):226–238.

Dahan A. Respiratory depression with opioid. *J Pain Palliat Care Pharmacother.* 2007;21(5):63–66.

Dahan A, Sarton E, Teppema L, et al. Anesthetic potency and influence of morphine and sevoflurane on respiratin in mu-opioid receptor knockout mice. *Anesthesiology.* 2001;94(5):824–832.

Daniell HW, Lentz R, Mazer NA. Open-label pilot study of testosterone patch therapy in men with opioid-induced androgen deficiency. *J Pain.* 2006;7(3):200–210.

Davis MP. The opioid bowel syndrome: a review of pathophysiology and treatment. *J Opioid Manag.* 2005;1(3):153–161.

Davis MP, Weissman DE, Arnold RM. Opioid dose titration for severe cancer pain: a systematic evidence-based review. *J Palliat Med.* 2004;7(3):462–468.

de Souza Moreno V, Bicego KC, Szawaka RE, et al. Serotonergic mechanisms on breathing modulation in the rat locus coeruleus. *Pflugers Arch.* 2010;459(3):357–368.

Downing GM, Kuziemsky C, Lesperance M, et al. Development and reliability testing of the Victoria Bowel Performance Scale (BPS). *J Pain Symptom Manage.* 2007;34(5):513–522.

Elliott JA, Horton E, Fibuch EE. The endocrine effects of long-term oral opioid therapy: a case report and review of the literature. *J Opioid Manag.* 2011;7(2):145–154.

Estfan B, Mahmoud F, Shaheen P, et al. Respiratory function during parenteral opioid titration for cancer pain. *Palliat Med.* 2007;21(2):81–86.

Farney RJ, Walker JM, Cloward TV, et al. Sleep-disordered breathing associated with long-term opioid therapy. *Chest.* 2003;123(2):632–639.

Feldman JL, Mitchell GS, Nattie EE. Breathing: rhythmicity, plasticity, chemosensitivity. *Annu Rev Neurosci.* 2003;26:239–266.

Ferris FD, Kerr IG, Sone M, et al. Transdermal scopolamine use in the control of narcotic-induced nausea. *J Pain Symptom Manage.* 1991;6(6):380–393.

Finley JC, Katz DM. The central organization of carotid body afferent projections to the brainstem of the rat. *Brain Res.* 1992;572(1–2):108–116.

Foley KM. The relationship of pain and symptom management to patient requests for physician-assisted suicide. *J Pain Symptom Manage.* 1991;6(5):289–297.

Forrow L, Smith HS. Palliative care. In Bajwa ZH, Warfield CA, eds. *Principles and Practice of Pain Medicine.* 2nd ed. New York: McGraw-Hill, 2004;492–502.

Frank L, Kleinman L, Farup C, et al. Psychometric validation of a constipation symptom assessment questionnaire. *Scand J Gastroenterol.* 1999;34(9):870–877.

Gordon S, Coletti D, Bergman S, et al. LNS5662 (Flavonol-PgP Modulator) ameliorates CNS effects of oxycodone in an acute pain model. *J Pain.* 2007;8(4):S45.

Grossman A. Brain opiates and neuroendocrine function. *Clin Endocrinol Metab.* 1983;12(3):725–746.

Guilleminault C, Cao M, Yue HJ, et al. Obstructive sleep apnea and chronic opioid use. *Lung.* 2010;188(6):459–468.

Hagen N, Swanson R. Strychnine-like multifocal myoclonus and seizures in extremely high-dose opioid administration treatment strategies. *J Pain Symptom Manage.* 1997;14(1):51–58.

Hajiha M, DuBord MA, Liu H, et al. Opioid receptor mechanisms at the hypoglossal motor pool and effects on tongue muscle activity in vivo. *J Physiol.* 2009;587(Pt 11):2677–2692.

Harrington KL, Haskvitz EM. Managing a patient's constipation with physical therapy. *Phys Ther.* 2006;86(11):1511–1519.

Harris SN, Sevarina FB, Sinatra RS, et al. Nausea prophylaxis using transdermal scopolamine in the setting of patient-controlled analgesia. *Obstet Gynecol.* 1991;78(4):673–677.

Hasler WL, Heldsinger A, Chung OY. Erythromycin contracts rabbit colon myocytes via occupation of motilin receptors. *Am J Physiol.* 1992;262(1 Pt 1):G50–G55.

Inturrisi CE. Clinical pharmacology of opioids for pain. *Clin J Pain.* 2002;18(4 Suppl):S3–S13.

Jansen JP, Lorch D, Langan J, Lasko B, Hermanns K, Kleoudis CS, Snidow JW, Pierce A, Wurzelmann J. A randomized, placebo-controlled phase 3 trial (Study SB-767905/012) of alvimopan for opioid-induced bowel dysfunction in patients with non-cancer pain. *J Pain* 2011;12(2):185–193.

Kalso E, Edwards JE, Moore RA, et al. Opioids in chronic non-cancer pain: systematic review of efficacy and safety. *Pain.* 2004;112(3):372–380.

Kalyani RR, Gavini S, Dobs AS. Male hypogonadism in systemic disease. *Endocrinol Metab Clin North Am.* 2007;36(2):333–348.

Kamei J, Ohsawa M, Hayashi SS, et al. Effect of chronic pain on morphine-induced respiratory depression in mice. *Neuroscience.* 2011;174:224–233.

Katz N, Hale M, Morris D, Stauffer J. Morphine sulphate and naltrexone hydrochloride extended release capsules in patients with chronic osteoarthritis pain. *Postgrad Med* 2010;122(4):112–128.

Katz N, Mazer NA. The impact of opioids on the endocrine system. *Clin J Pain.* 2009;25(2):170–175.

Kokko H, Hall PD, Afrin LB. Fentanyl associated syndrome of inappropriate antidiuretic hormone secretion. *Pharmacotherapy.* 2002;22(9):1188–1192.

Kotelko DM, Rottman RL, Wright WC, et al. Transdermal scopolamine decreases nausea and vomiting following cesarean section in patients receiving epidural morphine. *Anesthesiology.* 1989;71(5):675–678.

Kubin L, Alheid GF, Zuperku EJ, et al. Central pathways of pulmonary and lower airway vagal afferents. *J Appl Physiol.* 2006;101(2):618–627.

Kurz A, Sessler DI. Opioid-induced bowel dysfunction: pathophysiology and potential new therapies. *Drugs.* 2003;63(7):649–671.

Lalley PM. Opioidergic and dopaminergic modulation of respiration. *Respir Physiol Neurobiol.* 2008;164(1–2):160–167.

Lehmann KA. Opioids: overview on action, interaction and toxicity. *Support Care Cancer.* 1997;5(6):439–444.

Lewis SJ, Heaton KW. Stool form scale as a useful guide to intestinal transit time. *Scand J Gastroenterol.* 1997;32(9):920–924.

Librach SL, Bouvette M, De AC, et al. Consensus recommendations for the management of constipation in patients with advanced, progressive illness. *J Pain Symptom Manage.* 2010;40(5):761–773.

Longstreth GF, Thompson WG, Chey WD, et al. Functional bowel disorders. *Gastroenterology.* 2006;130(5):1480–1491.

Loper KA, Ready LB, Dorman BH. Prophylactic transdermal scopolamine patches reduce nausea in postoperative patients receiving epidural morphine. *Anesth Analg.* 1989;68(2):144–146.

Lundberg JM, Hökfelt T, Fahrenkrug J, et al. Peptides in the cat carotid body (glomus caroticum): VIP-,enkephalin-, and substance P-like immunoreactivity. *Acta Phsyiol Scand.* 1979a;107(3):279–281.

Lundberg JM, Hökfelt T, Kewenter J, et al. Substance P-, VIP-, and enkephalin-like immunoreactivity in the human vagus nerve. *Gastroenterology.* 1979b;77(3):468–471.

Marquis P, De La Loge C, Dubois D, et al. Development and validation of the Patient Assessment of Constipation Quality of Life questionnaire. *Scand J Gastroenterol.* 2005;40(5):540–551.

Martino PF, Davis S, Opansky C, et al. The cerebellar fastigial nucleus contributes to CO_2 H+ ventilator sensitivity in awake goats. *Respir Physiol Neurobiol.* 2007;157(2–3):242–251.

McKay LC, Evans KC, Frackowiak RS, et al. Neural correlates of voluntary breathing in humans. *J Appl Phsiol.* 2003;95(5):1170–1178.

McNicol E, Horowicz-Mehler N, Risk R, et al. Management of opioid side effects in cancer related and chronic noncancer pain: a systematic review. *J Pain.* 2003;4(5):231–256.

Mehendale S, Yuan CS. Opioid-induced gastrointestinal dysfunction. *Dig Dis.* 2006;24(1–2):105–112.

McMillan SC, Williams FA. Validity and reliability of the Constipation Assessment Scale. *Cancer Nurs.* 1989;12(3):183–188.

Moore TJ, Cohen MR, Furberg CD. Serious adverse drug events reported to the Food and Drug Administration, 1998–2005. *Arch Intern Med.* 2007;167(16):1752–1729.

Mulkey DK, Wenker IC. Astrocyte chemoreceptors: mechanisms of H+ sensing by astrocytes in the retrotrapezoid nucleus and their possible contribution to respiratory drive. *Exp Phsyiol.* 2011;96(4):400–406.

Münstedt K, Muller H, Blauth-Eckmeyer E, et al. Role of dexamethasone dosage in combination with 5-HT3 antagonists for prophylaxis of acute chemotherapy-induced nausea and vomiting. *Br J Cancer.* 1999;79(3–4):637–639.

Olesen AE, Drewes AM. Validated Tools for Evaluating Opioid-Induced Bowel Dysfunction. *Adv Ther.* 2011;28(4):279–294.

O'Mahony S, Coyle N, Payne R. Current management of opioid-related side effects. *Oncology (Williston Park).* 2001;15(1):61–73.

Oyamada Y, Ballantyne D, Muckenhoff K, et al. Respiration-modulated membrane potential and cehmosensitivity of licus coeruleus in the in vitro brainstem-spinal cord of the neonatal rat. *J Physiol.* 1998;513(Pt 2):381–398.

Paice JA, Penn RD, Ryan WG. Altered sexual function and decreased testosterone in patients receiving intraspinal opioids. *J Pain Symptom Manage.* 1994;9(2):126–131.

Pappagallo M. Incidence, prevalence, and management of opioid bowel dysfunction. *Am J Surg.* 2001;182(5A Suppl):11S–18S.

Pappagallo M, Stewart W, Woods M. Constipation symptoms in long-term users in opioid analgesic therapy. *Poster abstracts.* American Pain Society Annual Meeting, Fort Lauderdale, Florida, October 21–24, 1999.

Paton JF, Deuchars J, Li YW, et al. Properties of solitary tract neurones responding to peripheral arterial chemoreceptors. *Neuroscience.* 2001;105(1):231–248.

Pattison KT. Opioids and the control of respiration. *Br J Anaesth.* 2008; 100(6):747–758.

Pattison KT, Governo RJ, MacIntosh BJ, et al. Opioids depress cortical centers responsible for the volitional control of respiration. *J Neurosci.* 2009;29(25):8177–8186.

Poole SL, Deuchars J, Lewis DI, et al. Subdivision-specific responses of neurons in the nucleus of the tractus solitaries to activation of mu-opioid receptors in the rat. *J Neurophysiol.* 2007;98(5):3060–3071.

Portenoy RK, Coyle N. Controversies in the long-term management of analgesic therapy in patients with advanced cancer. *J Pain Symptom Manage.* 1990;5(5):307–319.

Rajagopal A, Vassilopoulou-Sellin R, Palmer JL, et al. Hypogonadism and sexual dysfunction in male cancer survivors receiving chronic opioid therapy. *J Pain Symptom Manage.* 2003;26(5):1055–1061.

Ruan X. Sustained-release morphine sulphate with sequestered naltrexone for moderate to severe pain: a new opioid analgesic formulation and beyond. *Expert Opin Pharmacother* 2011;12(7):999–1001.

Ruangkittisakul A, Ballanyi K. Methylxanthine reversal of opioid-evoked inspiratory depression via phosphodiesterase-4 blockade. *Respir Physiol Neurobiol.* 2010;172(3):94–105.

Sabatowski R, Schwalen S, Rettig K, et al. Driving ability under long-term treatment with transdermal fentanyl. *J Pain Symptom Manage.* 2003;25(1):38–47.

Sakaue S, Sunagawa M, Tanigawa H, et al. A single administration of morphine suppresses the reduction of the systemic immune activity caused by acute inflammatory pain in rats. *Masui.* 2011;60(3):336–342.

Saurer TB, Carrigan KA, Ijames SG, et al. Suppression of natural killer cell activity by morphine is mediated by the nucleus accumbens shell. *J Neuroimmunol.* 2006a;173(1–2):3–11.

Saurer TB, Ijames SG, Lysle DT. Neuropeptide Y Y1 receptors mediate morphine-induced reductions of natural killer cell activity. *J Neuroimmunol.* 2006b;177(1–2):18–26.

Schindler SD, Ortner R, Peternell A, et al. Maintenance therapy with synthetic opioids and driving aptitude. *Eur Addict Res.* 2004;10(2):80–87.

Shvarev Y, Berner J, Bilkei-Gorzo A, et al. Acute morphine effects on respiratory activity in mice with target deletion of the tachykinin 1 gene (Tac1-/-). *Adv Exp Med Biol.* 2010;669:129–132.

Slatkin NE, Rhiner M, Bolton TM. Donepezil in the treatment of opioid-induced sedation: report of six cases. *J Pain Symptom Manage.* 2001;21(5):425–438.

Smith HS. Editorial: Conventional Practice for Medical Conditions for Chronic Opioid Therapy. *Pain Physician.* 2012;15(3S):ES1–ES7.

Smith HS, Elliott JA. Opioid-Induced Androgen Deficiency (OPIAD). *Pain Physician.* 2012;15(3S):ES145–ES156.

Smith HS. A receptor-based paradigm of nausea and vomiting. *J Cancer Pain Symptom Palliat.* 2005;1(1):11–23.

Smith HS. Balancing hedonic tone. *J Cancer Pain Symptom Palliat.* 2006;2(2):35–37.

Smith HS. Morphine sulphate and naltrexone hydrochloride extended release capsules for the management of chronic, moderate-to-severe pain, while reducing morphine-induced subjective effects due to tampering by crushing. *Expert Opin Pharmcother.* 2011;12(7):1111–25.

Staats PS, Markowita J, Schein J. Incidence of constipation associated with long-acting opioid therapy: a comparative study. *South Med J.* 2004;97(2):129–134.

Strasser F, Palmer JL, Schover LR, et al. The impact of hypogonadism and autonomic dysfunction on fatigue, emotional function, and sexual desire in male patients with advanced cancer: a pilot study. *Cancer.* 2006;107(12):2949–2957.

Su CF, Liu MY, Lin MT. Intraventricular morphine produces pain relief, hypothermia, hyperglycemia and increased prolactin and growth hormone levels in patients with cancer pain. *J Neurol.* 1987;235(2):105–108.

Sykes N. Constipation and diarrhea. In Doyle D, Hanks G, MacDonald N, eds. *Oxford Textbook of Palliative Medicine.* New York: Oxford University Press, 1998; 513–521.

Tarkkila P, Torn K, Tuominen M, et al. Premedication with promethazine and transdermal scopolamine reduces the incidence of nausea and vomiting after intrathecal morphine. *Acta Anaesthesiol Scand.* 1995;39(7):983–986.

Terg R, Coronel E, Sorda J, et al. Efficacy and safety of oral naltrexone treatment for pruritus of cholestasis, a crossover, double-blind, placebo-controlled study. *J Hepatol.* 2002;37(6):717–722.

Twycross RG. Ethical and clinical aspects of pain treatment in cancer patients. *Acta Anaesthesiol Scand Suppl.* 1982;26(Suppl 74):83–90.

Vanegas G, Ripamonti C, Sbanotto A, et al. Side effects of morphine administration in cancer patients. *Cancer Nurs.* 1998;21(4):289–297.

Van Seventer R, Smit JM, Schipper RM, et al. Comparison of TTS-fentanyl with sustained-release oral morphine in the treatment of patients not using opioids for mild-to-moderate pain. *Curr Med Res Opin.* 2003;19(6):457–468.

Varma MG, Wang JY, Berian JR, et al. The constipation severity instrument: a validated measure. *Dis Colon Rectum.* 2008;51(2):162–172.

Walker JM, Farney RJ, Rhondeau SM, et al. Chronic opioid use is a risk factor for the development of central sleep apnea and atxic breathing. *J Clin Sleep Med.* 2007;3(5):455–462.

Wamsley JK. Opioid receptors: autoradiography. *Pharmacol Rev.* 1983;35(1):69–83.

Wakasa Y, Fujiwara A, Umeuchi H, et al. Inhibitory effects of TRK-820 on systemic skin scratching induced by morphine in rhesus monkeys. *Life Sci.* 2004;75(24):2947–2957.

Wan Q, Douglas SD, Wang X, et al. Morphine upregulates functional expression of neurokinin-1 receptor in neurons. *J Neurosci Res.* 2006;84(7):1588–1596.

Wang D, Teichtahl H, Drummer O, et al. Central sleep apnea in stable methadone maintenance treatment patients. *Chest.* 2005;128(3):1348–1356.

Webster L, Cochella S, Dasqupta N, et al. An analysis of the Root Causes for Opioid-Related Overdose Deaths in the United States. *Pain Med.* 2011;12(Suppl 2):S26–S35.

Webster L, Andrews M, Stoddard G. Modafinil treatment of opioid-induced sedation. *Pain Med.* 2003;4(2):135–140.

Webster LR, Choi Y, Desai H, Webster L, Grant BJ. Sleep-disordered breather and chronic opioid therapy. *Pain Med.* 2008;9(4):425–432.

Weil JV, McCullough RE, Kline JS, et al. Diminished ventilator response to hypoxia and hypercapnia after morphine in normal man. *N Engl J Med.* 1975;292(21):1103–1106.

Welters ID, Menzebach A, Goumon Y, et al. Morphine suppresses complement receptor expression, phagocytosis, and respiratory burst in neutrophils by a nitric oxide and mu(3) opiate receptor-dependent mechanism. *J Neuroimmunol.* 2000;111(1-2):139–145.

Wharton J, Polak JM, Pearse AG, et al. Enkephain-, VIP- and substance P-like immunoreactivity in the carotid body. *Nature.* 1980;284(5753):269–271.

Wikström B, Gellert R, Ladefoged SD, et al. Kappa-opioid system in uremic pruritus: multicenter, randomized, double-blind, placebo-controlled clinical studies. *J Am Soc Nephrol.* 2005;16(12):3742–3747.

Wilwerding MB, Loprinzi CL, Mailiard JA, et al. A randomized, crossover evaluation of methylphenidate in cancer patients receiving strong narcotics. *Support Care Cancer.* 1995;3(2):135–138.

Wirz S, Klaschik E. Management of constipation in palliative care patients undergoing opioid therapy: is polyethylene glycol an option? *Am J Hosp Paliat Care.* 2005; 22(5):375–381.

Wirz S, Wartenberg HC, Nadstawek J. Less nausea, emesis, and constipation comparing hydromorphone and morphine? A prospective open-labeled investigation on caner pain. *Support Care Cancer.* 2008;16(6):999–1009.

Wolfhagen FH, Sternieri E, Hop WC, et al. Oral naltrexone treatment for cholestatic pruritus: a double-blind, placebo-controlled study. *Gastroenterology.* 1997;113(4):1264–1269.

Wong BS, Camilleri M. Lubiprostone for the treatment of opioid-induced bowel dysfunction. *Expert Opin Pharmacother* 2011;12(6):983–90.

Yamamoto A, Sugumoto Y. Involvement of peripheral mu opioid receptors in scratching behaviour in mice. *Eur J Pharamcol.*2010;649(1–3):336–341.

Yancey-Wrona J, Dallaire B, Bilsky E, et al. 6β-naltrexol, a peripherally selective opioid antagonist that inhibits morphine-induced slowing of gastrointestinal transit: an exploratory study. *Pain Med.* 2011;12(12):1727–1737.

Young-McCaughan S, Miaskowski C. Definition of and mechanism for opioid-induced sedation. *Pain Manage Nurs.* 2001a;2(3):84–97.

Young-McCaughan S, Miaskowski C. Measurement of opioid-induced sedation. *Pain Manage Nurs.* 2001b;2(4):132–149.

Yu J. Airway mechanosensors. *Respir Phsiol Neurobiol.* 2005;148(3):217–243.

Zebraski SE, Kochenash SM, Raffa RB. Lung opioid receptors: pharmacology and possible target for nebulized morphine in dyspnea. *Life Sci.* 2000;66(23):2221–2231.

Zutler M, Holty JE. Opioids, sleep, and sleep-disordered breathing. *Curr Pharm Des.* 2011;17(15):1443–1449.

Chapter 5d

Optimizing Pharmacologic Outcomes: Opioid-Induced Hyperalgesia

Lucy Chen and Jianren Mao

Despite the extensive effort in search of new pharmacological tools for pain management, opioids remain the most efficacious pain medication to treat acute pain, chronic pain, and cancer-related pain. Opioid analgesics act on three major classes of opioid receptors including μ, k, δ (mu, kappa, and delta receptors). Activation of opioid receptors produces analgesia, euphoria, respiratory depression, decreased gastrointestinal motility, and cardiovascular effects. Exposure to opioids, however, can also lead to the development of opioid tolerance and opioid-induced hyperalgesia (OIH). The congregative effects of opioid tolerance and OIH can reduce the opioid analgesic efficacy, making it a significant challenge in chronic pain management. The concept of OIH is related to a state of nociceptive sensitization caused by exposure to opioids, resulting in a paradoxical reduced response to opioid therapy. This chapter will review recent evidence of OIH from both preclinical and clinical studies and discuss issues relevant to clinical diagnosis and management of OIH.

Evidence for OIH in Preclinical Studies

Original preclinical studies showed that there was a progressive reduction in baseline nociceptive threshold, as assessed using a foot-withdrawal test, in rats receiving repeated intrathecal morphine administration (10–20 mmg) over a seven-day period (Mao et al. 1994). This was followed by a number of animal studies that demonstrated a similar phenomenon. For example, (1) the reduced baseline nociceptive threshold was observed in animals receiving subcutaneous fentanyl boluses using the Randall-Sellitto test in which a constantly increasing pressure was applied to a rat's hindpaw. The decreased baseline nociceptive threshold lasted five days after the cessation of four fentanyl bolus injections (Celerier et al. 2000); (2) the reduced baseline nociceptive threshold was detected in animals with repeated heroin administration as well (Laulin et al. 2002); (3) rats exposed to morphine also developed a latent sensitization of visceral hyperalgesia with a shift of the morphine dose-response curve to the right (Lian et al. 2010); (4) exposure to methadone induced hyperalgesia in rats, which was not prevented by a weak NMDA receptor antagonist (memantine)

(Hay et al. 2010); and (5) a partial μ-receptor agonist buprenophine produced a dose-related OIH (Wala et al. 2011).

These findings indicate that repeated opioid administration can lead to a progressive and lasting reduction of baseline nociceptive threshold, referred as OIH (Mao et al. 2002a; Mao et al. 2002b; Mao 2006). This phenomenon differs from previous preclinical observations in which a large dose of intrathecal morphine resulted in hyperalgesic response (Woolf 1981; Yaksh et al. 1986) because OIH developed in response to a clinically relevant dose. Of interest to note is that OIH was observed in animals even when an opioid infusion continues via an implanted osmotic pump, suggesting the involvement of active cellular mechanisms in the process (Vanderah et al. 2001).

Thus, a prolonged opioid treatment can result in not only a loss of the opioid antinociceptive effect, a negative sign of system adaptation (desensitization), but also activation of a pro-nociceptive system manifested as the reduced nociceptive threshold, a positive sign of system adaptation (sensitization). Although both opioid tolerance and OIH are initiated by opioid administration, two opposing cellular mechanisms, that is, a desensitization process versus a sensitization process, are involved in the process. Therefore, it is important to understand the neural and cellular mechanisms underlying the development of OIH and their interaction with the mechanism of opioid tolerance, because clinical approaches to resolving opioid tolerance and OIH are quite different. This issue will be discussed later in this chapter.

Proposed Cellular Mechanisms of OIH

A considerable number of recent studies have explored the neurobiological basis of OIH, revealing a divergent range of cellular elements contributory to OIH.

N-methyl-D-aspartate (NMDA) Receptor and the Related Intracellular Pathways

NMDA receptors have long been implicated in the cellular mechanism of OIH (Mao et al. 2002a; Mao et al. 2002b; Mao 2006; Zhao and Joo 2008). A recent study indicates that the periaqueductal gray may be a site of systemic morphine action on NMDA receptors and protein kinase C (PKC) in relation to the development of OIH (Ghelardini et al. 2008). In addition, calcium/calmodulin-dependent protein kinase IIα also has been involved in the initiation and maintenance of OIH (Chen et al. 2010). Magnesium is an endogenous blocker at NMDA receptor-coupled calcium channels. In one study, intraperitoneal magnesium prevented or retarded the development of fentanyl-induced OIH in rats (Van Elstraete et al. 2006). In animal study of remifentanil-induced postoperative hyperalgesia, there was a marked increase in NR2B phosphorylation at Tyr1472 in the superficial spinal cord dorsal horn, which was attenuated by the pretreatment of the NMDA receptor antagonist ketamine (Gu et al. 2009). Pretreatment with ketamine diminished morphine-induced OIH in a mouse model of orthopedic pain (Minville et al. 2010). Systemic lidocaine also prevented remifentanil-induced OIH through the inhibition of PKCg membrane translocation in the rat's spinal cord dorsal horn (Cui et al. 2009). Co-administration of dextromethorphan (10 mg/kg), an NMDA receptor antagonist, with morphine produced anti-nociception and inhibited morphine-induced OIH (Gupta et al. 2011).

G-proteins

Inhibitory G-proteins played a role in OIH induced by a low opioid dose (Bianchi et al. 2011) and GPR3, an orphan G-protein-coupled receptor, contributed to the development of neuropathic pain and morphine-induced OIH (Ruiz-Medina et al. 2011). Another study showed that G-inhibitory protein-mu receptor coupling might be necessary for morphine-induced acute OIH because, when a compound that inhibits Gβg dimmer-dependent signaling was administered, low dose morphine-induced acute OIH was completely prevented (Bianchi et al. 2009).

5-HT Receptor

5-HT receptors also have been involved in the cellular mechanism of OIH because the 5HT3 antagonist ondansertron given systemically or intrathecally prevented and reversed OIH (Liang et al. 2011).

Neurokinin-1 (NK-1) Receptor

NK-1 receptors have been shown to be critically involved in modulation of fentanyl-induced OIH through the ascending and descending pathways (Rivat et al. 2009). A possible mechanism of NK-1 involvement is that NK-1-expressing neurons may play a critical role in morphine-induced neuroplastic changes. Ablation of NK-1-expressiing cells may eliminate the ascending limb of a spinal-bulbospinal loop that results in descending facilitation (Vera-Portocarrero et al. 2007).

Neuropeptide FF (NPFF)

NPFF has been proposed to play a role in pain modulation. When the potent and selective NPFF receptor antagonist RF9 was co-administered with heroin, paradoxical heroin-induced OIH was completely prevented (Simonin et al. 2006).

Nitric oxide (NO) and NO Synthase

Deletion of the inducible NO synthase gene attenuated remifentanil-induced OIH. Of interest is that in NO synthase mutant mice, remifentanil was still effective in enhancing incisional pain, but its pronociceptive effect was significantly attenuated as compared to wild-type mice (Celerier et al. 2006), suggesting a possible differential effect of opioid on anti-nociception and OIH.

TRPV1 Receptor

A recent study suggests that TRPV1 is an essential peripheral mechanism in the expression of OIH (Vardanyan et al. 2009). This finding suggests that opioid-related long-term potentiation in the spinal cord may be induced by a pre-synaptic event in which TRV1-expressing primary afferents played a significant role (Zhou et al. 2010).

Calcium Channels

Intrathecal administration of nifedipine, an L-type calcium channel blocker, antagonized morphine-induced OIH. Furthermore, pretreatment with the selective PKC inhibitor chelerythrine resulted in prevention of OIH, whereas the PKA inhibitor KT 5720 had no effect (Esmaeili-Mahani et al. 2008; Esmaeili-Mahani et al. 2007). Gabapentin, a proposed inhibitor of the $\alpha2\delta$ subunit of voltage-gated calcium channels, prevented a delayed fentanyl-induced OIH in a dose-dependent manner (Van Elstraete et al. 2008). When combined with ketamine, gabapentin produced the anti-hyperalgesic effect as well as an additive effect on the prevention of OIH (Van Elstraete et al. 2011; Wei and Wei, 2011).

Miscellaneous Findings

Fifty percent nitrous oxide (N2O) was shown to prevent high dose fentanyl-induced OIH (Bessiere et al. 2007). OIH was found to be associated with the increased expression of c-Fos or zif268 proteins in the amygdala receiving projections from the ascending spino-parabrachio-amygdaloid nociceptive pathway (Hamlin et al. 2007). In another study, spinal NADPH oxidase, a source of endogenous superoxide, is also implicated in the development of OIH and morphine anti-nociceptive tolerance (Doyle et al. 2010). It has been reported that variants of the Abcb1b gene and the beta2-AR gene may be partially responsible for the inter-strain differences in OIH (Liang et al. 2006a; Liang et al. 2006b). Gene expression studies also showed the involvement of opioid-induced SDF1/CXCR4 signaling in long-lasting OIH (Wilson et al. 2011).

Opioid Receptor-Independent Mechanisms

An interesting observation is that dynorphin A, a kappa-opioid receptor, given into the centromedial amygdala resulted in the decreased tail-flick latency, which was blocked by the NMDA receptor antagonist MK-801 but not kappa-opioid receptor antagonist nor-binaltorphimine (Terashvili et al. 2007). In addition, OIH appears to be present in opioid receptor triple knock-out (KO) mice that lack all three genes encoding mu, delta, and kappa opioid receptors, although the opioid anti-nociceptive effects were abolished in these mice (Juni et al. 2007). Similar findings of OIH are reported in opioid receptor triple knock-out mice after fentanyl bolus or infusion and the NMDA receptor antagonist MK-801 reversed OIH under this condition (Waxman et al. 2009).

Sex Differences

It has been reported that both low and high dose morphine induced OIH but the onset of OIH was earlier and OIH lasted longer in female rats. NMDA receptor antagonist reversed the low dose morphine-induced OIH in both male and female rats but reversed high dose morphine-induced OIH only in male rats, suggesting that the neural substrate contributing to this phenomenon is morphine dose-dependent (Juni et al. 2010). Ovariectomy without estrogen replacement treatment diminished this sex difference in OIH (Juni et al. 2008).

The increasing number of preclinical studies in the area of OIH indicates that (1) there is an enormous and growing interest in the field with regard to the cellular mechanisms of OIH, and (2) the current evidence points to a progressive sensitization process within the central nervous system that involves a constellation of cellular elements such as NMDA receptors similar to those contributory to the mechanisms of pathological pain.

Evidence for OIH in Human Studies

While preclinical studies can measure changes in baseline nociceptive threshold in a controlled setting, it is difficult to assess whether changes in pain threshold occur clinically following opioid administration (Mao 2006). It is indeed challenging to distinguish pharmacological tolerance from OIH when the outcome of opioid therapy is primarily based on subjective pain scores. Despite the challenge, an increasing number of anecdotal case reports and clinical studies have suggested that OIH is likely to be a significant factor in clinical opioid therapy (Forero et al. 2011; Vorobeychik et al. 2008; Cortinas Saenz et al. 2008; Siniscalchi et al. 2008; Okon and George 2008; Axelrod and Reville 2007; Singler et al. 2007; Hallett and Chalkiadis 2012).

In a large-scale study of 1,620 patients, remifentanil was used for general anesthesia and the incidence of post-operative remifentanil-induced hyperalgesia was reported to be 16.1%. This study found that age (a higher rate in patients <16y old), sex (male >female), operation duration (higher in duration >2h), and remifentanil dose (higher in dose >30 mg/kg) are the factors that have had an impact on the incidence of OIH (Ma et al. 2011). On the other hand, heroin or opioid addicts not only demonstrated OIH, but also had prolonged symptoms of OIH after detoxification from opioids for at least one month (Pud et al. 2006). In those chronic pain patients without opioid dependence, significantly lower pain threshold and lower pain tolerance were detected using pressure pain stimulation (Fishbain et al. 2011). It appears that the sensitivity of detecting OIH in the clinical setting may be influenced by the modality of sensory stimulation (Hay et al. 2009). A major caveat of these clinical observations is that OIH was not defined objectively, an issue that remains to be addressed.

In a prospective preliminary study of six patients with chronic low back pain, hyperalgesic response was detected after one month of oral morphine therapy in a cold pressor test but not in a heat pain test (Chu et al. 2006). In a prospective, randomized, placebo-controlled, two-way crossover study in healthy volunteers conducted by the same investigators, the development of OIH was quantified as changes in the average radius of the area of secondary hyperalgesia generated by electrical pain stimulation. A 23.6% increase in the area of secondary hyperalgesia over baseline was detected following the remifentanil infusion. The same study showed that endogenous opioids did not seem to have an effect on OIH because a single bolus of naloxone did not change the size of secondary hyperalgesic (Chu et al. 2011).

To date, a number of clinical studies have examined clinical approaches to preventing OIH in human subjects and the results remain inconclusive.

(1) Treatment with morphine (150 mg/kg) prior to remifentanil infusion did not prevent the development of remifentanil-induced OIH (McDonnell et al. 2008).

(2) Propofol infusion along with remifentanil both delayed and attenuated remifentanil-induced OIH (Singler et al. 2007).

(3) Intraoperative administration of 70% N2O appears to reduce postoperative OIH following an intra-operative remifentanil-propofol anesthesia regimen (Echevarria et al. 2011).

(4) Preventive administration of parecoxib significantly diminished OIH after withdrawal from remifentanil. In contrast, parecoxib given together with remifentanil did not prevent OIH, suggesting that pretreatment may be more meaningful in preventing OIH (Troster et al. 2006). Other NSAIDs administered preemptively also appears to prevent remifentanil-induced OIH (Tuncer et al. 2009).

(5) Intra-operative magnesium administration reduced post-operative opioid consumption and OIH in subjects receiving intra-operative remifentanil-based anesthesia (Lee et al. 2011a; Song et al. 2011). Intra-operative adenosine infusion also prevented acute opioid tolerance and remifentanil-induced OIH (Lee et al. 2011b).

(6) Continuous intra-operative infusion of ketamine, an NMDA receptor antagonist, significantly lowered postoperative VAS and morphine use (Hong et al. 2011).

(7) In a randomized, double-blind, placebo-controlled study of 90 patients who underwent total abdominal hysterectomy, cumulative morphine consumption was significantly greater in subjects with fentanyl alone than those with saline alone, ketamine alone, ketamine with fentanyl, or fentanyl with lornoxicam at three, six, and 12 hours postoperatively (Xuerong et al. 2008).

(8) In a double-blind, randomized, placebo-controlled study of 40 patients undergoing elective shoulder surgery, clonidine was given intra-operatively with a remifentanil/propofol-based anesthesia. The results showed that clonidine did not reduce postoperative morphine consumption and pain score in these patients (Schlimp et al. 2011). However, dexmedetomidine, another $\alpha 2$ receptor agonist, substantially reduced baseline opioid doses in hospitalized patients with OIH (Belgrade and Hall 2010).

Quantitative Sensory Testing (QST) and OIH

Despite the increasing effort, diagnostic tools for OIH are yet to be developed. However, many clinical studies have used QST as a useful tool to assess OIH (Chen et al. 2009; Bannister and Dickenson 2010). In a recent study, QST was used to compare pain threshold, pain tolerance, and the degree of temporal summation of second pain in response to thermal stimulation among three groups of subjects: Group 1 (no pain and no opioid), Group 2 (chronic pain but no opioid treatment), and Group 3 (both chronic pain and opioid therapy). Group 3 subjects displayed a decreased heat pain threshold and exacerbated temporal summation of second pain to thermal stimulation as compared with both group 1 and group 2 subjects. There were no differences in cold or warm sensation among all three groups. Among clinical factors, daily opioid dose consistently correlated with the decreased heat pain threshold and exacerbated temporal summation of second pain in group 3 subjects (Chen et al. 2009). Another study investigated the sensitivity to cold pain and the magnitude of diffuse noxious inhibitory control (DNIC) using QST in subjects with or without opioid therapy. Pain threshold, intensity and tolerance in response to cold pressor (1 degrees C) were measured. It was found that oral opioid use did not result in abnormal sensitivity to cold pain but altered pain modulation as detected by DNIC (Ram et al. 2008).

Opioid Regimen and OIH

Opioid regimen including the type of opioid analgesic and dose may influence the development of OIH. Anecdotal clinical observations have suggested that the degree of OIH may vary according to opioid analgesics (Compton et al. 2001). Although the exact relationship between the dose regimen and the development of OIH remains to be determined, it is conceivable that OIH would be more likely to develop in patients receiving high opioid doses with a prolonged treatment course, although OIH has been demonstrated in patients receiving a short course of highly potent opioid analgesics (Vinik and Kissin 1998). Moreover, patients with a pathological pain condition (e.g., neuropathic pain) treated with opioid therapy may be more susceptible to developing OIH, because both pathological pain and OIH may share a common cellular mechanism (Mao et al. 1995).

If OIH develops following exposure to one opioid, can switching to a different opioid diminish OIH (Sjogren et al. 1994)? If cross-pain sensitivity does not develop between different opioids, switching to a different opioid would be justified, a similar rationale for opioid rotation to overcome opioid tolerance. This issue remains to be investigated.

OIH and Pre-Emptive Analgesia

Despite the ongoing debate on the clinical effectiveness of preemptive analgesia in pain management, use of opioid analgesic as the sole agent for preemptive analgesia may not be desirable for several reasons. First, a large dose of intra-operative opioid could activate a pro-nociceptive mechanism leading to the development of postoperative OIH (Guignard et al. 2000). This may confound the assessment of postoperative pain and counteract the opioid analgesic effect. Second, preemptive analgesia calls for pre-emptive inhibition of neuroplastic changes mediated through multiple cellular mechanisms such as the central glutamatergic system. Paradoxically, opioid may activate the central glutamatergic system as discussed above. Third, the neural mechanism of opioid tolerance and OIH may interact with that of pathological pain and pathological pain could be exacerbated following opioid administration (Angst and Clark 2006; Baron and McDonald 2006). Nonetheless, this issue needs to be investigated in future studies.

Clinical Implications of OIH

Until recently, a decreased opioid analgesic effect following opioid therapy is often considered to result from pharmacological opioid tolerance (i.e., desensitization of the responsiveness of opioid receptor and its cellular mechanism) and/or a worsening clinical pain condition. Therefore, opioid dose escalation appears to be a logical approach to regain the analgesics effectiveness of opioid. This practice should be re-considered in light of the information on OIH. In the clinical setting, apparent opioid tolerance may result from pharmacological tolerance, worsening pain condition due to disease progression, or OIH. The important issue is how to distinguish the elements of apparent opioid tolerance and form differential diagnosis in the clinical settings (Mao 2002c). As listed in Table 5d.1, a number of issues should be taken into consideration.

Table 5d.1 Differential Diagnosis of OIH

	OIH	Opioid tolerance
QST Exacerbated temporal summation of second pain	Yes	No
Decreased pain threshold	Yes	No
Decreased pain tolerance	Yes	No
Opioid dose (the higher, the more likely)	Yes	Yes
Duration of opioid therapy (the longer, the more likely)	Yes	Yes
Dose escalation	Limited improvement in clinical pain and QST responses	Improvement in pain relief
Dose reduction	Improved opioid analgesia	Reduced opioid analgesia
Pain quality	Spontaneous, burning, diffuse pain similar to neuropathic pain	No change (from pre-existing pain)
Pain location	Possibly beyond the dermatome distribution of the pre-existing pain	No change (from pre-existing pain)
Pain intensity	Similar or greater than the pre-existed pain	Similar to the preexisted pain condition

(1) The quality, location, and distribution pattern of pain due to OIH would be different from a pre-existed pain condition. Because opioid analgesics are often administered systemically, changes in pain quality would be diffuse as compared to the preexisted pain condition. Since the mechanism of OIH has many in common with that of pathological pain such as neuropathic pain, changes in pain threshold, tolerability, and distribution patterns seen in OIH would be similar to those seen in neuropathic pain patients. Moreover, QST may be a useful tool to detect such changes.

(2) OIH could exacerbate a pre-existing pain condition. Therefore, overall pain intensity (VAS) would conceivably be increased above the level of pre-existed pain in the absence of disease progression. Opioid dose escalation could only transiently and minimally reduce pain intensity in such a setting, with a subsequent increase in pain intensity due to OIH.

(3) When a diagnosis is uncertain, a trial of opioid dose escalation or dose decrease may be used to differentiate tolerance from OIH. In an undertreated, worsening pain condition due to disease progress and/or pharmacological opioid tolerance, improved pain control may well be an outcome after a trial of opioid dose escalation. On the other hand, opioid dose escalation may exacerbate pain condition due to OIH, whereas a supervised opioid tapering may reduce OIH and improve clinical pain. In this regard, if a patient is on a low opioid dose regimen and complains of unsatisfactory pain relief, a trial of opioid dose escalation may be appropriate. If a patient is already on a megadose of opioid analgesic, further dose escalation is rarely justified and may exacerbate OIH.

(4) It is important to remember that the clinical outcome of opioid therapy is a dynamic balance among the opioid analgesic effect, OIH, and worsening pain due to disease progression. While any opioid dose escalation may transiently increase the analgesic effect, albeit being small in many cases, the real issue is whether the dose escalation may also exacerbate OIH that could quickly overtake the transient improvement in opioid analgesia. Therefore, clinical judgment is fundamentally important and all clinical conditions related to opioid therapy need to be taken into consideration in this decision making process.

Clinical Management of OIH

It is important to review various aspects of a differential diagnosis when the decreased opioid analgesic effect is encountered during a course of opioid therapy. If the increased nociceptive input (e.g., disease progression) or psychological issues are ruled out as the primary contributor to a state of increased pain, differentiating between pharmacologic tolerance and OIH should be considered. It seems reasonable to have a trial of opioid dose escalation at this point. If pain improves, the lack of opioid analgesic efficacy is more likely due to tolerance. However, if pain worsens or does not proportionally respond to the dose escalation, OIH could be the cause. This clinical diagnosis process could be aided by using QST and considering other clinical features of OIH as discussed above and listed in Table 5d.1.

If OIH is suspected, either dose decrease or taper-off would be a reasonable approach. Alternatively, opioid rotation could be a feasible step if opioid therapy is considered to be necessary regardless of OIH. Patients may get better pain relief with a different opioid medication, often at a lower equalanalgesic dosage. Adjuvant nonopioid pain medications have been highly recommended in combination with opioid treatment to reduce the amount of opioid usage, minimize opioid side effects, and reduce the risk of opioid tolerance and OIH. Lastly, one should also consider the history of the patient's pain and its response to opioids. A patient who was previously on a stable opioid regimen and now complains of worsening pain is much different from the one whose pain never was improved with that opioid regimen. In the latter case, instead of having continued dose escalation, the patient would be better off if that opioid is weaned off, a nonopioid regimen is considered, and/or a different opioid is used for rotation.

Summary

OIH should be considered when the adjustment of opioid dose is contemplated if (a) prior opioid dose escalation failed to provide the expected analgesic effect and (b) there is unexplainable pain exacerbation following an initial period of effective opioid analgesia. Although in some cases increasing opioid dose leads to some improvement in pain management, in other cases less opioid may lead to more effective pain reduction. This goal may be accomplished by initiating a trial of opioid tapering, opioid rotation, adding adjunctive medications, or combining opioid with a clinically available N-methyl-D-aspartate receptor antagonist. Continuing opioid therapy with endless dose escalations in the absence of clinical evidence of improved pain management is neither scientifically sound nor clinically justified.

References

Angst MS, Clark JD. Opioid-induced hyperalgesia: A qualitative systematic review. *Anesthesiology*. 2006;104(3):570–587.

Axelrod DJ, Reville B. Using methadone to treat opioid-induced hyperalgesia and refractory pain. *J Opioid Manag*. 2007;3(2):113–114.

Bannister K, Dickenson AH. Opioid hyperalgesia. *Curr Opin Support Palliat Care*. 2010;4(1):1–5.

Baron MJ, McDonald PW. Significant pain reduction in chronic pain patients after detoxification from high-dose opioids. *J Opioid Manag*. 2006;2(5):277–282.

Belgrade M, Hall S. Dexmedetomidine infusion for the management of opioid-induced hyperalgesia. *Pain Med*. 2010;11(12):1819–1826.

Bessiere B, Richebe P, Laboureyras E, Laulin JP, Contarino A, Simonnet G. Nitrous oxide (N2O) prevents latent pain sensitization and long-term anxiety-like behavior in pain and opioid-experienced rats. *Neuropharmacology*. 2007;53(6):733–740.

Bianchi E, Galeotti N, Menicacci C, Ghelardini C. Contribution of G inhibitory protein alpha subunits in paradoxical hyperalgesia elicited by exceedingly low doses of morphine in mice. *Life Sci.* 2011;89(25–26):918–925.

Bianchi E, Norcini M, Smrcka A, Ghelardini C. Supraspinal gbetagamma-dependent stimulation of PLCbeta originating from G inhibitory protein-mu opioid receptor-coupling is necessary for morphine induced acute hyperalgesia. *J Neurochem.* 2009;111(1):171–180.

Celerier E, Gonzalez JR, Maldonado R, Cabanero D, Puig MM. Opioid-induced hyperalgesia in a murine model of postoperative pain: Role of nitric oxide generated from the inducible nitric oxide synthase. *Anesthesiology.* 2006;104(3):546–555.

Celerier E, Rivat C, Jun Y, et al. Long-lasting hyperalgesia induced by fentanyl in rats Preventive effect of ketamine. *Anesthesiology.* 2000;92(2):465–472.

Chen L, Malarick C, Seefeld L, Wang S, Houghton M, Mao J. Altered quantitative sensory testing outcome in subjects with opioid therapy. *Pain.* 2009;143(1–2):65–70.

Chen Y, Yang C, Wang ZJ. Ca2+/calmodulin-dependent protein kinase II alpha is required for the initiation and maintenance of opioid-induced hyperalgesia. *J Neurosci.* 2010;30(1):38–46.

Chu LF, Dairmont J, Zamora AK, Young CA, Angst MS. The endogenous opioid system is not involved in modulation of opioid-induced hyperalgesia. *J Pain.* 2011;12(1):108–115.

Chu LF, Clark DJ, Angst MS. Opioid tolerance and hyperalgesia in chronic pain patients after one month of oral morphine therapy: A preliminary prospective study. *J Pain.* 2006;7(1):43–48.

Compton P, Charuvastra VC, Ling W. Pain intolerance in opioid-maintained former opiate addicts: Effect of long-acting maintenance agent. *Drug Alcohol Depend.* 2001;63(2):139–146.

Cortinas Saenz M, Geronimo Pardo M, Cortinas Saenz ML, Hernandez Vallecillo MT, Ibarra Marti ML, Mateo Cerdan CM. Acute opiate tolerance and postoperative hyperalgesia after a brief infusion of remifentanil managed with multimodal analgesia. *Rev Esp Anestesiol Reanim.* 2008;55(1):40–42.

Cui W, Li Y, Li S, et al. Systemic lidocaine inhibits remifentanil-induced hyperalgesia via the inhibition of cPKCgamma membrane translocation in spinal dorsal horn of rats. *J Neurosurg Anesthesiol.* 2009;21(4):318–325.

Doyle T, Bryant L, Muscoli C, et al. Spinal NADPH oxidase is a source of superoxide in the development of morphine-induced hyperalgesia and antinociceptive tolerance. *Neurosci Lett.* 2010;483(2):85–89.

Echevarria G, Elgueta F, Fierro C, et al. Nitrous oxide (N(2)O) reduces postoperative opioid-induced hyperalgesia after remifentanil-propofol anaesthesia in humans. *Br J Anaesth.* 2011;107(6):959–965.

Esmaeili-Mahani S, Shimokawa N, Javan M, et al. Low-dose morphine induces hyperalgesia through activation of G alphas, protein kinase C, and L-type ca 2+ channels in rats. *J Neurosci Res.* 2008;86(2):471–479.

Esmaeili-Mahani S, Fereidoni M, Javan M, Maghsoudi N, Motamedi F, Ahmadiani A. Nifedipine suppresses morphine-induced thermal hyperalgesia: Evidence for the role of corticosterone. *Eur J Pharmacol.* 2007;567(1–2):95–101.

Fishbain DA, Lewis JE, Gao J. Are psychoactive substance (opioid)-dependent chronic pain patients hyperalgesic? *Pain Pract.* 2011;11(4):337–343.

Forero M, Chan PS, Restrepo-Garces CE. Successful reversal of Hyperalgesia/Myoclonus complex with low-dose ketamine infusion. *Pain Pract.* 2012;12(2):154–158.

Ghelardini C, Galeotti N, Vivoli E, et al. Molecular interaction in the mouse PAG between NMDA and opioid receptors in morphine-induced acute thermal nociception. *J Neurochem.* 2008;105(1):91–100.

Gu X, Wu X, Liu Y, Cui S, Ma Z. Tyrosine phosphorylation of the N-methyl-D-aspartate receptor 2B subunit in spinal cord contributes to remifentanil-induced postoperative hyperalgesia: The preventive effect of ketamine. *Mol Pain.* 2009;5:76.

Gupta LK, Gupta R, Tripathi CD. N-methyl-D-aspartate receptor modulators block hyperalgesia induced by acute low-dose morphine. *Clin Exp Pharmacol Physiol.* 2011;38(9):592–597.

Guignard B, Bossard AE, Coste C, et al. Acute opioid tolerance: Intraoperative remifentanil increases postoperative pain and morphine requirement. *Anesthesiology.* 2000;93(2):409–417.

Hallett BR, Chalkiadis GA. Suspected opioid-induced hyperalgesia in an infant. *Br J Anaesth.* 2012;108(1):116–118.

Hamlin AS, McNally GP, Osborne PB. Induction of c-fos and zif268 in the nociceptive amygdala parallel abstinence hyperalgesia in rats briefly exposed to morphine. *Neuropharmacology.* 2007;53(2):330–343.

Hay JL, Kaboutari J, White JM, Salem A, Irvine R. Model of methadone-induced hyperalgesia in rats and effect of memantine. *Eur J Pharmacol.* 2010; 626(2–3):229–233.

Hay JL, White JM, Bochner F, Somogyi AA, Semple TJ, Rounsefell B. Hyperalgesia in opioid-managed chronic pain and opioid-dependent patients. *J Pain.* 2009;10(3):316–322.

Hong BH, Lee WY, Kim YH, Yoon SH, Lee WH. Effects of intraoperative low dose ketamine on remifentanil-induced hyperalgesia in gynecologic surgery with sevoflurane anesthesia. *Korean J Anesthesiol.* 2011;61(3):238–243.

Juni A, Cai M, Stankova M, et al. Sex-specific mediation of opioid-induced hyperalgesia by the melanocortin-1 receptor. *Anesthesiology.* 2010;112(1):181–188.

Juni A, Klein G, Kowalczyk B, Ragnauth A, Kest B. Sex differences in hyperalgesia during morphine infusion: Effect of gonadectomy and estrogen treatment. *Neuropharmacology.* 2008;54(8):1264–1270.

Juni A, Klein G, Pintar JE, Kest B. Nociception increases during opioid infusion in opioid receptor triple knock-out mice. *Neuroscience.* 2007;147(2):439–444.

Laulin JP, Maurette P, Corcuff JB, Rivat C, Chauvin M, Simonnet G. The role of ketamine in preventing fentanyl-induced hyperalgesia and subsequent acute morphine tolerance. *Anesth Analg.* 2002;94(5):1263–9, table of contents.

Lee C, Song YK, Jeong HM, Park SN. The effects of magnesium sulfate infiltration on perioperative opioid consumption and opioid-induced hyperalgesia in patients undergoing robot-assisted laparoscopic prostatectomy with remifentanil-based anesthesia. *Korean J Anesthesiol.* 2011a;61(3):244–250.

Lee C, Song YK, Lee JH, Ha SM. The effects of intraoperative adenosine infusion on acute opioid tolerance and opioid induced hyperalgesia induced by remifentanil in adult patients undergoing tonsillectomy. *Korean J Pain.* 2011b;24(1):7–12.

Lian B, Vera-Portocarrero L, King T, Ossipov MH, Porreca F. Opioid-induced latent sensitization in a model of non-inflammatory viscerosomatic hypersensitivity. *Brain Res.* 2010;1358:64–70.

Liang DY, Li X, Clark JD. 5-hydroxytryptamine type 3 receptor modulates opioid-induced hyperalgesia and tolerance in mice. *Anesthesiology.* 2011;114(5):1180–1189.

Liang DY, Liao G, Wang J, et al. A genetic analysis of opioid-induced hyperalgesia in mice. *Anesthesiology.* 2006a;104(5):1054–1062.

Liang DY, Liao G, Lighthall GK, Peltz G, Clark DJ. Genetic variants of the P-glycoprotein gene Abcb1b modulate opioid-induced hyperalgesia, tolerance and dependence. *Pharmacogenet Genomics.* 2006b;16(11):825–835.

Ma JF, Huang ZL, Li J, Hu SJ, Lian QQ. Cohort study of remifentanil-induced hyperalgesia in postoperative patients. *Zhonghua Yi Xue Za Zhi.* 2011;91(14):977–979.

Mao J. Opioid-induced abnormal pain sensitivity. *Curr Pain Headache Rep.* 2006;10(1):67–70.

Mao J, Sung B, Ji RR, Lim G. Chronic morphine induces downregulation of spinal glutamate transporters: Implications in morphine tolerance and abnormal pain sensitivity. *J Neurosci.* 2002a;22(18):8312–8323.

Mao J, Sung B, Ji RR, Lim G. Neuronal apoptosis associated with morphine tolerance: Evidence for an opioid-induced neurotoxic mechanism. *J Neurosci.* 2002b;22(17):7650–7661.

Mao J. Opioid-induced abnormal pain sensitivity: Implications in clinical opioid therapy. *Pain.* 2002c;100(3):213–217.

Mao J, Price DD, Mayer DJ. Mechanisms of hyperalgesia and morphine tolerance: A current view of their possible interactions. *Pain.* 1995;62(3):259–274.

Mao J, Price DD, Mayer DJ. Thermal hyperalgesia in association with the development of morphine tolerance in rats: Roles of excitatory amino acid receptors and protein kinase C. *J Neurosci.* 1994;14(4):2301–2312.

McDonnell C, Zaarour C, Hull R, et al. Pre-treatment with morphine does not prevent the development of remifentanil-induced hyperalgesia. *Can J Anaesth.* 2008;55(12):813–818.

Minville V, Fourcade O, Girolami JP, Tack I. Opioid-induced hyperalgesia in a mice model of orthopaedic pain: Preventive effect of ketamine. *Br J Anaesth.* 2010;104(2):231–238.

Okon TR, George ML. Fentanyl-induced neurotoxicity and paradoxic pain. *J Pain Symptom Manage.* 2008;35(3):327–333.

Pud D, Cohen D, Lawental E, Eisenberg E. Opioids and abnormal pain perception: New evidence from a study of chronic opioid addicts and healthy subjects. *Drug Alcohol Depend.* 2006;82(3):218–223.

Ram KC, Eisenberg E, Haddad M, Pud D. Oral opioid use alters DNIC but not cold pain perception in patients with chronic pain - new perspective of opioid-induced hyperalgesia. *Pain.* 2008;139(2):431–438.

Rivat C, Vera-Portocarrero LP, Ibrahim MM, et al. Spinal NK-1 receptor-expressing neurons and descending pathways support fentanyl-induced pain hypersensitivity in a rat model of postoperative pain. *Eur J Neurosci.* 2009;29(4):727–737.

Ruiz-Medina J, Ledent C, Valverde O. GPR3 orphan receptor is involved in neuropathic pain after peripheral nerve injury and regulates morphine-induced antinociception. *Neuropharmacology.* 2011;61(1–2):43–50.

Schlimp CJ, Pipam W, Wolrab C, Ohner C, Kager HI, Likar R. Clonidine for remifentanil-induced hyperalgesia: A double-blind randomized, placebo-controlled study of clonidine under intra-operative use of remifentanil in elective surgery of the shoulder. *Schmerz.* 2011;25(3):290–295.

Simonin F, Schmitt M, Laulin JP, et al. RF9, a potent and selective neuropeptide FF receptor antagonist, prevents opioid-induced tolerance associated with hyperalgesia. *Proc Natl Acad Sci U S A.* 2006;103(2):466–471.

Singler B, Troster A, Manering N, Schuttler J, Koppert W. Modulation of remifentanil-induced postinfusion hyperalgesia by propofol. *Anesth Analg.* 2007;104(6): 1397–403, table of contents.

Siniscalchi A, Piraccini E, Miklosova Z, Taddei S, Faenza S, Martinelli G. Opioid-induced hyperalgesia and rapid opioid detoxification after tacrolimus administration. *Anesth Analg.* 2008;106(2):645–6, table of contents.

Sjogren P, Jensen NH, Jensen TS. Disappearance of morphine-induced hyperalgesia after discontinuing or substituting morphine with other opioid agonists. *Pain.* 1994;59(2):313–316.

Song JW, Lee YW, Yoon KB, Park SJ, Shim YH. Magnesium sulfate prevents remifentanil-induced postoperative hyperalgesia in patients undergoing thyroidectomy. *Anesth Analg.* 2011;113(2):390–397.

Terashvili M, Wu HE, Schwasinger E, Tseng LF. Paradoxical hyperalgesia induced by mu-opioid receptor agonist endomorphin-2, but not endomorphin-1, microinjected into the centromedial amygdala of the rat. *Eur J Pharmacol.* 2007;554(2–3):137–144.

Troster A, Sittl R, Singler B, Schmelz M, Schuttler J, Koppert W. Modulation of remifentanil-induced analgesia and postinfusion hyperalgesia by parecoxib in humans. *Anesthesiology.* 2006;105(5):1016–1023.

Tuncer S, Yalcin N, Reisli R, Alper Y. The effects of lornoxicam in preventing remifentanil-induced postoperative hyperalgesia. *Agri.* 2009;21(4):161–167.

Vanderah TW, Ossipov MH, Lai J, Malan TP,Jr, Porreca F. Mechanisms of opioid-induced pain and antinociceptive tolerance: Descending facilitation and spinal dynorphin. *Pain.* 2001;92(1–2):5–9.

Van Elstraete AC, Sitbon P, Benhamou D, Mazoit JX. The median effective dose of ketamine and gabapentin in opioid-induced hyperalgesia in rats: An isobolographic analysis of their interaction. *Anesth Analg.* 2011;113(3):634–640.

Van Elstraete AC, Sitbon P, Mazoit JX, Conti M, Benhamou D. Protective effect of prior administration of magnesium on delayed hyperalgesia induced by fentanyl in rats. *Can J Anaesth.* 2006;53(12):1180–1185.

Van Elstraete AC, Sitbon P, Mazoit JX, Benhamou D. Gabapentin prevents delayed and long-lasting hyperalgesia induced by fentanyl in rats. *Anesthesiology.* 2008;108(3):484–494.

Vardanyan A, Wang R, Vanderah TW, et al. TRPV1 receptor in expression of opioid-induced hyperalgesia. *J Pain.* 2009;10(3):243–252.

Vera-Portocarrero LP, Zhang ET, King T, et al. Spinal NK-1 receptor expressing neurons mediate opioid-induced hyperalgesia and antinociceptive tolerance via activation of descending pathways. *Pain.* 2007;129(1–2):35–45.

Vinik HR, Kissin I. Rapid development of tolerance to analgesia during remifentanil infusion in humans. *Anesth Analg.* 1998;86(6):1307–1311.

Vorobeychik Y, Chen L, Bush MC, Mao J. Improved opioid analgesic effect following opioid dose reduction. *Pain Med.* 2008;9(6):724–727.

Yaksh TL, Harty GJ, Onofrio BM. High dose of spinal morphine produce a nonopiate receptor-mediated hyperesthesia: Clinical and theoretic implications. *Anesthesiology.* 1986;64(5):590–597.

Wala EP, Holtman JR,Jr. Buprenorphine-induced hyperalgesia in the rat. *Eur J Pharmacol.* 2011;651(1–3):89–95.

Waxman AR, Arout C, Caldwell M, Dahan A, Kest B. Acute and chronic fentanyl administration causes hyperalgesia independently of opioid receptor activity in mice. *Neurosci Lett.* 2009;462(1):68–72.

Wei X, Wei W. Role of gabapentin in preventing fentanyl- and morphine-withdrawal-induced hyperalgesia in rats. *J Anesth.* 2012;26(2):236–241.

Wilson NM, Jung H, Ripsch MS, Miller RJ, White FA. CXCR4 signaling mediates morphine-induced tactile hyperalgesia. *Brain Behav Immun.* 2011;25(3):565–573.

Woolf CJ. Intrathecal high dose morphine produces hyperalgesia in the rat. *Brain Res.* 1981;209(2):491–495.

Xuerong Y, Yuguang H, Xia J, Hailan W. Ketamine and lornoxicam for preventing a fentanyl-induced increase in postoperative morphine requirement. *Anesth Analg.* 2008;107(6):2032–2037.

Zhao M, Joo DT. Enhancement of spinal N-methyl-D-aspartate receptor function by remifentanil action at delta-opioid receptors as a mechanism for acute opioid-induced hyperalgesia or tolerance. *Anesthesiology.* 2008;109(2):308–317.

Zhou HY, Chen SR, Chen H, Pan HL. Opioid-induced long-term potentiation in the spinal cord is a presynaptic event. *J Neurosci.* 2010;30(12):4460–4466.

Chapter 5e

Optimizing Pharmacologic Outcomes: Principles of Opioid Rotation

Howard S. Smith and Bill H. McCarberg

With gradual escalation of the opioid dose in most patients, a favorable balance between analgesia and side effects can be achieved. However, some patients experience intolerable side effects before adequate analgesia is reached or, more rarely, do not benefit at all. Several strategies can be employed to reduce toxicity and improve pain control, including more aggressive treatment of side effects, use of coanalgesics or intravenous or anesthetic procedures, and use of nonpharmacologic interventions. An alternative approach is to change to another opioid in an attempt to allow titration to adequate pain control while limiting side effects.

The practice of changing from one opioid to another, referred to as *opioid rotation*, is most commonly undertaken when adequate analgesia is limited by the occurrence of problematic side effects. The principle of rotation is based on the observation that a patient's response can vary from opioid to opioid, both for analgesia and adverse effects. Importantly, an inadequate response or the occurrence of intolerable side effects with one opioid does not necessarily predict a similar response to another (Inturrisi 2002).

Clinical Experience

The reported use of opioid rotation varies widely, ranging in frequency from less than 10% to up to 80% of patients (Cherny et al. 1995; Fainsinger 1998; Hawley et al. 1998; Kloke et al. 2000). Vadalouca and colleagues performed a retrospective review and reported that the incidence of switching opioids in cancer patients ranged from 12% to 42% (Vadalouca et al. 2008). With the release of a number of new opioids and opioid formulations in recent years, it is likely that opioid rotation has become more frequent. A review of palliative care by Muller-Busch and colleagues (2005) showed that in some units, rotation from one long-acting opioid to another occurred less frequently than expected based on the published literature. This suggests that many problems can be managed by adaptation of dosage, route change, or the use of coanalgesics and adjuvants. Although a recent review found that opioid rotation results in clinical improvement in at least 50% of patients with chronic pain presenting with a poor response to a particular opioid (Mercadante and Bruera 2006), a

Cochrane review (Quigley 2004) revealed that there are no randomized controlled studies for opioid rotation. The evidence to support the practice is largely anecdotal or based on uncontrolled studies, but switching appears to be a useful maneuver.

The most common aims of opioid rotation are to improve pain control, reduce toxicity, or both. Other indications for opioid rotation include patient preference/convenience, convenience of route, wish for a reduction in invasiveness, problems with drug availability and cost (Cherny et al. 2001). Additional reasons may include attempts to improve bioavailability; attempts to improve patient adherence or compliance; or changing patient clinical condition (e.g., patient can no longer keep down enteral medications, problematic drug-drug interactions, patient has developed progressive renal failure).

Possible Mechanisms

A reason for opioid rotation's success has not been determined, and there is little hard evidence that it does, in fact, work. However, several theories have surfaced to explain why it might.

Toxicity

The accumulation of toxic metabolites may lead to severe side effects in patients on chronic opioid therapy. For example, the primary metabolite of morphine, morphine-6-glucuronide (M6G), is an active compound that is considerably more potent than its parent compound. M6G accumulates in patients with renal failure and is a common cause of opioid-related toxicity in such patients (Osborne et al. 1986). The metabolites of other opioids (e.g., dextropropoxyphene and tramadol) also accumulate in renal failure and will contribute to toxicity in the absence of dose reduction. Still other opioids (e.g., fentanyl and alfentanil) are metabolized in the liver to inactive products and are therefore safer to use in patients with renal failure than morphine. Thus, in a patient with renal impairment, rotating from morphine to an opioid with pharmacodynamics not dependent on renal function should allow for the clearance of toxic metabolites while simultaneously enabling the maintenance or improvement of pain control.

Pain Pathophysiology

The mechanism of pain may influence a patient's pattern of response to different opioids. For example, there is a perception that patients with neuropathic pain may be less responsive to opioids than patients with nociceptive pain. However, recent studies have demonstrated that patients with some types of neuropathic pain respond well to opioids (Eisenberg et al. 2006), and that opioid therapy should not be withheld from patients with neuropathic pain based on the assumption that this type of pain will be unresponsive to opioids.

Pharmacogenetics

Considerable evidence is accumulating to suggest genetic variability between individuals and in their ability to metabolize and respond to drugs. For example, codeine is ineffective as an analgesic in about 10% of the Caucasian population due to genetic polymorphisms in the enzyme necessary to O-methylate codeine to morphine, the active metabolite. Other polymorphisms can lead to enhanced metabolism and thus increased sensitivity to codeine's effects (Eichelbaum and Evert 1996). Genetic variability in the expression or density of opioid receptors, receptor affinity, or secondary messenger activation may explain the interindividual variation seen in patients' response to morphine. Similarly, variability in the expression of the enzymes responsible for the metabolism of different opioids may contribute to differences in dose requirements and toxicity. In the future, pharmacogenetic mapping may allow us to predict which opioid will be best suited to a particular individual (Roses 2000).

The scientific rationale for opioid switching may be appreciated in the genetic variation of certain candidate genes that help define an individual patient's unique pharmacokinetics/pharmacodynamics/μ opioid receptor (MOR), signaling efficiency.

Genetic variation in the multidrug-resistance gene MDR-1 (which encodes for P-glycoprotein, a membrane-bound drug transporter that regulates transfer of opioids across the blood–brain barrier by actively pumping opioids out of the central nervous system [CNS]) may account for the genetic variability in P-glycoprotein activity (Marzolini 2004; Ross et al. 2006). The mutation resulting in the G2677T/A genotype of P-glycoprotein has been demonstrated to alter drug levels (Kim et al. 2001) and drug-induced side effects (Yamauchi et al. 2002), though no such studies exist for opioid effects (Ross et al. 2006).

Investigators have identified more than 100 polymorphisms in the human MOR gene (Oprm), with some variants exhibiting altered binding affinities to different opioids (Surratt et al. 1994; Pil and Tytgat 2001; Ross et al. 2006). The best-known polymorphism in the Oprm is the A118G nucleotide substitution, which codes for the amino acid change of asparagine to aspartic acid. It is unclear whether genetic variation in various polymorphisms contributes to variation in the effects of different opioids.

Ross et al. (2005) found a significant difference in genotype and allelic frequency for the T8622C polymorphism in the b-arrestin-2 gene, which encodes for b-arrestin (an intracellular protein involved in regulating MOR phosphorylation, desensitization, and internalization); this variation is of unclear clinical significance.

Microarray analysis performed by Matsuoka and colleagues revealed that the mRNA expression levels of arrestin b 1 (ARRB1) were significantly down-regulated by morphine treatment. Real-time RT-PCR analysis against independent samples confirmed the results (P=0.003) and changes during treatment were negatively correlated with the plasma morphine concentration (R=0.42) (Matsuoka et al. 2012). The plasma concentration of morphine and the required dose of morphine were significantly lower for the A/A genotype of COMT (vs. A/G+G/G, P=0.008 and 0.03). Matsuoka and colleagues suggested that changes in the expression of ARRB1 may be a novel pharmacodynamic biomarker and the COMT 472G®A genotype may be a predictive biomarker of the response to morphine treatment (Matsuoka et al. 2012).

Genetic variation in the transcription factor hepatic nuclear factor 1 a (HNF-1a) may result in up to 10-fold variability in the expression of uridine diphosphate-glucuronosyl transferase 2B7 (UGT2B7) mRNA in human liver biopsies (Toide et al. 2002; Ross et al. 2006). UGT2B7 is the enzyme that catalyzes morphine glucuronidation (Coffman et al. 1997), and multiple single nucleotide polymorphisms in the promoter region of UGT2B7 have been reported which are of unknown significance (Duguay et al. 2004).

Ross et al. (2005) compared opioid switchers who did not tolerate morphine with controls who responded to morphine. Their study revealed significant differences in the genotype of the signal transducer and activator of the transcription 6 (STAT-6) gene between switchers and controls. STAT-6 recognition sites may exist in the Oprm gene. STAT-6 may interact with Oprm, altering Oprm expression and affecting different opioid responses (Ross et al. 2005).

Polymorphic variations in the catechol-O-methyltransferase (COMT) gene (which encodes for COMT, an enzyme that metabolizes catecholamines and thus may affect CNS neurotransmitters) have been demonstrated to influence μ opioid neurotransmitter responses to pain stressors (Zubieta et al. 2003) and to affect inter-individual variation in pain sensitivity (Diatchenko et al. 2005; Ross et al. 2006). Furthermore, Rakvag et al. (2005) found a correlation between COMT genotype and morphine dose requirements in cancer patients.

Drug Interactions

The metabolism of many opioids is dependent on the cytochrome P450 system. Moreover, many drugs commonly used in palliative care are inducers, inhibitors, or substrates for cytochrome P450 isoforms 3A4 and 2D6 (see Table 5e.1). Therefore, comedication with known P450 inhibitors or inducers will affect opioid metabolism and thus dose requirements and toxicity. Any beneficial or deleterious outcome following rotation may reflect changing drug interactions (Bernard and Bruera 2000).

Incomplete Cross-Tolerance

Incomplete cross-tolerance is the mechanism of action most commonly thought to explain the perceived benefits of opioid rotation (Crews et al. 1993; Fallon 1997; Mercadante et al. 1999). Analgesic tolerance is defined as a state of adaptation in which exposure to a drug induces changes that result in a diminution of one or more of the drug's effects over time. Incomplete cross-tolerance has been postulated as the mechanism whereby a patient remains tolerant to the side effects but not to the analgesic effect of an opioid in rotating from one opioid to another. Incomplete cross-tolerance describes patients who are tolerant to high doses of the first opioid yet have a lower tolerance to the new opioid. It is a result of the rate and magnitude of tolerance to side effects being different from the rate and magnitude of tolerance to pain. A patient will benefit from a change of opioid only if the cross-tolerance to the analgesic effect is

Table 5e.1 Interaction Between Analgesics, Inducers, and Inhibitors of the Cytochrome P450 System

Cytochrome	Substrate	Inhibitor	Inducer
3A4	Alfentanil	Fluconazole	Carbamazepine
	Fentanyl	Ketoconazole	Phenytoin
		Itraconazole	Erythromycin
		Metronidazole	Omeprazole
		Norfloxacin	Cyclophosphamide
		Fluoxetine	Dexamethasone
		Fluvoxamine	Rifampin
		Sertraline	Phenobarbitol
		Clarithromycin	St John's Wort
		Erythromycin	
		Cannabinoids	
2D6	Oxycodone	Cimetidine	Phenytoin
	Methadone	Paroxetine	Carbamazepine
	Tramadol	Desipramine	Phenobarbitol
	Codeine	Fluoxetine	
	Morphine	Haloperidol	
		Sertraline	
		Celecoxib	

less than the cross-tolerance to the adverse effects. Postulated mechanisms for incomplete cross-tolerance include preferential binding to different receptor subtypes and/or the use of different secondary messenger systems by different opioids, perhaps related to differences in their chemical structure and receptor binding properties (Fallon 1997).

General Issues

In principle, opioid rotation is an attractive way to achieve a desired benefit, yet many factors (e.g., pharmacokinetics, mixed pain syndromes, opioid side effects, opioid titration, patient preferences) can make this approach difficult. Conversion tables are often inaccurate, opioid choices are limited by formulations and availability, new drug interactions can occur, and there may be increased costs. All of these factors should be considered prior to rotating opioids. Before discarding the current treatment because of adverse side effects or a lack of efficacy, consider readjusting the opioid dose, adding adjuvant analgesics (thus sparing opioids), and giving specific treatments for the side effects.

At the same time, through observational studies and clinician experience, opioid rotation is often considered a first-line treatment option when pain control is lacking despite dose increases or when side effects limit titrations. These experiences have been corroborated by experiments in mice showing marked variability in response to morphine (Abbadie and Pasternak 2001). Gene splicing has elucidated at least 15 splice variants of the MOR gene (MOR-1), which have variable affinity to different opioids and distinct regional distributions (Pasternak et al. 2004). Although studies of specific gene splice variants are not possible in humans, the complexity of the human genome suggests even more inter-individual variation.

When the clinician is selecting a specific opioid to switch to, multiple factors may be considered, including: opioid metabolism (Smith 2009; Smith 2011), comorbid conditions, past history of opioids/medications tried and how well they were tolerated (where there were any adverse effects), the patient's cardiac/pulmonary/hepatic/renal function, the patient's living environment (e.g., outpatient living alone, long-term facility), patient prognosis, and any issues such as any balance or gait disturbances and history of cognitive difficulties or delirium. It is also vitally important that the clinician prescribing the new opioid that the patient is being switched to be very familiar with that opioid (particularly for opioids such as methadone and buprenorphine) or appropriate consultation should be obtained.

Guidelines for opioid rotation have been published based largely on case reports or retrospective analyses of patients with cancer pain (Hanks et al. 2001; Kefalianakis et al. 2002; Indelicato and Portenoy 2002). Although morphine remains the gold standard in palliative treatment, there are no studies providing evidence on the preferred selection of a baseline opioid or on indications for switching to alternative opioids. If patients with problems on one opioid are rotated, many symptoms appear to improve regardless of the direction of the switch. One guideline that has been widely used for opioid rotation is presented in Table 5e.2. Two articles with current recommendations with respect to opioid rotation are Knotkova et al. (2009) and Fine et al. (2009).

Table 5e.2 Dose Conversion Guidelines

- Calculate the equianalgesic dose of the new opioid based on an equianalgesic table.
- If switching to any opioid other than methadone or fentanyl, decrease the equianalgesic dose by 25% to 50%.
- If switching to methadone, reduce the dose by 75% to 90%.
- If switching to transdermal fentanyl, do not reduce the equianalgesic dose.
- Consider further changes in the adjusted equianalgesic dose based on medical condition and pain.
  - If the patient is elderly or has significant cardiopulmonary, hepatic, or renal disease, consider further dose reduction.
  - If the patient has severe pain, consider a lesser dose reduction.
- Calculate a rescue dose of 5% to 15% of the total daily opioid dose and administer at an appropriate interval.
- Reassess and titrate the new opioids.

Reproduced with permission from Indelicato RA, Portenoy RK. Opioid rotation in the management of refractory cancer pain. *J Clin Oncol* 2002;20:348–352.

Dose Conversion

Conversion doses should be based on an equianalgesic table that provides values for the relative potencies among different opioids (Table 5e.3). However, several limitations of equianalgesic tables must be acknowledged. Most conversion

Table 5e.3 Equianalgesic Conversion Table

Name	Equianalgesic Dose		Comments	Precautions and Contraindications
	Oral	Parenteral		
Morphine	30 mg	10 mg	Standard of comparison for opioid analgesics.	Clearance of parent drug and active metabolite is prolonged in renal failure
Hydromorphone	7.5 mg	1.5 mg	Exact dose equivalence unclear	
Oxycodone	20–30 mg	N/A	Variable oxycodone:morphine dose equivalence	Clearance is prolonged in hepatic failure
Methadone	20 mg (single dose)	10 mg	Long plasma half-life (24-36 hours), unique characteristics, considerable interindividual difference in pharmacokinetics, cannot be titrated in the same manner as other opioids	Accumulates with repeated dosing, unpredictable pharmacology in individual patients, use with caution
Oxymorphone	10–15 mg	1 mg		
Buprenorphine	N/A	0.3-0.6 mg	Limited availability Available in 7-day transdermal formulations (see manufacturers recommendations for morphine dose equivalence range)	
Fentanyl	N/A	100 mcg	Available in transdermal preparation (see manufacturers recommendations for morphine dose equivalence range)	"Safe" in patients with renal impairment
Alfentanil	N/A	1 mg	Lipophilic opioid more potent than fentanyl	As per fentanyl

tables are based on studies in which opioid-naïve individuals were given single low-dose opioids, without attention to side effects, organ failure, polypharmacy, complications, or the reason for rotation. These studies also failed to take into account the inter-individual variations that play a prominent role in determining the real conversion for each individual. The variation in published conversion ratios is also a problem. Oxycodone, fentanyl, and methadone show the largest differences among the available conversion tables (Anderson et al. 2001). Small variations in conversion ratios can lead to large differences in calculated equianalgesic doses, especially at higher doses. For example, reported morphine-to-oxycodone ratios have ranged from 1:1 to 2:1.

Methadone deserves special consideration in dose conversion. It has many advantages, including low cost, good oral and rectal absorption, no active metabolites, low tolerance development, and long duration of effect. At the same time, however, its half-life is long and unpredictable, with large inter-individual variations. This can result in delayed toxicity. Moreover, methadone has been linked to prolongation of the QTc (see chapter 5a). The conversion dose varies depending on the dose of the original opioid used. At morphine equivalence of less than 90mg, a conversion of 5:1 (morphine: methadone) is recommended. At morphine equivalence of 90 to 300mg, a conversion of 6:1 is suggested. For doses of morphine over 300mg, a rotation of 8:1 is recommended (Bruera and Sweeney 2002). In some individuals, steady-state blood levels are not achieved for four days; therefore dose adjustments should be made every four to five days. Despite the many advantages of methadone, the variable conversion ratios and its unpredictable half-life make this a difficult medication to use unless the provider is experienced with it.

Once the equianalgesic dose of the new opioid has been calculated, the dose should be adjusted due to incomplete cross-tolerance. When switching, it is prudent to decrease the equianalgesic dose by 25% to 50%—with two exceptions. First, if the new opioid is methadone, the dose should be reduced by 75% to 90%. Second, if the new opioid is transdermal fentanyl, the equianalgesic dose should not be reduced. The dose should be further adjusted based on medical conditions and pain characteristics.

Supplemental Medication During Conversion

Because it is difficult to predict a patient's response to a new opioid, care should always be taken to achieve analgesia without excessive dosing. Especially as incomplete cross-tolerance is unpredictable, rotating to a percentage of the equianalgesic dose is prudent. This may in turn result in underdosing, resulting in increased pain; therefore, short-acting breakthrough medication must be made available. After the steady state of the new opioid is achieved and the usage of the breakthrough medication is known, increases in the new opioid can be appropriately calculated.

Change of Route

In addition to a change of drug, opioid rotation may also involve a change in route of drug delivery (e.g., a rotation from oral morphine to rectal morphine or subcutaneous fentanyl). Some believe that a change of route rather than a change of opioid is the most logical means of instigating an opioid rotation (McQuay 1999); the issue is whether changing the route allows for a dose increase and effective analgesia without an increase in side effects. This may hold true for those drugs with active metabolites that undergo extensive first-pass metabolism when given orally. Kalso et al. (1996) published a small, double-blind crossover study in which patients were randomized to receive epidural and subcutaneous morphine. There was no difference in effectiveness or acceptability between arms, and both treatments provided better pain relief with fewer adverse effects compared to the prestudy oral morphine treatment. Enting and colleagues (2002) evaluated the efficacy of parenteral opioids (morphine, fentanyl, and sufentanil) in 100 patients who had failed conventional opioids (codeine, tramadol, morphine, methadone, and transdermal fentanyl). The authors reported an improved balance between analgesia and side effects in 71% of the patients. Furthermore, there was no difference between the patients who changed opioid and route and those who changed route alone.

Key Points for Opioid Rotation

- Utilize an opioid equianalgesic table that is appropriate/relevant for your practice, and use it consistently.
- In deciding on an alternative opioid, consider all patient factors, for example: What is the best route of drug delivery in this patient? Which drug is most convenient for the patient/treating team? Is cost going to be an issue? Is the new drug available in the community?
- In rotating opioids, consider all medical factors that may be relevant (e.g., renal function, liver function, age, comorbidities), and adjust equianalgesic dose based on these factors.
- In rotating to an opioid other than methadone or fentanyl, decrease the equianalgesic dose by 25% to 50%.
- In rotating to methadone, reduce the dose by 75% to 90%.
- In rotating to transdermal fentanyl, maintain the equianalgesic dose.
- In rotating because of uncontrolled pain, consider a lesser dose reduction than usual.
- Ensure that appropriate rescue/breakthrough doses are available. Use 5% to 15% of the total daily opioid dose as a guide, and reassess and retitrate the new opioid.

Although the above recommendations encourage the utilization of an opioid equianalgesic conversion table, health care providers must keep in mind that there is significant variability among opioids and significant differences

Table 5e.4 Recommendations for a new paradigm for opioid rotation	
Step 1	Begin a downward titration of the original opioid by reducing the current dose by about 10–30% while beginning the new opioid at a dose that would normally be used in an opioid-naïve patient or at the lowest available dose for the formulation.
Step 2	Slowly reduce the dose of the original total daily opioid dose by about 10–25% per week while increasing the dose of the new daily opioid dose by about 10–20% based on clinical need and safety. The complete switch can generally occur within 3–4 weeks
Step 3	Provide sufficient immediate-release opioid throughout the rotation to prevent withdrawal and/or increased pain if the dosing changes prove insufficient. (This minimizes the risk of potentially fatal patient self-medicating due to inadequate analgesia).

(Webster and Fine 2012a)

among patients. Clinicians need to practice medicine and actively decide the most appropriate opioid dose to start with, tailoring their decisions to specific individual patients, rather than simply robotically calculating an opioid dose and prescribing that amount without deciding whether any adjustments are needed. Subsequent close patient follow-up and careful opioid titration should ensue in attempts to achieve optimal analgesia with minimal adverse effects.

An increasing number of deaths have occurred in the last few years associated with current opioid prescribing practices (Bohnert et al. 2011; Dhalla et al. 2009; Paulozzi et al. 2006; Moore et al. 2007). Webster and Fine performed a focused literature review which suggested that widely used opioid rotation practices may be an important contributor to the increasing incidence of opioid-related fatalities (Webster et al. 2011; Webster and Fine 2012a). They further noted that the entire current "system of opioid rotation" appears to be flawed, in particular: 1.) not taking into account large variations in interpatient pharmacokinetics/pharmacodynamics (PK/PD), and responses to opioids; 2.) inadequate prescriber knowledge, experience and competence with respect to issues surrounding the appropriate prescribing of opioids; and 3.) an over-reliance on mathematical calculations based on outdated/limited equianalgesic dose tables (Webster et al. 2011; Webster and Fine 2012a; Webster and Fine 2012b) In efforts to minimize adverse effects of opioid rotation, Webster and Fine proposed a new paradigm for opioid rotation (Table 5e.4) (Webster and Fine 2012b).

Acknowledgment

The authors would like to thank Janet R. Hardy, MD, BSc, MBChB, FRACP, for her help in the preparation of this chapter.

References

Abbadie C, Pasternak GW. Differential in vivo internalization of MOR-1 and MOR-1C by morphine. *Neuroreport*. 2001;12(14):3069–3072.

Anderson R, Saiers JH, Abram S, et al. Accuracy in equianalgesic dosing: conversion dilemmas. *J Pain Symptom Manage*. 2001;21(5):397–406.

Bernard S, Bruera E. Drug interactions in palliative care. *J Clin Oncol*. 2000;18(8):1780–1799.

Bohnert AS, Valenstein M, Bair MJ, et al. Association between opioid prescribing patterns and opioid overdose-related deaths. *J Am Med Assoc*. 2011;305(13):1315–1321.

Bruera E, Sweeney C. Methadone use in cancer patients with pain: a review. *J Palliat Med*. 2002;5(1):127–138.

Cherny NJ, Chang V, Frager G, et al. Opioid pharmacotherapy in the management of cancer pain. *Cancer*. 1995;76(7):1283–1293.

Cherny N, Ripamonti C, Pereira J, et al. Expert Working Group of the European Association of Palliative Care Network: Strategies to manage the adverse effects of oral morphine: an evidence-based report. *J Clin Oncol*. 2001;19(9):2542–2554.

Coffman BL, Rios GR, King CD, et al. Human UGT2B7 catalyzes morphine glucuronidation. *Drug Metab Dispos*. 1997;25(1):1–4.

Crews JC, Sweeney NJ, Denson DD. Clinical efficacy of methadone in patients refractory to other mu-opioid receptor agonist analgesics for management of terminal cancer pain. *Cancer*. 1993;72(7):2266–2272.

Dhalla IA, Mamdani MM, Sivilotti ML, et al. Prescribing of opioid analgesics and related mortality before and after the introduction of long-acting oxycodone. *CMAJ*. 2009;181(12):891–896.

Diatchenko L, Slade GD, Nackley AG, et al. Genetic basis for individual variations in pain perception and the development of a chronic pain condition. *Hum Mol Genet*. 2005;14(1):135–143.

Duguay Y, Baar C, Skorpen F, et al. A novel functional polymorphism in the uridine diphosphate-glucuronosyltransferase 2B7 promoter with significant impact on promoter activity. *Clin Pharmacol Ther*. 2004;75(5):223–233.

Eichelbaum M, Evert B. Influence of pharmacogenetics on drug disposition and response. *Clin Exp Pharmacol Physiol*. 1996;23(10–11):983–985.

Eisenberg E, McNicol E, Carr DB. Opioids for neuropathic pain. *Cochrane Database Syst Rev*. 2006;3. DOI: 10.1002/14651858.CD006146.

Enting R, Oldenmenger W, van der Rijt C, et al. A prospective study evaluating the response of patients with unrelieved cancer pain to parenteral opioids. *Cancer*. 2002;94(11):3049–3056.

Fainsinger R. Opioids, confusion and opioid rotation. *Palliat Med*. 1998;12(6):463–464.

Fallon M. Opioid rotation: does it have a role? *Palliat Med*. 1997;11(3):177–178.

Fine PG, Portenoy RK; Ad Hoc Expert Panel on Evidence Review and Guidelines for Opioid Rotation. Establishing "best practices" for opioid rotation: conclusions of an expert panel. *J Pain Symptom Manage*. 2009;38(3):418–425.

Hanks GW, Conno F, Cherny N, et al. Morphine and alternative opioids in cancer pain: the EAPC recommendations. *Br J Cancer*. 2001;84(5):1695–1700.

Hawley P, Forbes K, Hanks GW. Opioids, confusion and opioid rotation. *Palliat Med.* 1998;12(1):63–64.

Indelicato RA, Portenoy RK. Opioid rotation in the management of refractory cancer pain. *J Clin Oncol.* 2002;20(1):348–352.

Inturrisi CE. Clinical pharmacology of opioids for pain. *Clin J Pain.* 2002; 18(4 Suppl):S3–13.

Kalso E, Heiskanen T, Rantio M, et al. Epidural and subcutaneous morphine in the management of cancer pain: a double-blind cross-over study. *Pain.* 1996;67(2–3):443–449.

Kefalianakis F, Kugler M, van der Auwera R, et al. Die Opioid Rotation in der Schmerztherapie. *Anaesthesist.* 2002;51(1):28–32.

Kloke M, Rapp M, Bosse B, et al. Toxicity and/or insufficient analgesia by opioid therapy: risk factors and the impact of changing the opioid. A retrospective analysis of 273 patients observed at a single center. *Support Care Cancer.* 2000;8(6):479–486.

Kim RB, Leake BF, Choo EF, et al. Identification of functionally variant MDR1 alleles among European Americans and Africans Americans. *Clin Pharmacol Ther.* 2001;70(2):189–199.

Knotkova H, Fine PG, Portenoy RK. Opioid rotation: the science and the limitations of the equianalgesic dose table. J Pain Symptom Manage. 2009;38(3):426–439.

McQuay H. Opioids in pain management. *Lancet.* 1999;353(9171):2229–2232.

Marzolini C, Paus E, Buclin T, et al. Polymorphisms in human MDR1 (P-glycoprotein): recent advances and clinical relevance. *Clin Pharmacol Ther.* 2004;75(1):13–33.

Matsuoka H, Arao T, Makimura C, et al. Expression changes in arrestin β and genetic variation in catechol-O-methyltransferase are biomarkers for the response to morphine treatment in cancer patients. *Oncol Rep.* 2012;27(5):1393–1399.

Mercadante S, Bruera E. Opioid switching: a systematic and critical review. *Cancer Treat Rev.* 2006;32(4):304–315.

Mercadante S, Casuccio A, Calderone L. Rapid switching from morphine to methadone in cancer patients with poor response to morphine. *J Clin Oncol.* 1999;17(10):3307–3312.

Moore TJ, Cohen MR, Furberg CD. Serious adverse drug events reported to the Food and Drug Administration, 1998–2005. *Arch Intern Med.* 2007;167(16):1752–1759.

Muller-Busch HC, Lindena G, Tietz K, et al. Opioid switch in palliative care, opioid choice by clinical need and opioid availability. *Eur J Pain.* 2005;9(5):571–579.

Osborne R, Joel S, Slevin M. Morphine intoxication in renal failure: the role of morphine-6-glucuronide. *Br Med J.* 1986;292(6535):1548–1549.

Paulozzi LJ, Budnitz DS, Xi Y. Increasing deaths from opioid analgesics in the United States. *Pharmacoepidemiol Drug Saf.* 2006;15(9):618–627.

Pasternak DA, Pan L, Xu J, et al. Identification of three alternatively spliced variants of the rat mu opioid receptor gene: dissociation of affinity and efficacy. *J Neurochem.* 2004;91(4):881–890.

Pil J, Tytgat J. The role of the hydrophilic Asn230 residue of the mu-opioid receptor in the potency of various opioid agonists. *Br J Pharamacol.* 2001;134(3):496–506.

Quigley C. Opioid switching to improve pain relief and drug tolerability. Cochrane Database Syst Rev. 2004;3. DOI: 10.1002114651858.CD004847.

Rakvag TT, Klepstad P, Baar C, et al. The Va1158Met polymorphism of the human catechol-O-methyltransferase (COMT) gene mat influence morphine requirements in cancer pain patients. *Pain.* 2005;116(1–2):73–78.

Roses A. Pharmacogenetics and future drug development and delivery. *Lancet.* 2000;355(9212):1358–1361.

Ross JR, Rutter D, Welsh K, et al. Clinical response to morphine in cancer patients and genetic variation in candidate genes. *Pharmacogenomics.* 2005;5(5):324–336.

Ross JR, Riley J, Quigley C, et al. Clinical pharmacology and pharmacotherapy of opioid switching in cancer patients. *Oncologist.* 2006;11(7):765–773.

Smith HS. The metabolism of opioid agents and the clinical impact of their active metabolites. *Clin J Pain.* 2011;27(9):824–838.

Smith HS. Opioid metabolism. *Mayo Clin Proc.* 2009;84(7):613–624.

Surratt CK, Johnson PS, Moriwaki A, et al. Mu opiate receptor. Charged transmembrane domain amino acids are critical for agonist recognition and intrinsic activity. *J Biol Chem.* 1994;269(32):20548–20533.

Toide K, Takahashi Y, Yamazaki H, et al. Hepatocyte nuclear factor-1 alpha is a causal factor responsible for interindividual differences in expression of UDP-glucuronosyltransferase 2B7 mRNA in human livers. *Drug Metab Dispos.* 2002;30(6):613–615.

Vadalouca A, Moka E, Argyra E, et al. Opioid rotation in patients with cancer: a review of the current literature. *J Opioid Manag.* 2008;4(4):213–250.

Webster LR, Fine PG. Overdose Deaths Demand a New Paradigm for Opioid Rotation. *Pain Med.* 2012a;13(4):571–574.

Webster LR, Fine PG. Review and critique of opioid rotation practices and associated risks of toxicity. *Pain Med.* 2012b;13(4):562–570.

Webster LR, Cochella S, Dasgupta ND, et al. An analysis of the root causes for opioid-related overdose deaths in the United States. *Pain Med.* 2011;12(Suppl 2):S26–S35.

Yamauchi A, Ieiri I, Kataoka Y, et al. Neurotoxicity induced by tacrolimus after liver transplantation: relation to genetic polymorphisms of the ABCBI (MDR1) gene. *Transplantation.* 2002;74(4):571–572.

Zubieta JK, Heitzeg MM, Smith YR, et al. COMT va1158met genotype affects mu-opioid neurotransmitter responses in pain stressor. *Science.* 2003;299(5610):1240–1243.

Chapter 5f

Optimizing Pharmacologic Outcomes: Individualization of Therapy

Howard S. Smith

The success of opioid therapy ultimately depends on individualization of the dose through titration. The goal of titration is to identify a dose associated with a favorable balance between analgesia and side effects.

An "analgesic ladder" approach to the selection of analgesic drugs for cancer pain has been popularized by the World Health Organization and is now widely accepted as a broad guideline and educational tool (WHO 1996). No such universally accepted and validated simplistic guideline or stepwise algorithm exists for persistent noncancer pain; however, similar principles of therapy exist, including initiating treatment conservatively with progressive titration of doses and the addition of more aggressive strategies in the face of a lack of responsiveness.

According to the analgesic ladder, selection of an analgesic should be guided by the usual severity of pain: patients with mild to moderate pain usually are first treated with acetaminophen or a nonsteroidal anti-inflammatory drug (NSAID). This is combined with one or more adjuvant drugs if a specific indication for one exists. These adjuvants include drugs selected to treat a side effect of the analgesic (e.g., laxatives) and drugs with analgesic effects (the so-called adjuvant analgesics).

Patients with moderate to severe pain (including those with insufficient relief after a trial of acetaminophen or an NSAID) are treated with an opioid conventionally used for moderate pain (Table 5f.1). This opioid usually is combined with acetaminophen or an NSAID and may be coadministered with an adjuvant drug if indicated. The most common approach in the United States involves

Table 5f.1 WHO Step 2 Analgesic Agents					
Oral Agents	**Bioavailability**	**Half-life (hr)**	**Onset (min)**	**Peak Effect (min)**	**Duration (hr)**
Codeine	40% (12–84%)	2.5–3.5	30–60	45–60	4–6
Dihydrocodeine	20%	3–4	30	45–60	3–4
Tramadol	75%	6	30	180	4–6
Hydrocodone	39%	3.8 (2–4.5)	20–30	1.3 (1–2)	3–6

the administration of a combination product containing an opioid plus either acetaminophen or aspirin. The dose of this drug is increased as needed until the maximum safe dose of the aspirin or acetaminophen is reached. For acetaminophen, this maximal safe dose is usually considered to be 4g/day, or lower (e.g., 2 to 3g/day) in patients with known hepatopathy or heavy alcohol use.

Patients with severe pain (including those who fail to achieve adequate relief after appropriate administration of drugs on the second rung of the analgesic ladder) receive an opioid conventionally selected for severe pain (Table 5f.2). This treatment may also be combined with acetaminophen, an NSAID, or an adjuvant drug as indicated.

The analgesic-ladder approach to drug selection must be individualized. Some patients with generally moderate pain should be considered for treatment with a long-acting opioid typically used for the third rung of the ladder, particularly if the convenience of the formulation or the likelihood of progressive pain provides a justification for this strategy.

In the United States, the opioids conventionally used for moderate pain include codeine, hydrocodone, dihydrocodeine, and oxycodone plus acetaminophen (oxycodone is also commonly administered as a single entity for severe pain).

The unique, centrally acting analgesic tramadol can also be used to manage cancer pain at the second rung of the analgesic ladder (Grond et al. 1999). The

Table 5f.2 WHO Step 3 Opioids

Oral Agents	Bio-availability	Half-life (hr)	Onset (min)	Peak Effect (min)	Duration (hr)
Morphine Sulfate IR	25–35% (15–64%)	2–3	20–30	60–90	3–6
Oxycodone IR	75% (60–87%)	2–3.5	20–30	60–120	3–6
Hydromorphone IR	37–62%	2.5 (2–3)	30	1–2	3–6
Oxymorphone IR	10%	7.3–9.4	15–23	45–90	4–6
Methadone	80%	(12–150)	30–90	2–4	Analgesia 6–8 For suppressing opioid withdrawal (24–48)
Levorphanol	Uncertain	11–16 Chronic dosing (up to 30)	20–60	1–2	3–6

* SS – steady state
IR – Immediate Release/Short-Acting

analgesic mechanism of this drug involves a mixture of mu agonism and inter-action with analgesic monoaminergic pathways in the central nervous system. Tramadol is also available in an extended-release formulation.

The opioids conventionally used in the United States for severe pain include morphine, hydromorphone, fentanyl, oxycodone (used as a single entity), levorphanol, methadone, and oxymorphone. All these drugs should be viewed as alternatives in practice. Although morphine has been considered the first-line drug for severe pain, there is now a large clinical experience that establishes very substantial individual variation in the response to different opioids (Portenoy 2007). For every patient, therefore, the overall balance between analgesia and side effects, as well as the pattern of side effects, can vary dramatically from opioid to opioid. This phenomenon justifies sequential trials of different opioid drugs—a technique known as opioid rotation—to identify the opioid that yields the most favorable balance between analgesia and side effects (Bruera et al. 1996; Portenoy 2007).

There is no standard correct dose for any opioid analgesic for a given patient or indication. Individual dose titration remains the only useful way to determine an appropriate analgesic dose. Opioid analgesic doses should be increased as appropriate for necessary analgesia within the constraints of an acceptable adverse-effect profile. Initial dosing for moderate to severe pain should be conservative, especially in the elderly or those with renal impairment.

When pain is inadequately controlled and there are no treatment-limiting side effects, the opioid dose should be increased as soon as steady-state serum levels are reached. In the case of short-half-life opioids such as morphine and oxycodone, a half-life of about two hours would provide steady-state levels within approximately 10 hours. In this setting, upward dose titration could occur rapidly without concern for accumulative toxicity. Pharmaceutically altered drugs, such as extended-release morphine, have a longer period to steady state (i.e., two to three days) and must be titrated more slowly and carefully.

Many clinicians use very conservative dose increments in escalating opioid therapy. This, unfortunately, can lead to treatment failure. Doses should be increased to response. The size of the increase is usually selected as either the total quantity of rescue drug consumed during the previous day or a percentage of the current total daily dose. Appropriate dose increments should be based on the clinical scenario, but may be 25% to 50% of the dose and can be increased every five half-lives. This percent increase applies no matter what the prior dose. The increment can be larger (75% to 100% of the total daily dose) if pain is severe or smaller if the patient is already experiencing opioid toxicity or is predisposed to adverse effects because of advanced age or coexisting major organ dysfunction. Caution is also reasonable if the patient has limited prior opioid exposure. However, when dealing with patients with severe acute pain or cancer pain or palliative care patients, it may be better to err slightly in the direction of too much opioid rather than too little. Initially, sedation may be advantageous for anxious patients or those with sleep deficits.

With palliative care patients in particular, there is no ceiling dose during this process of dose finding. The absolute dose is immaterial as long as side effects do not supervene. Occasional patients require opioid doses equivalent to many grams of morphine per day.

In most cases, titration identifies a dose that yields a favorable balance between analgesia and side effects, and the opioid requirement remains stable for a prolonged period. In the absence of progressive disease, patients may find the same dose effective for many months or years. This phenomenon belies the inevitability of tolerance as a problem in the long-term administration of opioid drugs (Nghiemphu and Portenoy 2000). There may be multiple reasons for an apparent increase in opioid requirements after a patient has been stable on the same does for many months or years (Table 5f.3). Moreover, when the

---

Table 5f.3 Reasons for Apparent Requiring of Increasing Opioid Dose during Opioid Therapy

1. INCREASING PHYSICAL PAIN
• Increasing nociception
  • Tumor growth
  • Inflammation
• New Pathology
• Development of neuropathic mechanisms
  • Nerve injury related to tumor
  • Nerve injury related to Cancer or AIDS therapy

2. INCREASING TOTAL PAIN OR SUFFERING
• Psychological or psychiatric processes
  • Increasing anxiety or depression
  • Delirium
  • Conditioned pain behavior
• Decline in psychologic benefit of medication
• Spiritual suffering
• Emotional suffering
• Socioeconomic suffering

3. PHARMACOLOGIC
• Pharmacokinetic
  • Decreased opioid bioavailability, Increased opioid metabolism
  • Increased protein binding (decreased free fraction of opioid analgesic)
  • Decreased Elimination
• Pharmacodynamic
  • Decreased receptor availability (downregulation)
  • Decreased opioid intrinsic affinity for receptor, and/or receptor availability
  • Decreased opioid receptor efficiency
• Analgesic Tolerance

4. PSEUDOTOLERANCE
• Increased or excessive physical activity
• Noncompliance
• Drug interactions
• Opioid misuse/diversion

Adapted from Portenoy, 2007

patient's pain does increase again, this declining efficacy of the opioid regimen can often be attributed to one or more overt processes that could potentially increase pain even if tolerance were not occurring. Progression of the disease is usually identified as the most likely etiology.

Thus, although analgesic tolerance to opioid drugs can occur and limit therapy, it seldom appears to be the primary reason for declining effects (Portenoy 2007). When pain increases during long-term therapy, the development of tolerance should not be assumed. Rather, recurrent pain should signal the need to reevaluate the nature of the pain. Dose titration should start again and should continue until the favorable balance between analgesia and side effects is regained or the therapy is determined to be ineffective because of treatment-limiting toxicity (Portenoy 2007).

Opioids, though effective for neuropathic pain (Eisenberg 2005) may not be as effective for neuropathic pain as they are for somatic pain (Figure 5f.1) (Smith 2012; Smith 2011a). This may be due in part from MOR desensitization secondary to neuropathic pain that appears to involve protein kinase A. It has been demonstrated that the MOR and the NMDA receptors coexist at certain postsynapses and that both receptors show an electrophysiological interaction in individual neurons (Rodr´guez-Muñoz et al. 2011). Therefore, it is conceivable that PKA may be partly responsible for the dissociation of NR1 subunits from MORs, which occurs as a result of NMDAR activation leading to MOR Serine phosphorylation and uncoupling from G-proteins (Rodr´guez-Muñoz et al. 2011; Smith 2012; Smith, 2011a) (Figure 5f.2).

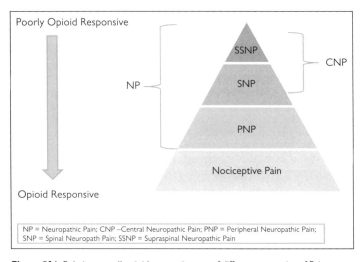

Poorly Opioid Responsive

SSNP

CNP

NP

SNP

PNP

Nociceptive Pain

Opioid Responsive

NP = Neuropathic Pain; CNP –Central Neuropathic Pain; PNP = Peripheral Neuropathic Pain;
SNP = Spinal Neuropath Pain; SSNP = Supraspinal Neuropathic Pain

Figure 5f.1 Relative overall opioid responsiveness of different categories of Pain

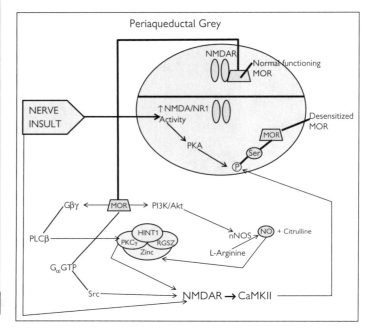

Figure 5f.2 Schematic of potential mechanisms whereby neuropathic pain may promote desensitized or reduced MOR analgesic signaling

If one opioid is not providing effective analgesia, switching to a different opioid may help certain patients achieve adequate analgesia. Multiple opioids have been successfully utilized to treat neuropathic pain including morphine (Raja et al. 2002), methadone (Raja et al. 2002), hydromorphone (Moulin et al. 2010), levorphanol (Rowbotham et al. 2003), and transdermal fentanyl (Agarwal et al. 2007). However, all opioids are not created equally, and although definitive evidence does not exist, it is conceivable that some opioids (or opioid-like analgesic agents) may be relatively more effective at providing analgesia for patients with neuropathic pain than others (Smith 2012; Smith 2011a). Agents that may conceivably be particularly effective against neuropathic pain may include oxycodone, methadone, buprenorphine, tapentadol, and tramadol (Smith 2012; Smith 2011a).

It is possible that the interaction of different opioids with different G-protein subtypes may be partly responsible for the different analgesic responses of different individuals and/or different pain states. Therefore, if one opioid agent does not provide adequate analgesia it is still worthwhile proceeding with a trial of a different opioid agent (preferably one with different G-protein interactions).

Table 5f.4 Different G-protein Subtype Interactions of Different Opioids (Data from Sánchez-Blázquez et al., 2001.)

Opioid	G-Protein Subtype				
	G_i	G_o	G_z	G_q	G_{ll}
Morphine	G_{i2}	—	G_z	—	—
Methadone	G_{i1} G_{i2} G_{i3}	G_{o1}	G_z	—	G_{ll}
Buprenorphine	G_{i2} G_{i3}	G_{o2}	G_z	G_q	—

In particular, it is conceivable that the interaction/participation of G_o- and Gq_{11}-proteins may lead to analgesic effects that are especially beneficial in certain neuropathic pain states (Smith 2011a). Methadone and buprenorphine interact with these G-protein subtypes but morphine does not. Methadone and buprenorphine are also significantly different from each other. Buprenorphine and methadone demonstrate significant difference in activation of G proteins, $G\text{-}a_{i1}$, $G\text{-}a_{o1}$, and G-al1 are necessary for methadone-induced analgesia, but not buprenorphine-induced analgesia, whereas buprenorphine-induced analgesia requires $G\text{-}a_{o2}$ and $G\text{-}a_q$ but methadone does not (Sánchez-Blázquez et al. 2001). (Table 5f.4).

Opioid-induced Block of Sodium Channels

One specific property of opioids which may contribute to the reason why some opioids may be particularly well-suited to provide analgesia in various neuropathic pain states may be the ability of various opioids to inhibit voltage-gated sodium channels. It is becoming appreciated that various different mu-opioid receptor agonists may differ significantly in their ability/potency to inhibit voltage-gated sodium channels as well as the individual sodium channel type that they inhibit (Table 5f.5).

Meperidine appears to be the best studied opioid with respect to blocking voltage-gated sodium channels and it has been shown to block skeletal muscle sodium channel Nav 14 in a state-dependent manner via the local anesthetic (LA)-binding site (Lampert et al. 2010). Leffler has shown that buprenorphine may also act as a potent local anesthetic and block voltage-gated sodium channels via the local anesthetic binding site (Leffler et al. 2012). The potency of buprenorphine to block sodium channels is significantly higher than that of meperidine, lidocaine, or even bupivacaine when evaluated under identical experimental conditions (Leffler et al. 2012; Leffler et al. 2010; Leffler et al. 2007). Buprenorphine blocked the generation of action potentials in isolated C-fibers with a higher potency and with slower onset and offset kinetics versus lidocaine (Kistner et al. 2010). This is likely due in part to the high lipophilicity of buprenorphine (octanol: water partition coefficient roughly 2,000 versus about

Table 5f.5 – Potency of opioids to inhibit Na+ Channels

Opioid	Voltage-gated Na+ Channel	Rough Relative Potency to Block Na+ Channel
Buprenorphine	Nav 1.4	+++++
Meperidine	Nav 1.4	++++
Fentanyl	Nav 1.2	+++
Sufentanil	Nav 1.2	+++
Tramadol	Nav 1.2	++
Morphine	Nav 1.7	+
Remifentanil	—	—

Table 5f.6 Therapeutic Options When an Opioid Regimen Fails

Approach	Options
Try to open the therapeutic window	More aggressive side effect management
Try to find an opioid with a more favorable balance between analgesia and side effects	Opioid rotation
Use a pharmacologic approach to reduce the systemic opioid requirement	• Coadminister an NSAID or an adjuvant analgesic • Consider intraspinal opioid therapy
Use a nonpharmacologic approach to reduce the systemic opioid requirement	• Anesthetic approaches, (e.g., nerve blocks) • Surgical approaches, (e.g., cordotomy) • Physiatric approaches, (e.g., an orthotic) • Psychological approaches, (e.g., biofeedback, cognitive behavioral therapy) • Neuromodulation approaches, (e.g. spinal cord stimulation, peripheral nerve stimulation) • Alternative medicine approaches, (e.g., acupuncture)

Adapted from Portenoy, 2007

200 for norbuprenorphine versus about 39 for meperidine), since lipophilicity is a major factor for potency of local anesthetics acting on sodium channels (Yanagidate and Strichartz 2007).

Haeseler et al. (2006) found that sufentanil, fentanyl, and tramadol (but not morphine) block neuronal Nav 1.2 in a state dependent manner. Morphine does appear to block neuronal excitability in an opioid-receptor independent manner (Brodin and Skoglund 1990; Mizuta et al. 2008); likely via tonic block of the tetrodotoxin (TTX) sensitive sodium channel Nav 1.7 (Leffler et al. 2012).

Some patients will not attain a favorable balance between analgesia and side effects during dose titration. Strategies for the management of such patients, which are based entirely on clinical experience, may not only include switching to a different opioid (opioid rotation), but also switching to a different route (e.g., intrathecal opioids), more aggressive treatment of side effects, addition of other analgesic therapy (e.g., adjuvant analgesics), addition of pharmacologic agents that may reduce tolerance effects (e.g., NMDA antagonists), and/or addition of nonpharmacologic approaches (e.g., neuromodulation) (Table 5f.6) (Portenoy 2007). There are numerous options, ranging from more sophisticated side-effect management to invasive analgesic therapies. Therapeutic decision making must be based on a careful reassessment of the patient. The goals of care must be considered in balancing the risks and benefits of any intervention (Portenoy 2007). Clinicians need to weigh the risk/benefit ratio and weigh all the considerations of chronic opioid therapy as well as choosing specific opioid analgesic agents. In patients with HIV-related pain, theoretic possibilities may exist that certain opioids (e.g., morphine may have the potential to actually promote nociceptive processes and/or HIV infectivity (Smith 2011b); whereas treatment with other opioids (e.g., buprenorphine) may be less apt to do this and may potentially also provide improved analgesia (Palma et al. 2011).

References

Agarwal S, Polydefkis M, Block B, Haythornthwaite J, Raja SN. Transdermal fentanyl reduces pain and improves functional activity in neuropathic pain states. *Pain Med.* 2007;8(7):554–562.

Brodin P, Skoglund LA. Dose-response inhibition of rat compound nerve action potential by dextropropoxyphene and codeine compared to morphine and cocaine *in vitro. Gen Pharmacol* 1990; 21(4):551–553.

Bruera E, Pereira J, Watanabe S, et al. Opioid rotation in patients with cancer pain: a retrospective comparison of dose ratios between methadone, hydromorphone, and morphine. *Cancer.* 1996;78(4):852–857.

Eisenberg E, McNicol ED, Carr DB. Efficacy and safety of opioid agonists in the treatment of neuropathic pain of nonmalignant origin: systematic review and meta-analysis of randomized controlled trials. *JAMA.* 2005;293(24):3043–3052.

Grond S, Radbruch L, Meuser T, et al. Assessment and treatment of neuropathic cancer pain following WHO guidelines. *Pain.* 1999;79(1):15–20.

Haeseler G, Foadi N, Ahrens J, Dengler R, Hecker H, Leuwer M. Tramadol, fentanyl and sufentanil but not morphine block voltage-operated sodium channels. *Pain.* 2006; 126(1–3):234–244.

Kistner K, Zimmermann K, Ehnert C, Reeh PW, Leffler A. The tetrodotoxin-resistant Na+ channel Na (v)1.8 reduces the potency of local anesthetics in blocking C-fiber nociceptors. *Pflugers Arch.* 2010; 459(5):751–763.

Lampert A, O'Reilly AO, Reeh P, Leffler A. Sodium channelopathies and pain *Pflugers Arch.* 2010; 460(2):249–263.

Leffler A, Frank G, Kistner K, Niedermirtl F, Koppert W, Reeh PW, Nau C. Local Anesthetic-like Inhibition of Voltage-gated Na+ Channels by the Partial μ-opioid Receptor Agonist Buprenorphine. *Anesthesiology.* 2012;116(6):1335–1346.

Leffler A, Reckzeh J, Nau C. Block of sensory neuronal Na+ channels by the secre-olytic ambroxol is associated with an interaction with local anesthetic binding sites. *Eur J Pharmacol.* 2010; 630(1–3):19–28.

Leffler A, Reiprich A, Mohapatra DP, Nau C. Use-dependent block by lidocaine but not amitriptyline is more pronounced in tetrodotoxin (TTX)-Resistant Nav1.8 than in TTX-sensitive Na+ channels. *J Pharmacol Exp Ther.* 2007; 320(1):354–364.

Mizuta K, Fujita T, Nakatsuka T, Kumamoto E. Inhibitory effects of opioids on compound action potentials in frog sciatic nerves and their chemical structures. *Life Sci.* 2008(5–6); 83:198–207.

Moulin DE, Richarz U, Wallace M, Jacobs A, Thipphawong J. *J Pain Palliat Care Pharamcother.* 2010;24(3):200–212.

Nghiemphu LP, Portenoy RK. Opioid tolerance: a clinical perspective. In Bruera EB, Portenoy RK, eds. *Topics in Palliative Care*, vol. 5. New York: Oxford University Press, 2000; 197–212.

Palma J, Cowan A, Geller EB, Adler MW, Benamar K. Differential antinociceptive effects of buprenorphine and methadone in the presence of HIV-gp120. *Drug Alcohol Depend.* 2011; 118(2–3):497–499.

Portenoy RK. Supportive and palliative care. In Straus DJ, ed. *Educational Review Manual in Medical Oncology.* New York: Castle Connolly Graduate Medical Publishing, 2007; 361–408.

Raja SN, Haythornthwaite JA, Pappagallo M, Clark MR, Travison TG, Sabeen S, Royall RM, Max MB. Opioids versus antidepressants in postherpetic neuralgia: a randomized, placebo-controlled trial. *Neurology.* 2002;59(7):1015–1021.

Rodríguez-Muñoz M, Sánchez-Blázquez P, Vicente-Sánchez A, Berrocoso E, Garzón J. The Mu-Opioid Receptor and the NMDA Receptor Associate in PAG Neurons: Implications in Pain Control. *Neuropsychopharmacology.* 2012;37(2):338–349.

Rowbotham MC, Twilling L, Davies PS, Reisner L, Taylor K, Mohr D. Oral opioid therapy for chronic peripheral and central neuropathic pain. *N Engl J Med.* 2003;348(13):1223–1232.

Sánchez-Blázquez P, Gómez-Serranillos P, Garzón J. Agonists determine the pattern of G-protein activation in mu-opioid receptor-mediated supraspinal analgesia. *Brain Res Bull.* 2001;54(2):229–235.

Smith HS. Opioids and Neuropathic Pain. *Pain Physician.* 2012; 15(3S):ES93–ES110.

Smith HS. Opioids and Neuropathic Pain. Presented at the Capital District Pain Conference; Albany, NY. September, 2011a.

Smith HS. Treatment Considerations in Painful HIV-Related Neuropathy. *Pain Physician.* 2011b;14(6):E505–E524.

Yanagidate F, Strichartz GR. Local anesthetics. *Handb Exp Pharmacol.* 2007:95–127.

World Health Organization (WHO). *Cancer Pain Relief, with a Guide to Opioid Availability*, 2nd ed. Geneva: World Health Organization, 1996.

Chapter 6

Opioid Therapy for Cancer Pain

Mellar P. Davis and Howard S. Smith

The classic guideline for analgesic use in cancer pain was formulated by the World Health Organization (WHO). The core of this guideline is a three-step analgesic ladder that matches pain severity to analgesia to potency. This same three-step analgesic ladder is recommended for nociceptive and neuropathic pain management. Good pain relief is defined as a two-point decrease in pain severity on a numerical rating scale (NRS) (Farrar et al. 2001). By following the analgesic ladder, 76% of patients reported a 30% reduction in pain severity and 12% reported satisfactory pain relief (Zech et al. 1995; Grond et al. 1999). Despite the success of the analgesic ladder, significant under-treatment of chronic pain is experienced by many patients receiving active anti-tumor treatment for solid tumors; it is even more of a problem for those with advanced disease (Higginson and Hearn 1997).

Cancer Pain Syndromes

Numerous pain syndromes have been described, and three-quarters are a direct effect of the neoplasm (Portenoy 2011). A smaller but important proportion of syndromes are a result of therapies to manage cancer, and a still smaller group arise from co-morbid disease (Portenoy 2011).

The most common syndromes are nociceptive pain derived from metastatic bone lesions; however, many individuals with cancer suffer from multiple types of pain: somatic, visceral, and neuropathic pain syndromes related to malignancy or treatment as well as multiple foci. Only a small proportion of bone metastases become painful; although the cause of bone pain is unknown, it is likely that pain is due to multiple factors (Smith 2003; Jimenez-Andrade et al. 2010; Yoneda et al. 2011; Anborgh et al. 2010). However, 85% of patients with bone metastases will experience pain (Laird et al. 2011). Laboratory models of cancer induced bone pain indicate that the pain mechanism of bone metastases is distinct from both inflammatory and neuropathic pain (Luger et al. 2002; Jimenez-Andrade et al. 2010). Descriptors used for bone pain include dull, sore, hurting, aching, and heavy. Most (75%) have breakthrough pain with weight bearing. Those with breakthrough pain have greater average daily pain and greater interference with activity. The time from pain onset to maximum intensity is five minutes, and, because of this, oral potent opioids are less effective than for chronic pain.Individuals with bone metastases and breakthrough pain experience on average four episodes per day (Laird et al. 2011).

The spine is the most common site of bone metastasis. While pain may occur at any site along the vertebral column, epidural cord compression is most common in the thoracic spine. Several specific syndromes characterized by pain referral patterns or associated features have been described with vertebral metastases. Tumor invasion of C1 or C2 vertebra causes progressive neck pain to radiate over the posterior vertex, which worsens by flexion of the neck. Metastases to C7 or T1 vertebra cause focal pain, which can be referred to the inferior interscapular region; a lesion at T12 or L1 can refer pain to the ipsilateral sacroiliac joint or iliac crest. The reversed pain pattern may not be recognized by physicians, and therefore imaging may be obtained from the wrong location (Portenoy 2007).Hence, clinicians need a thorough understanding of pain syndromes particularly referred pain patterns.

Cancer pain may be one or more of the following:

Somatic: Related to cancer (invasion of joints, bone and soft tissue), related to cancer treatment (e.g., radiation-induced osteonecrosis), or related to paraneoplastic phenomena (e.g., hypertrophic osteoarthropathy).

Visceral: Related to cancer induced intestinal obstruction (peritoneal carcinomatosis and parenchymal invasion) or cancer treatment (radiation-induced chronic pelvic pain and radiation enteritis). Paraneoplastic pseudo-obstruction is an example of paraneoplastic visceral pain.

Neuropathic: Related to cancer invasion of the plexus (brachial, lumbar, celiac, hypogastric) or cancer treatment (postmastectomy syndrome, chemotherapy-induced polyneuropathies, radiation-induced plexopathy).

Breakthrough pain can occur with any cancer pain syndrome.By definition, it is at least a two-point rise in pain severity over the average daily pain (Laird et al. 2011).Two types of breakthrough pain have been described: spontaneous and incident (with voluntary or involuntary activity).Pain that increases spontaneously just before another around-the-clock dose is end-of-dose failure pain. This particular flare of pain is related to suboptimal around-the-clock analgesics and is not considered a breakthrough pain.

Cancer Pain Management: Primary Therapies

Interventions targeted to the etiology of the pain can have analgesic consequences and should be considered in every case. An extensive literature review of the potential analgesic benefits of radiotherapy (Falkmer et al. 2003) is complemented by a small number of studies documenting the potential utility of chemotherapy for pain control (Burris et al. 1997; Ernst et al. 2003). To realize the potential benefits of primary therapy the pain assessment must include a competent examination and appropriate imaging studies, which together clarify the extent of disease and the etiology of the pain. Baseline and breakthrough pain intensity, pain interference, and the quality and radiating nature of pain should be documented before starting analgesics or interventional therapies. Once the underlying problem has been characterized, decision making is further influenced by numerous other factors such as the availability, safety, and efficacy of treatment, and the potential of treatment to prolong life or reduce the likelihood of further complications and the overriding goals of care.

Opioid therapy provides adequate pain relief to more than three-quarters of patients with cancer pain (Grond et al. 1991; Jacox et al. 1994; WHO 1996). This success rate justifies the widely held view that long-term opioids are the first-line approach for moderate to severe cancer pain (The Ad Hoc Committee 1992; Jacox et al. 1994; WHO 1996; American Pain Society 2003).

Principles governing the proper use of opioids in severe chronic cancer pain management are to (1) use oral morphine or enteral/transdermal equivalent opioids for severe pain as the opioid of choice; (2) prescribe around-the-clock (ATC) medication (in pre-emptive reduction of pain); (3) select analgesics using the WHO's three-step analgesic ladder based on severity; (4) individualize prescribing based upon pain patterns, comorbidities, and comedications; and (5) pay attention to details and conduct frequent reassessments (Walsh 2000; Caraceni et al. 2011; Klepstad et al. 2011). Recommendations are also available from the European Association for Palliative Care (EAPC) (Caraceni et al. 2012) and the National Institute for Health and Clinical Excellence (NICE) (Bennett et al. 2012).

Successful management of cancer pain requires the strategic use of opioids based upon both the temporal nature and intensity of the pain; that is, the right opioid must be prescribed at the right dose and the right time (Walsh 2000; Inturrisi 2002; Walsh et al. 2004). The WHO's three-step analgesic ladder does not provide specific guidance on dosing strategies for temporal pain patterns. Cancer pain has two main temporal patterns, continuous and intermittent. Intermittent pain is referred to as breakthrough pain, and, as mentioned, is defined as a transitory episode of pain superimposed on an otherwise controlled baseline pain.

Dosing Strategies

Acute Pain

Acute pain is managed by small, frequent doses of potent opioids, given until a response is elicited. The dose that effectively managed the acute pain episode is referred to as the acute opioid dose. Once relieved, the acute pain episode is followed by maintenance ATC dosing of the opioid based upon the acute opioid dose. This strategy reduces the risk of overdose, produces rapid analgesia (usually within an hour), and determines the dose needed to maintain analgesia (Upton et al. 1997). The dose at which a significant reduction of pain occurs is divided by three and given as a continuous hourly infusion. If intravenous access is not available, then subcutaneous morphine (2mg), fentanyl (40µg), or hydromorphone (0.4mg) can be given every five minutes until pain subsides. Subcutaneous morphine has a delay to maximum concentration relative to intravenous morphine, which explains the longer dosing interval (Stuart-Harris et al. 2000). Patients on chronic morphine prior to an episode of acute pain will need to have the acute opioid dose added to the around-the-clock in order to maintain analgesic dose. The previous 24-hour oral ATC dose and rescue doses for nonincident breakthrough pain are added, divided by three (oral-to-parenteral dose ratio), and then divided by 24 and added to the preexisting maintenance dose for the intravenous hourly dose.

Although respiratory depression has not been reported with acute opioid dosing strategies (Davis et al. 2004), it would be important to be knowledge-able about naloxone in case of unexpected reactions. Naloxone 0.4mg/mL is diluted 1 to 10 in water for injection, which results in a 40μg/mL solution. One milliliter (40μg) is given intravenously or subcutaneously every three minutes until the patient is arousable and has a respiration rate of 10 or more breaths per minute (Wasiak 2002). If respiratory depression has occurred from a sustained-release opioid or methadone, the dose that reversed respiratory depression should be infused hourly, since naloxone has a short half-life (Watson et al. 1998; Wasiak 2002). Titration of small doses of naloxone can reverse opioid-induced respiratory depression without inducing withdrawal symptoms or reversing analgesia.

Chronic Pain

Around-the-clock or fixed-schedule dosing is preferred for continuous or frequently recurring pain. An as-needed dose (referred to as rescue dose) is usually combined with the fixed regimen to treat breakthrough pain (Zeppetella 2011). Rescue dosing alone should be considered at the start of therapy in relatively opioid-naïve patients, in patients with rapidly changing pain (e.g., after radiotherapy to a painful bone lesion), and in patients with intermittent pain separated by pain-free intervals. This is particularly appropriate with methadone because of the risk of late toxicity from drug accumulation.

For the patient with limited prior opioid exposure (e.g., the use of an acetaminophen-oxycodone combination product in several doses per day), the starting dose of an opioid conventionally used for severe pain is usually the oral equivalent to morphine sulfate five to 10 mg every four hours. Pain severity does not predict the effective opioid dose. Therefore, graded opioid doses based on pain severity should not be done. When a patient is switched to a new opioid, the initial dose is calculated from an equianalgesic table; this calculation is revised based on the specific drug, the patient's medical status, and the degree of pain at the time of the switch (Indelicato and Portenoy 2002). Because individual variability is significant and there is the possibility of incomplete cross-tolerance, the dose of the new drug should be reduced by 30% to 50% in most circumstances between opioids.

The two exceptions to this are (1) methadone, which has a potency greater than anticipated and is linear to the morphine dose; it should be reduced by 75% to 90% or should have a graduated linear analgesic equivalent scale

(Mercadante and Caraceni 2011) and (2) transdermal fentanyl, which is typically administered at the calculated equianalgesic dose based on the conversions in the package insert.This may be conservative.Oral morphine equivalents to transdermal fentanyl are 70 – 100 to 1. The dose of the new opioid should be reduced relatively more when the patient is medically frail or is taking high doses (>200 -300 mg) of morphine per day) and it should be reduced relatively less if the ongoing pain is severe.

There are few studies involving rescue dosing, therefore, the selection of a drug, dose, and dosing interval is usually based on clinical experience. With most opioids, the rescue drug is usually the same drug as that administered on an ATC basis (e.g., short-acting oxycodone is used as needed for breakthrough pain when sustained-release oxycodone is the baseline opioid). Dosages of baseline and/or rescue doses will need to be adjusted to response (Zeppetella 2011). There is no evidence, however, that results are better with this approach than when a different short-acting drug is used to supplement the baseline opioid. When methadone or transdermal fentanyl is being used, depending on the clinical circumstance, an alternative short-acting opioid, such as morphine, is typically co-administered. Also, oral transmucosal fentanyl citrate (OTFC) or the fentanyl buccal tablets, a less expensive opioid, can be selected for use with transdermal fentanyl in those who cannot afford recently released and licensed fentanyl pharmaceuticals. There is a poor correlation between chronic and breakthrough doses when using fentanyl oral, buccal, or nasal preparations.In certain circumstances methadone alone is appropriate for ATC and rescue dosing.

With the exception of OTFC and the fentanyl buccal tablet, the size of the rescue dose is usually 5% to 15% of the total daily dose or an increment of the four-hourly dose (25% to 100%) (Hanks et al. 2001; Zeppetella 2011).The dosing interval in the ambulatory population is usually one to two hours, as needed. Dosing oral or nasal formulations of fentanyl should begin with the lowest available dose and titrated to response.No more than four fentanyl doses for breakthrough pain should be used per day.

Chronic pain requires ATC opioid dosing. For the frail elderly or those with significantly diminished organ function/reserves, parenteral morphine 0.5 mg/h is used; otherwise, 1 mg/h is a reasonable starting dose in the opioid-naïve (Walsh et al. 2004). Alternatively, fentanyl 10µg/h or hydromorphone 0.2 mg/h could be substituted for morphine (Walsh et al. 2004). Starting doses for oral morphine are either 5 mg every four hours or 15 mg of the sustained-release form every 12 hours. Mild drowsiness, dizziness, or mental clouding commonly occur at the start of therapy, but resolve in most patients over several days. Laxatives and stool softeners should be started proactively for constipation except in those with an ileostomy (Larkin et al. 2008). Nausea and vomiting are not uncommon at the start of morphine administration, but usually resolve over several days. Either metoclopramide 10 mg four times daily or haloperidol 1 mg every four hours as needed will relieve nausea in most (Hanks et al. 2001; Laugsand et al. 2011). Analgesia and side effects should be evaluated 12 to 24 hours after initiating opioids. Although corticosteroids may lead to analgesic effects in certain specific instances, in advanced cancer patients coadministration of corticosteroids and opioids does not reduce opioid consumption (Mercadante et al. 2007). However, they seem to reduce the intensities of some opioid-induced adverse effects (especially gastrointestinal symptoms), and a transient improvement in the patient's general condition may be seen (Mercadante et al. 2007).

If pain persists despite starting ATC morphine, the rescue doses are added to the ATC dose and the total opioid daily dose is increased by 30% to 50%. Adding the rescue doses only to the ATC dose will not relieve pain, since the patient has already had this dose over the previous 24 hours (Walsh et al. 2004). Rescue doses for incident pain should not be added to the ATC dose. For example, if the patient has received 100mg of sustained-release morphine twice daily as well as 4 doses of 20mg of oral morphine for breakthrough pain (280mg over 24 hours) and still has persistent chronic, severe pain, the dose should be titrated to 200mg twice daily and the rescue dose adjusted to 30mg every two to four hours as needed. If chronic pain is controlled but incident pain severe the breakthrough opioid dose should be titrated 50 to 100% but not added to the ATC dose. In general, 10% to 20% of the total daily dose should be available every two to four hours as needed for breakthrough pain (Mercadante et al. 2010).End-of-dose failure, like nonincident breakthrough pain, is a sign of an ineffective ATC dose, and the ATC dose will need to be adjusted in a similar fashion. End-of-dose failure can also be managed by shortening the interval (8 hours rather than 12 hours for sustained-release morphine, 48 hours rather than 72 hours for transdermal fentanyl) or by increasing the dose by 50% and maintaining the dosing interval. Those with end-of-dose failure on immediate-release morphine should receive a 50% increase in the opioid dose, rather than a shortening of the interval (Walsh et al. 2004). The plasma half-life of morphine is two to three hours, and steady state is reached in five half-lives; hence, ATC doses should not be adjusted more than once daily and sustained release morphine every 48 hours. Increasing the ATC dose prior to reaching a steady state risks delayed opioid toxicity. If pain persists during the interval, the breakthrough dose is increased (50% if pain is only partially relieved by the rescue dose, 100% if there is no relief) (Hanks et al. 2001; Walsh et al. 2004).Taking frequent rescue doses of fentanyl (> six days) can result in delayed opioid toxicity. Dosing intervals should be four hours apart as a minimum (Fine 2010).

Pain Poorly Responsive to Opioids

Cancer pain generally responds in a predictable way to opioids. However, a small percentage (20%) of patients do not respond well to morphine, mainly due to the onset of dose-limiting toxicity (hallucinations, myoclonus, confusion, intractable nausea, and vomiting) (Hanks et al. 2001) before analgesia occurs. Certain pains are less responsive to opioids (neuropathic pain, colic, and tenemus).Opioid poorly responsive pain is defined as inadequately relieved pain by doses that cause intolerable side effects. Morphine and other opioids have wide

Table 6.1 Nonopioid/Adjuvant Analgesics

Medication	Dose	Interval
NSAIDS		
Ibuprofen	400–800 mg	3–4 times/day
Naproxen	250–500 mg	3 times/day
Ketorolac	10–45 mg	3–4 times/day
Corticosteroids		
Prednisone	10–20 mg	3–4 times/day
Dexamethasone	2–8 mg	8 am and noon
Antidepressants		
Amitriptyline	10–150 mg	at night
Nortriptyline	10–150 mg	at night
Duloxetine	60–120 mg	daily
Venlafaxine	150–225 mg	daily
Anticonvulsants		
Gabapentin	100–800 mg	3-4 times/day
Pregabalin	75–150 mg	twice daily
Valproic acid	500–1000 mg	twice daily
Topical anesthetic		
Lidoderm patch 5%	one patch	one daily

individual variations in pharmacological efficacy and tolerability and hence the therapeutic index (dose at which side effects occur versus the dose at which analgesia is experienced) is different for each individual and for each opioid. Differences in pharmacodynamics are related to the various μ receptor isotypes, receptor G protein interactions, beta-arrestin-2 receptor interactions, receptor desensitization, endocytosis, and resensitization (Davis and Pasternak 2005). Management of poorly responsive pain involves (1) switching or rotation of opioids; (2) opioid dose reduction (usually by 30%) with the addition of an adjuvant analgesic (Table 6.1); (3) opioid route conversion (usually to intrathecal or epidural infusions); and (4) surgery or radiation, which hopefully will reduce pain and allow for dose reduction (Hanks and Forbes 1997; Hanks et al. 2001; Walsh et al. 2004; Mercadante and Caraceni 2011; Bennett 2011; Kurita et al. 2011).

Common Dosing Errors

Common opioid dosing errors can be divided into (1) errors in strategy (lack of prescribing to pain pattern); (2) errors in titration (failure to match opioid dose to pain intensity); and (3) errors in route conversion or opioid rotation. Dosing errors occur in 27 to 70% of those prescribed opioids (Shaheen et al. 2010; Denison Davies et al. 2011). Potential lethal errors occur in 6% (Denison Davies 2011). Specific common errors are prescribing as-needed opioids only for continuous pain and not providing rescue doses for breakthrough pain with ATC medication (Shaheen et al. 2010; Denison Davies et al. 2011).Other common errors are incorrect dosing interval and using two long acting opioids simultaneously. Prescribing long-acting opioids for incident pain leads to opioid toxicity due to a carryover effect. Physicians (in our experience 15% to 20%) commonly prescribe multiple opioids due to the misconception that potent opioids have limitations in analgesic response related to dose (a dose "ceiling") or that by using two or more opioids in modest doses, better pain relief will occur which is safer and better than titrating one opioid (Kochhar et al. 2003; Davis et al. 2005; Shaheen et al. 2010). The use of multiple opioids has not been shown to improve pain relief but potentially increases the risk of drug interactions, dosing errors, and threatens compliance. If opioid-related side effects occur, all opioids are suspect and must be discontinued.

Additional problems include (1) physician use of adjuvant analgesics sparingly and often prescribing ineffective opioid rescue doses (<25% of the hourly dose); (2) titrating doses without regard to the baseline dose (increasing morphine from 100mg every 12 hours to 120mg every 12 hours); and (3) changing opioid dose, route, or timing while simultaneously adding an adjuvant analgesic. Only one change should be made at a time (Kochhar et al. 2003; Shaheen et al. 2010).The same opioid dose may be used when converting from oral to parenteral routes in opioids with high hepatic first pass clearance (Denison Davies et al. 2011).

Pain Management: Nonopioid and Adjuvant Analgesics

The term *nonopioid analgesic* is conventionally applied to acetaminophen and all nonsteroidal anti-inflammatory drugs (NSAIDs). The term *adjuvant analgesic* refers to any drug that has a primary indication other than pain but is known to be analgesic in specific circumstances (Bennett 2011). Both categories of analgesics are fundamental to the "analgesic ladder" approach to cancer pain management.Classes of adjuvant analgesics include antiepileptics (gabapentin, pregabalin), antidepressants (tricylic antidepressants, selective norepinephrine, serotonin reuptake inhibitors) and sodium channel blockers (lidocaine, bupivicaine).Adjuvants are used to improve pain control, limit opioid dose escalation, or allow opioid dose reduction and maintain analgesia ("opioid sparing").

Analgesic Strategies for Bone Pain

Radiation therapy is usually considered when bone pain is focal and poorly controlled with an opioid or is associated with impending fracture.A substantial degree of pain relief is experienced by 60 to 90% and total relief in 40%.Benefits are seen 10 to 14 days after beginning radiation in 70% (Delank et al. 2011). Multifocal bone pain that has been refractory to opioid therapy may benefit from co-administration of an NSAID, corticosteroid, or gabapentin. Adjuvant analgesics that may be useful for this indication include bisphosphonate compounds (Ernst et al. 1992; Hortobagyi et al. 1996), calcitonin (Serdengecti et al. 1986; Roth and Kolaric 1986), and bone-seeking radionuclides (e.g., strontium-89, Samarium-153) (Porter et al. 1993; Serafini et al. 1998; Falkmer et al. 2003; Smith et al. 2004). There have been no comparative trials of these adjuvant analgesics for bone pain; the selection of one over another is usually based on convenience, patient preference, and clinical indicators.Surgery, kyphoplasty, radiofrequency, ablation, and stereotactic radiation surgery may improve pain and opioid responses in sites that have previously been radiated (Delank et al. 2011; Qian et al. 2011).

Analgesic Strategies for Neuropathic Pain

Neuropathic pain is a consequence of insult to the nervous system.Patients with neuropathic pain have mechanical or thermal hyperalgesia, mechanical or thermal allodynia, or hyperpathia. Mechanisms initiating neuropathic pain include ectopic excitability, peripheral sensitization via upregulation of ion channels, phenotypic switch, central sensitization, decreased brain stem inhibition on dorsal lamina, structural reorganization, or increased facilitation via rostral ventromedial medulla (Scholz and Woolf 2002). Neuropathic pain is less responsive to opioids.Clinicians need to titrate opioids to higher doses and use adjuvant analgesics in order to achieve adequate analgesia. It may be useful to combine opioids with several adjuvant analgesics (e.g., antiepileptic drugs, antidepressants) or to utilize neuromodulation or destruction techniques.

Questionnaires developed to evaluate neuropathic pain include (1) the Neuropathic Pain Scale, which assesses different qualities of neuropathic pain and hence phenotype pain;this questionnaire is sensitive to changes in pain and can be used to follow treatment response (Galer and Jensen 1997; Lynch et al. 2003; Jensen et al. 2005) and (2) the Neuropathic Pain Symptom Inventory, consisting of 12 self-report items which the patient rates on a scale of 0 to 10 (Bouhassira et al. 2004).

Other questionnaires less sensitive to pain phenotype are (1) the Leeds Assessment of Neuropathic Symptoms and Signs (LANSS), consisting of five self-report items and two examiner-assessed sensory testing items (Bennett 2001), as well as the newer S-LANSS, which is a self-report version of the LANSS (Bennett et al. 2005); (2) the Neuropathic Pain Questionnaire (NPQ) (Krause and Backonja 2003), consisting of 12 items rated by patients, or its short form (NPQ-SF), with three of these items (Backonja and Krause 2003); and (3) the DN4, a clinician-administered tool with 10 items based on history and physical examination (Bouhassira et al. 2005).

The European Federation of Neurological Societies has published guidelines on neuropathic pain assessment (Cruccu et al. 2004). Multiple guidelines on the pharmacologic treatment of neuropathic pain have been published (Attal et al. 2006; Dworkin et al. 2007; Moulin et al. 2007). Recent reviews have updated the evidence (Vadalouca et al. 2012; Dworkin et al. 2010; Finnerup et al. 2010.

Medications that provide level A evidence for efficacy in the treatment of neuropathic pain include tricylic antidepressants, gabapentin, pregabalin, and opioids (Attal et al. 2006). Several guidelines suggest that opioids should not be used as first-line agents to treat neuropathic pain (Attal et al. 2006; Dworkin et al. 2010).In the consensus statement of the Canadian Pain Society, the recommended first-line agents to treat neuropathic pain are tricylic antidepressants and antiepileptic drugs (e.g., gabapentin, pregabalin). Second-line agents included serotonin–noradrenaline reuptake inhibitors (SNRIs) and topical lidocaine. In recent updates, both SNRIs and lidocaine are first line adjuvant analgesics (Dworkin et al. 2010).Opioids were included as second or third-line agents (Moulin et al. 2007; Dworkin et al. 2010). Others suggest that first-line medications for the treatment of neuropathic pain should include gabapentin (this was before pregabalin was clinically available), a 5% lidocaine patch, opioid analgesics, tramadol hydrochloride, or tricylic antidepressants (Dworkin et al. 2003). Opioids may be used more frequently in cancer-related neuropathic pain because neuropathic pain is frequently accompanied by nociceptive pain, which requires an opioid for analgesia.Combinations of an opioid plus a gabapentinoid are superior to single agents but are associated with higher risk of side effects (Dworkin et al. 2010).

Morphine sulfate is titrated for neuropathic pain beginning with 5 to 15 mg orally every four hours as needed. After one or two days, the total daily dosage is converted to a long-acting opioid analgesic, with continuation of a short-acting opioid as needed for breakthrough pain.Two dosing schemas have been used when combining an opioid with a gabapentinoid.Either the opioid or the gabapentinoid is titrated while the adjuvant or opioid dose in maintained respectively. Both the opioid and adjuvant analgesic should not be titrated simultaneously.

Pain Management: Nonpharmacologic Approaches

A small proportion of cancer patients will be unable to attain adequate analgesia from optimally administered pharmacotherapy. A large number of nonpharmacologic approaches may be considered when this occurs (Table 6.2). These approaches are reviewed elsewhere (Jacox et al. 1994; American Society of Anesthesiologists 1996; Portenoy 2000; Berger et al. 2002; Bruera and Portenoy 2003; Doyle et al. 2004; Delank et al. 2011) and may be broadly categorized. Interventional techniques include injection therapies (ethanol), neural blockade (e.g., celiac plexus block for painful pancreatic cancer), and implant therapies (spinal cord stimulation or neuraxial infusion) and ablative procedures (thermal or cryoablation). Another group of invasive approaches, neurosurgical therapies, involve surgical interruption of afferent neural pathways. With the advent of nondestructive procedures such as neuraxial analgesia, these procedures are now rarely performed.Acupuncture can be effective in relieving pain. Psychological therapies and cognitive-behaviour approaches range from education to mind-body therapies such as imagery, yoga, and hypnosis biofeedback. There are numerous psychotherapeutic approaches. Rehabilitative approaches

Table 6.2 Nonpharmacologic Interventions for Cancer Pain

Approach	Type	Examples
Interventional	Neural blockade	Celiac Plexus block
	Cordotomy and other lesions in brain	
	or spinal cord; neurolysis of peripheral nerve or root	
	Neuraxial infusion	Intraspinal infusion (ITDD)
	Intraventricular infusion of opioids	
Neuromodulation	Superficial	Transcutaneous electrical nerve stimulation, counterirritation
	Invasive	
		Spinal cord stimulation
		Peripheral nerve stimulation
		Deep brain stimulation
Physiatric	Orthoses/prostheses	Spinal or limb bracing techniques
	Physical/occupational	
	Therapeutic exercise therapy	Myofascial release techniques
	Modalities—Heat or cold	
Psychologic, other	Cognitive	Relaxation techniques, distraction, hypnosis
Psychoeducational		Individual and group therapy, family therapy
Complementary	Manual techniques ("hands-on" and "hands-off" strategies)	Therapeutic massage Acupuncture
	Pharmacologic	Herbal treatment

Adapted with permission (Portenoy, 2007)

include therapeutic exercise, occupational therapy, and the use of various modalities such as heat, cold, ultrasound, and topical stimulation. Finally, complementary modalities include a very broad array of treatments, some of which (therapeutic massage, a number of movement therapies, some nutritional interventions) are mainstream (Portenoy 2007).

Conclusion

Opioids are the analgesics of choice for moderate to severe cancer pain. When properly used, opioids control 80% of cancer pain. By prescribing the right dose of the right drug at the right time, one optimizes the relief of cancer pain. Patients who continue to have suboptimal analgesia benefit from adjuvant analgesics, interventional, and psychotherapeutic approaches.

Acknowledgment

The author would like to thank Michele Wells and Pam Gamier for their technical skills in preparing this manuscript.

References

American Pain Society. *Principles of Analgesic Use in the Treatment of Acute Pain and Cancer Pain.* 5th ed. Skokie, IL: American Pain Society, 2003.

American Society of Anesthesiologists' Task Force on Pain Management, Cancer Pain Section. Practice guidelines for cancer pain management. *Anesthesiology.* 1996;84(5):1243–1257.

Anborgh PH, Mutrie JC, Tuck AB, et al. Role of the metastasis-promoting protein osteopontin in the tumour microenvironment. *J Cell Mol Med.* 2010; 14(8):2037–2044.

Attal N, Cruccu G, Haanpää M, et al. EFNS guidelines on pharmacological treatment of neuropathic pain. *Eur J Neurol.* 2006;13(11):1153–1169.

Backonja MM, Krause SJ. Neuropathic pain questionnaire-short form. *Clin J Pain.* 2003;19(5):315–316.

Bennett MI. Effectiveness of antiepileptic or antidepressant drugs when added to opioids for cancer pain: systematic review. *Palliat Med.* 2011;25(5):553–559.

Bennett M. The LANSS Pain Scale: the Leeds Assessment of Neuropathic Symptoms and Signs. *Pain.* 2001;92(1-2):147–157.

Bennett MI, Graham J. Schmidt-Hansen M, et al. Prescribing strong opioids for pain in adult palliative care: summary of NICE guidance. *BMJ.* 2012;344:e2806.

Bennett MI, Smith BH, Torrance N, et al. The S-LANSS score for identifying pain of predominantly neuropathic origin: validation for use in clinical and postal research. *J Pain.* 2005;6(3):149–158.

Berger A, Portenoy RK, Weisman DE, eds. *Principles and Practice of Palliative Care and Supportive Oncology.* 2nd ed. Philadelphia: Lippincott, 2002.

Bouhassira D, Attal N, Alchaar H, et al. Comparison of pain syndromes associated with nervous or somatic lesions and development of a new neuropathic pain diagnostic questionnaire (DN4). *Pain.* 2005;114(1–2):29–36.

Bouhassira D, Attal N, Fermanian J, et al. Development and validation of the Neuropathic Pain Symptom Inventory. *Pain.* 2004;108(3):248–469.

Bruera EB, Portenoy RK (Eds.). *Cancer Pain.* London: Churchill Livingstone, 2003.

Burris HA 3rd, Moore MJ, Andersen J, et al. Improvements in survival and clinical benefit with gemcitabine as first-line therapy for patients with advanced pancreas cancer: a randomized trial. *J Clin Oncol.* 1997;15(6):2403–2413.

Caraceni A, Hanks G, Kaasa S, et al. Use of opioid analgesics in the treatment of cancer pain: evidence-based recommendations from the EPAC. *Lancet Oncol.* 2012;13(2):358–368.

Caraceni A, Pigni A, Brunelli C. Is oral morphine still the first choice opioid for moderate to severe cancer pain?A systematic review within the European Palliative Care Research Collaborative guidelines project.*Palliative Med* 2011; 25(5):402–409.

Cruccu G, Anand P, Attal N, et al. EFNS guidelines on neuropathic pain assessment. *Eur J Neurol.* 2004;11(3):153–162.

Davis MP, Weismann DE, Arnold RM. Opioid dose titration for severe cancer pain: a systematic evidence-based review. *J Palliat Med.* 2004;7(3):462–468.

Davis MP, Walsh D, Lagman R, et al. Controversies in pharmacotherapy of pain management. *Lancet Oncol.* 2005;6(9):696–704.

Davis M, Pasternak G. Opioid receptors and opioid pharmacodynamics. In Davis M, Glare P, Hardy J, eds. *Opioids in Cancer Pain.* New York: Oxford University Press, 2005.

Delank KS, Wendtner C, Eich HT, et al. The treatment of spinal metastases. *Deutsches Arzteblatt* 2011;108(5):71–80.

Denison Davies E, Schneider D, Child S, et al. A prevalence study of errors in opioid prescribing in a large teaching hospital. *Int J Clin Pract.* 2011;65(9):923–929.

Doyle D, Hanks GW, Cherny N, et al. (eds.): *Oxford Textbook of Palliative Medicine*, 3rd ed. Oxford: Oxford University Press, 2004.

Dworkin RH, Backonja M, Rowbotham MC, et al. Advances in neuropathic pain: diagnosis, mechanisms, and treatment recommendations. *Arch Neurol.* 2003;60(11):1524–1534.

Dworkin RH, O'Connor AB, Audette J. et al. Recommendations for the pharmacological management of neuropathic pain: an overview and literature update. *Mayo Clin Proc.* 2010;85(3 Suppl):S3–S14.

Dworkin RH, O'Connor AB, Backonja M, et al. Pharmacologic management of neuropathic pain: evidence-based recommendations. *Pain.* 2007;132(3):237–251.

Ernst DS, MacDonald RN, Paterson AH, et al. A double-blind, crossover trial of intravenous clodronate in metastatic bone pain. *J Pain Symptom Manage.* 1992;7(1):4–11.

Ernst DS, Tannock IF, Winquist EW, et al. Randomized, double-blind, controlled trial of mitoxantrone/prednisone and clodronate versus mitoxantrone/prednisone and placebo in patients with hormone-refractory prostate cancer and pain. *J Clin Oncol.* 2003;21(17):3335–3342.

Falkmer U, Jarhult J, Wersall P, et al. A systematic overview of radiation therapy effects in skeletal metastases. *Acta Oncol.* 2003;42(5–6):620–633.

Farrar JT, Young JP Jr, LaMoreaux, et al. Clinical importance of changes in chronic pain intensity measured on an 11-point numerical pain rating scale. *Pain.* 2001;94(2):149–158.

Fine PG, Narayana A, Passik S. Treatment of breakthrough pain with fentanyl buccal treatment in opioid tolerant patients with chronic pain: appropriate patient selection and management. *Pain Med* 2010;11(7):1024–1036.

Finnerup NB, Sindrup SH, Jensen TS. The evidence of pharmacological treatment of neuropathic pain. *Pain.* 2010;150(3):573–581.

Grond S, Zech D, Schug SA, et al. Validation of World Health Organization guidelines for cancer pain relief during the last days and hours of life. *J Pain Symptom Manage.* 1991;6(7):411–412.

Galer BS, Jensen MP. Development and preliminary validation of a pain measure specific to neuropathic pain: the Neuropathic Pain Scale. *Neurology.* 1997;48(2):332–338.

Grond S, Radbruch L, Meuser T, et al. Assessment and treatment of neuropathic cancer pain following WHO guidelines. *Pain.* 1999;79:15–20.

Hanks GW, Forbes K. Opioid responsiveness. *Acta Anaesthesiol Scand*. 1997;41(1 Pt 2):154–158.

Hanks GW, Conno F, Cherny N, et al. Morphine and alternative opioids in cancer pain: the EAPC recommendations. *Br J Cancer*. 2001;84(5):587–593.

Higginson IJ, Hearn J. A multicenter evaluation of cancer pain control by palliative care teams. *J Pain Symptom Manage*. 1997;14(1):29–35.

Hortobagyi GN, Theriault RL, Porter L, et al. Efficacy of pamidronate in reducing skeletal complications in patients with breast cancer and lytic bone metastases. *N Engl J Med*. 1996;335(24):1785–1791.

Indelicato RA, Portenoy RK. Opioid rotation in the management of refractory cancer pain. *J Clin Oncol*. 2002;20(1):348–352.

Inturrisi CE. Clinical pharmacology of opioids for pain. *Clin J Pain*. 2002;18(4 Suppl):S3–S13.

Jacox A, Carr DB, Payne R, et al. *Management of Cancer Pain*. AHCPR Publication No. 94–0592: Clinical Practice Guideline No. 9. Rockville, MD: US Department of Health and Human Services, Public Health Service, March 1994.

Jensen MP, Dworkin RH, Gammaitoni AR, et al. Assessment of pain quality in chronic neuropathic and nociceptive pain clinical trials with the Neuropathic Pain Scale. *J Pain*. 2005;6(9):98–106.

Jimenez-Andrade JM, Mantyh WG, Bloom AP, et al. Bone cancer pain. *Annals NY Acad Sci*. 2010;1198:173–181.

Jin SJ, Jung JY, Noh MH, et al. The population pharmacokinetics of fentanyl in patients undergoing living-donor liver transplantation. *Clin Pharmacol Ther*. 2011;90(3):423–431.

Klepstad P, Kaasa S, Borchgrevink PC. Starting step III opioids for moderate to severe pain in cancer patients: dose titration: a systematic review. *Palliat Med* .2011:25(5):424–430.

Kochhar R, Legrand SB, Walsh D, et al. Opioids in cancer pain: common dosing errors. *Oncology (Williston Park)*. 2003;17(4):571–575.

Krause SJ, Backonja MM. Development of a neuropathic pain questionnaire. *Clin J Pain*. 2003;19(5):306–314.

Kurita GP, Kaasa S, Sjøgren P; European Palliative Care research Collaborative (EPCRC). Spinal opioids in adult patients with cancer pain: a systematic review: a European Palliative Care research Collaborative (EPCRC) opioid guidelines project. *Palliat Med*. 2011;25(5):560–577.

Laird BJA, Walley J, Murray GD, et al. Characterization of cancer-induced bone pain: an exploratory study. *Support Care Cancer*. 2011;19(9):1393–1401.

Larkin PJ, Sykes NP, Centerio C, et al. The management of constipation in palliative care: clinical practice recommendations. *Palliat Med*. 2008;22(7):796–807.

Laugsand EA, Kaasa S, Klepstad P. Management of opioid-induced nausea and vomiting in cancer patients: systematic review and evidence-based recommendations. *Palliat Med*. 2011;25(5):442–453.

Lipton A, Goessl C. Clinical development of anti-RANKL therapies for treatment and prevention of bone metastasis. *Bone*. 2011;48(1):96–99.

Luger NM, Sabino MA, Schwei MJ, et al. Efficacy of systematic morphine suggests a fundamental difference in the mechanisms that generate bone cancer vs inflammatory pain. *Pain*. 2002;99(3):397–406.

Lynch ME, Clark AJ, Sawynok J. Intravenous adenosine alleviates neuropathic pain: a double blind placebo controlled crossover trial using an enriched enrollment design. *Pain.* 2003;103(1–2):111–117.

Mercadante S, Caraceni A. Conversion ratios for opioid switching in the treatment of cancer pain: a systematic review. *Palliat Med.* 2011;25(5):504–515.

Mercadante S, Villari P, Ferrera P, et al. The use of opioids for breakthrough pain in acute palliative care unit by using doses proportional to opioid basal regimen. *Clin J Pain.* 2010;26(4):306–309.

Mercadante SL, Berchovich M, Casuccio A, et al. A prospective randomized study of corticosteroids as adjuvant drugs to opioids in advanced cancer patients. *Am J Hosp Palliat Care.* 2007;24(1):13–19.

Moulin DE, Clark AJ, Gilron I, et al. Pharmacological management of chronic neuropathic pain—consensus statement and guidelines from the Canadian Pain Society. *Pain Res Manag.* 2007;12(1):13–21.

Portenoy RK. Treatment of cancer pain. *Lancet* 2011;377(9784):2236–2247.

Portenoy RK. *Contemporary Diagnosis and Management of Pain in Oncologic and AIDS Patients.* 3rd ed. Newtown, PA: Handbooks in Health Care, 2000.

Portenoy RK. Supportive and palliative care. In Straus DJ, ed. *Educational Review Manual in Medical Oncology.* New York: Castle Connolly Graduate Medical Publishing, 2007; 361–408.

Porter AT, McEwan AJ, Powe JE, et al. Results of a randomized phase III trial to evaluate the efficacy of strontium-89 adjuvant to local field external beam irradiation in the management of endocrine-resistant metastatic prostate cancer. *Int J Radiat Oncol Biol Phys.* 1993;25(5):805–813.

Qian Z, Sun Z, Yang H, et al. Kyphoplasty for the treatment of malignant vertebral compression fractures caused by metastases.*J Clin Neurosci.* 2011;18(6):763–767.

Roth A, Kolarić K. Analgesic activity of calcitonin in patients with painful osteolytic metastases of breast cancer. Results of a controlled randomized study. *Oncology.* 1986;43(5):283–287.

Scholz J, Woolf CJ. Can we conquer pain? *Nat Neurosci.* 2002;5:1062–1067.

Serafini AN, Houston SJ, Resche I, et al. Palliation of pain associated with metastatic bone cancer using samarium-153 lexidronam: a double-blind placebo-controlled clinical trial. *J Clin Oncol.* 1998;16(4):1574–1581.

Serdengecti S, Serdengecti K, Derman U, et al. Salmon calcitonin in the treatment of bone metastases. *Int J Clin Pharmacol Res.* 1986;6(2):151–155.

Shaheen P, LeGrand SB, Walsh D, et al. Errors in opioid prescribing: a prospective survey in cancer pain. *J Pain Symptom Manage.* 2010;39(4):702–711.

Smith H, Navani A, Fishman SM. Radiopharmaceuticals for palliation of painful osseous metastases. *Am J Hosp Palliat Care.* 2004;21(4):303–313.

Stone P, Minton O. European Palliative Care Research collaborative pain guidelines. Central side-effects management: what is the evidence to support best practice in the management of sedation, cognitive impairment and myoclonus? *Palliat Med.* 2010;25(5):431–441.

Stuart-Harris R, Joel SP, McDonald P, et al. The pharmacokinetics of morphine and morphine glucuronide metabolites after subcutaneous bolus injection and subcutaneous infusion of morphine. *Br J Clin Pharmacol.* 2000;49(3):207–214.

Smith HS. Novel analgesic approaches to painful bone metastases. In Smith HS, ed. *Drugs for Pain.* Philadelphia: Hanley & Belfus, 2003.

The Ad Hoc Committee on Cancer Pain of the American Society of Clinical Oncology. Cancer pain assessment and treatment curriculum guidelines. *J Clin Oncol.* 1992;10(2):1976–1982.

Upton RN, Semple TJ, Macintyre PE. Pharmacokinetic optimisation of opioid treatment in acute pain therapy. *Clin Pharmacokinet.* 1997;33(3):225–244.

Vadalouca A, Raptis E, Moka E, et al. Pharmacological treatment of neuropathic cancer pain: a comprehensive review of the current literature. *Pain Pract.* 2012;12(3):219–251.

Walsh D. Pharmacological management of cancer pain. *Semin Oncol.* 2000;27(1):45–63.

Walsh D, Rivera N, Davis MP, et al. Strategies for pain management: Cleveland Clinic Foundation guidelines for opioid dosing for cancer pain. *Support Cancer Ther.* 2004;1(3):157–164.

Wasiak J, Clavisi O. Is subcutaneous or intramuscular naloxone as effective as intravenous naloxone in the treatment of life-threatening heroin overdose? *Med J Aust.* 2002;176(10):495.

Watson WA, Steele MT, Muelleman RL, et al. Opioid toxicity recurrence after an initial response to naloxone. *J Toxicol Clin Toxicol.* 1998;36(1–2):11–17.

World Health Organization (WHO). *Cancer Pain Relief, with a Guide to Opioid Availability.* 2nd ed. Geneva: World Health Organization, 1996.

Yoneda T, Hata K, Nakanishi M, et al. Involvement of acidic microenvironment in that pathophysiology of cancer-associated bone pain. *Bone.* 2011;48(1):100–105.

Zeppetella G. Opioids for the management of breakthrough cancer pain in adults: A systematic review undertaken as part of an EPCRC opioid guidelines project. *Palliat Med.* 2011;25(5):516–524.

Zech DF, Grond S, Lynch J, et al. Validation of World Health Organization Guidelines for cancer pain relief: a 10-year prospective study. *Pain.* 1995;63(1):65–76.

Chapter 7

Evidence for the Use of Long-Term Opioid Therapy in Persistent Noncancer Pain

Howard S. Smith, Gary McCleane, and Gary Thompson

Since 1871, the pendulum of "opiophobia" versus "opiophilia" has swung back and forth for health care providers. Times change, from periods marked by opiophobia when opioids are withheld from terminally ill cancer patients because of irrational fears of addiction, to others where opiophilia leads to increased opioid abuse and diversion along with an increase in the medical use of opioids for persistent noncancer pain. Recent times have seen a swing toward more extensive use of opioids. Opioid therapy for chronic pain was described as an "extension of the basic principles of good medical practice" in a consensus statement jointly published by the American Pain Society and the American Academy of Pain Medicine (American Academy of Pain Medicine 2004).

Practicing in the middle of the road by employing the appropriate use of opioids in the context of good medical practice, as well as focusing appropriate attention on the risk assessment and management of opioid abuse (being cognizant of potential abuse, addiction, and diversion), has become known as balance (WHO 2000; Zacny et al. 2003; DEA 2004).

The practice of pain medicine should be patient-centered, and guided by sound clinical judgment sculpted by evidence-based medicine, consensus guidelines, pragmatism, and clinical experience. Although it may be optimal for every patient with pain to be assessed and managed by an interdisciplinary dream team of experts including addiction medicine specialists, this is clearly not a realistic goal. Therefore, it is the authors' belief that the complexity of the issues surrounding the patient should dictate the involvement of different levels of health care professionals. For example, a simple, straightforward patient who has been classified as being at low risk for substance misuse can be managed by a primary care physician alone. However, the complex and difficult patient with multiple chemical dependency issues may best be followed by an interdisciplinary pain team and an addiction medicine specialist (see Figure 7.1).

Clinical Use of Opioids

Kalso and colleagues (2004) reviewed data from 1145 patients initially randomized in 15 placebo-controlled trials of potent opioids used in the treatment

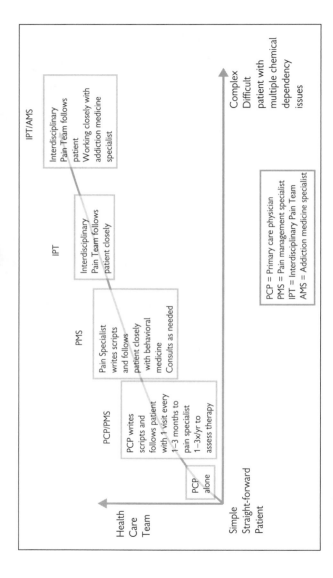

Figure 7.1. Suggested uses of health care team professional

of severe pain; these opioids were analyzed for efficacy and safety in chronic noncancer pain. Four studies tested intravenous opioids in neuropathic pain in a crossover design, with 115 of 120 patients completing the protocols. Using either pain intensity difference or pain relief as the endpoint, all four studies reported average pain relief of 30% to 60% with opioids. Eleven studies (1025 patients) compared oral opioids with placebo for four days to eight weeks. Six of the 15 trials that were included had an open-label follow-up of six to 24 months. The mean decrease in pain intensity in most studies was at least 30% with opioids and was comparable in neuropathic and musculoskeletal pain. Roughly 80% of patients noted at least one adverse effect. The most common adverse effects were constipation (41%), nausea (32%), and somnolence (29%). Only 44% of 388 patients on open-label treatments were still on opioids after therapy for between seven and 24 months. Adverse effects and lack of efficacy were two common reasons for discontinuation.

Watson and colleagues (2004) surveyed 102 patients with persistent noncancer pain in a neurologic practice followed by a neurologist every three months for a year or more (median eight years, range one to 22 years). They reported that approximately one-third of patients (34 out of 102) had a change in their pain status from either severe or moderate pain, as measured by (1) a 0-to-10 numerical rating scale as follows: mild=1–3, moderate=4–7, and severe=8–10; (2) a category scale (absent, mild, moderate, severe, very severe); and (3) the consideration of pain with movement. The investigators queried patients as to whether they were satisfied with pain relief despite adverse events. Forty-five patients (44%) answered that they were satisfied and 57 (56%) replied that they were not satisfied with their pain relief. However, of the 86 patients assessed for disability, 47 (54%) patients had significant improvement in their disability status on opioids. Also, there was some pain improvement on opioids in 78 (91%) of 102 patients, and these patients chose to continue opioid therapy for some analgesia despite adverse effects.

Eisenberg and colleagues (2005) examined 22 studies that met inclusion criteria and were classified as short-term (less than 24 hours; n=14) or intermediate-term (median 28 days; range of 8 to 56 days; n=8) trials. They reported contradictory results in the short-term trials. However, all 8 intermediate-term trials demonstrated opioid efficacy for spontaneous neuropathic pain. A fixed-effects model meta-analysis of 6 intermediate-term trials showed mean post-treatment scores of pain intensity (on a visual analogue scale) after opioids to be 14 units lower on a scale from 0 to 100 than after placebo (95% confidence interval [CI] -18 to -10; p 0.001). As the mean initial pain intensity recorded from 4 of the intermediate-term trials ranged from 46 to 69, this 14-point difference was considered to correspond to a 20% to 30% greater reduction with opioids than with placebo.

Analysis of data from large, randomized clinical trials has revealed that a roughly 30% reduction in pain intensity may be the threshold for patients to describe a reduction in chronic pain as meaningful (Farrar et al. 2000; Farrar et al. 2001). When the number needed to harm (NNH) is considered, the most common adverse event was nausea (NNH, 3.6; 95% CI, 2.9 to 4.8), followed by constipation (NNH, 4.6; 95% CI, 3.4 to 7.1), drowsiness (NNH, 5.3; 95% CI, 3.7 to 8.3), vomiting (NNH, 6.2; 95% CI, 4.6 to 11), and dizziness (NNH, 6.7; 95% CI,

4.8 to 10.0) (Eisenberg et al. 2005). Eisenberg and colleagues (2005) concluded that although short-term studies provide only equivocal evidence regarding the efficacy of opioids in reducing the intensity of neuropathic pain, intermediate-term studies demonstrate significant efficacy of opioids over placebo. They also concluded that further randomized, controlled trials are needed in order to establish the long-term efficacy of opioids for neuropathic pain, the safety of long-term opioids (including addiction potential), and the effects of opioids on quality of life.

In 2007, Martell and colleagues performed a systemic review and meta-analysis in which they concluded that opioids may be efficacious for short-term pain relief but that long-term efficacy (>16 weeks) was unclear (Martell et al. 2007). Additionally, Deshpande and colleagues performed a Cochrane Review of opioids for low-back pain that same year and found that tramadol was more effective than placebo for pain relief but the benefits of opioids for long-term management of chronic low back pain remain questionable and further research is needed (Deshpande et al. 2007).

Deyo and colleagues analyzed electronic data for 6 months before and after an index visit for back pain in a managed care plan (Deyo et al. 2011). They found that prescription of opioids was common among patients with back pain. The prevalence of psychologic distress, unhealthy lifestyles, and health care utilization increased incrementally with duration of use. Coprescribing sedative-hypnotics was common (Deyo et al. 2011).

Altman and Smith published that at least in certain subpopulations, the judicious use of chronic opioid therapy may reduce pain and improve function for osteoarthritis and chronic low back pain (Altman and Smith 2010).

Stein and colleagues (2010) have reviewed what they describe as the "second generation" of guidelines on the use of opioids in noncancer pain. They feel that the evidence base for long-term administration of opioids is weak, and that opioids have no superior effects compared with other analgesics. The recent Cochrane Database Systematic Review (2010) by Noble and colleagues examined 26 studies involving 4893 participants receiving oral, transdermal and/or intrathecal opioids. It is worth quoting their conclusion:

"Many patients discontinue long-term opioid therapy (especially oral opioids) due to adverse events or insufficient pain relief; however, weak evidence suggests that (many) patients who are able to continue (an opioid therapy on a) long-term (basis) experience clinically significant pain relief. Whether quality of life or functioning improves (as a result of chronic opioid therapy) is inconclusive."

Issues for Long-Term Opioid Treatment of Persistent Noncancer Pain

In spite of available guidelines for opioid therapy, controversies persist. Chronic opioid therapy (COT) for persistent noncancer pain is an area that is not easily amenable to algorithms and black-or-white doctrines; rather, this gray zone is better approached with individualized sound clinical judgment, balanced and appropriate approaches, and common sense. Many issues remain unresolved. For example, while Fine and colleagues (2010) have shown that buccal administration of fentanyl can produce useful alleviation of breakthrough pain in patients with chronic, noncancer pain, should immediate release opioids such as buccal fentanyl be used in those with noncancer pain, or should their use be limited to those with cancer pain? Do treatment agreements formed between the prescriber and the patient have any value when considering initiation of opioid therapy, and should patients receiving opioids for noncancer pain have routine urine monitoring to detect misuse of the opioid? The answer to these questions typifies the problems formulating an evidence-based approach. Starrels and colleagues (2010) examined 102 studies of which only 11 met inclusion criteria. They concluded that the evidence for patient agreements and urine testing was weak.

Additionally, the particular practice and its environment may influence these decisions in the minds of some clinicians. For example, some clinicians feel that a lower degree or intensity of unscheduled pill counts, urine drug testing, and other COT monitoring efforts should be used for a cancer pain or palliative medicine clinic than for a chronic noncancer pain clinic. Although opioid misuse clearly exists in cancer pain or palliative medicine clinics, the incidence is significantly lower than in chronic noncancer pain clinics (perhaps at least in part due to the higher average age of the patients being treated in cancer pain/palliative medicine clinics).

So the issues that remain when considering long term opioid therapy are whether effectiveness of the opioid is likely to be as good as or better than with other analgesics, whether the risk of adverse events with opioid use justifies their prescription, and what type of ongoing assessment of therapy is instituted.

Therefore, COT should optimally be undertaken in conjunction with the following:

1. Appropriate interdisciplinary medical care and documentation,
2. Other appropriate pharmacologic approaches,
3. Any appropriate physical medicine approaches,
4. Any appropriate behavioural medicine approaches,
5. Attention to comorbidities,
6. Establishment of an appropriate clinician–patient relationship, and
7. Appropriate monitoring and follow-up.

References

Altman RD, Smith HS. Opioid therapy for osteoarthritis and chronic low back pain. *Postgrad Med.* 2010;122(6):87–97.

American Academy of Pain Medicine, American Pain Society. The use of opioids for the treatment of chronic pain. Pain Consultants of Atlanta Web site. www.painmd.org/productpub/statements/pdfs/opioids.pdf. Accessed August 4, 2004.

Eisenberg E, McNicol ED, Carr DB. Efficacy and safety of opioid agonists in the treatment of neuropathic pain of nonmalignant origin: systematic review and meta-analysis trials. *JAMA.* 2005;293(24):3043–3052.

Deshpande A, Furlan A, Mailis-Gagnon A, et al. Opioids for chronic low-back pain. *Cochrane Database Syst Rev.* 2007;(3): DOI: 10.1002/14651858. CD004959.

Deyo RA, Smith DH, Johnson ED, et al. Opioids for back pain patients: primary care prescribing patterns and use of services. *J Am Board Fam Med.* 2011;24(6):7217–727.

Farrar JT, Portenoy RK, Berlin JA, et al. Defining the clinically important difference in pain outcome measures. *Pain.* 2000;88(3):287–294.

Farrar JT, Young JP Jr, LaMoreaux L, et al. Clinical importance of changes in chronic pain intensity measured on an 11-point numerical pain rating scale. *Pain.* 2001;94(2):149–158.

Fine PG, Messina J, Xie F, Rathmell J. Long-term safety and tolerability of fentanyl buccal tablet treatment of breakthrough pain in opioid-tolerant patients with chronic pain: an 18 month study. *J Pain Symptom Manage* 2010;40(5):747–760.

Kalso E, Edwards JE, Moore RA, et al. Opioids in chronic non-cancer pain: a systematic review of efficacy and safety. *Pain.* 2004;112(3):372–380.

Martell BA, O'Connor PG, Kerns RD, et al. Systemic review: opioid treatment for chronic back pain: prevalence, efficacy, and association with addiction. *Ann Intern Med.* 2007;146(2)116–127.

Noble, M, Treadwell J, Tregear S et al. Long-term opioid management for chronic noncancer pain. *Cochrane Database Syst Rev* 2010;1:DOI: 10.1002/14651858. CD006605.

Starrels J, Becker W, Alford D, Kapoor A, Williams A, Turner B. Systematic review: treatment agreements and urine drug testing to reduce opioid misuse in patients with chronic pain. *Ann Intern Med* 2010;152(11):712– 720.

Stein C, Reinecke H, Sorgatz H. Opioid use in chronic noncancer pain: guidelines revisited. *Curr Opin Anaesthesiol* 2010;23(5):598–601.

US Drug Enforcement Administration (DEA). Joint statement from 21 health organizations and the Drug Enforcement Administration. Promoting pain relief and preventing abuse of pain medications: a critical balancing act. Biomedical Computing Group, University of Wisconsin Medical School Web site. www.medsch.wisc.edu/Consensus2.pdf. Accessed August 4, 2004.

Watson CP, Watt-Watson JH, Chipman ML. Chronic noncancer pain and the long term utility of opioids. *Pain Res Manage.* 2004;9(1):19–24.

World Health Organization (WHO). Achieving Balance in National Opioids Control Policy: Guidelines for Assessment. Geneva: WHO, 2000.

Zacny J, Bigelow G, Compton P, et al. College on Problems of Drug Dependence taskforce on prescription opioid non-medical use and abuse: position statement. *Drug Alcohol Depend.* 2003;69(3):215–232.

Chapter 8

Pre-Opioid Prescribing Period

Howard S. Smith

As noted in the previous chapter, the use of opioids for the management of persistent noncancer pain (PNCP) remains controversial, and many issues surround the use of chronic opioid therapy (COT) for this type of pain. Overall, the use of COT in patients with PNCP may provide many with significant analgesia and minimal side effects for many years. However, the use of COT in other patients may result in a less favorable outcome. Therefore, when making the decision to prescribe opioids for this type of pain, the following factors should be kept in mind:

- COT may not be optimal for all patients.
- COT does not provide good or excellent analgesia in all patients.
- COT is not devoid of side effects.
- COT should be monitored in an effort to assess efficacy, function, side effects, and aberrant drug behavior.
- COT can be successfully withdrawn in selected patients who may do better without opioids.
- The prescription of COT for PNCP is an art that may be used alone or in conjunction with other therapeutic options. COT is not typically used as a first-line agent for patients with PNCP who have not tried previous treatments (McCleane and Smith 2007).

A practical method for classifying issues surrounding COT (although artificial and not precise) is to categorize issues into three phases, similar to the three phases of delivering an anesthetic (i.e., induction, maintenance, and emergence). In COT, these phases might be identified as initiation (i.e., determining whether to use COT), maintenance (i.e., interassessment period), and reassessment (i.e., increasing the dose, continuing the same dose, decreasing the dose, or tapering off the dose). This chapter focuses primarily on the initiation phase of COT, referred to as the pre-opioid prescribing period, but it is also relevant to the maintenance and reassessment phases.

The Pre-Opioid Prescribing Period

The pre-opioid prescribing period (POPP) is the period during which the physician determines whether opioids should be prescribed and, if the decision to prescribe such an agent is made, which (if any) necessary controls are to be put in place prior to initiating therapy. Activities that surround the initiation phase (and in some cases the maintenance phase) include discussions with the patient and other relevant parties (e.g., the patient's family or other health care providers), assessments, and documentation. The following are other specific activities associated with this period:

- Obtaining and documenting informed consent (see chapter 11),
- Executing opioid contracts or treatment agreements (see chapter 11),
- Executing goal-directed therapy agreements (see below),
- Evaluating the potential for substance abuse with one or more of many available screening tools (see chapter 10),
- Performing a urine drug test (see chapter 13),
- Performing a psychological assessment (this may be an informal assessment by the provider), and
- Developing a sense of the doctor–patient relationship.

Evaluating Patient Factors

Whether to initiate COT for PNCP must be determined on a case-by-case basis, as must the timing of initiation. The various factors of which the clinician should be cognizant and that could potentially enter into the health care provider's decision-making process may include the patient's age, prognosis, documentation of diagnosis, previous treatments, willingness to be involved in treatment (e.g., to be a participant), willingness to change (e.g., behavior), pain duration and intensity, history of substance use and mental health issues, patient and clinician goals, and the particular physician–patient relationship.

The clinician must have a reasonable, dynamic picture of the intensity of the patient's pain, as well as its impact on the social (e.g., family, relationships, recreational activities), emotional (e.g., mood) and functional (e.g., physical functioning, activities of daily living, occupational issues, etc.) domains before initiating opioid therapy. It is also vital that the clinician continue to evaluate the patient's status in each of these domains. If the patient does not improve or begins to deteriorate during COT, it may be appropriate at some point to change to a different opioid, to taper the medication slowly to a lower dose, or to discontinue COT completely and attempt an alternative treatment.

Although there may not be any specific need for psychological/psychiatric evaluations or psychological testing prior to the initiation of COT with every patient, the clinician should know the patient and have an established provider–patient relationship before initiating COT for PNCP.

Establishing Realistic Expectations for Long-Term Opioid Therapy

Quality of life has been defined as "the extent to which our hopes and ambitions are matched by experience" (Ruta et al. 1994). To improve a patient's quality of life via medical care would be to narrow the gap between a patient's hopes and expectations and what actually happens (Ruta et al. 1994). In efforts to produce optimal outcomes, expectations should match reality (or at least be in the same ballpark).

Therefore, it is important to discuss goals/expectations of COT before instituting treatment. If the patient's goal is to be pain free but the prescriber's goal is to provide analgesia sufficient for the patient to return to work, then both the patient and the prescriber will most likely be dissatisfied with COT. In order to set reasonable goals and expectations, the prescriber should spend time and effort attempting to obtain a comprehensive picture of the patient's baseline quality of life, pain intensity and impact on life, distress level, level of physical functioning, and social and emotional state and functioning. In some selected cases it may be appropriate to ask the physical medicine and rehabilitation department to perform a functional-capacity evaluation on a particular patient in order to document baseline physical function (especially if the goal is to increase physical function). Also, informed consent for COT and risk management plans/monitoring should be discussed, as well as the consequences of not adhering to the agreements/plans.

Goal-Directed Therapy Agreements

Perhaps one of the most important principles in initiating and maintaining COT for PNCP is to know where you are and where you are going. Goal-directed therapy agreements (GDTA) may be helpful in initiating COT for PNCP (Smith 2005). Clinicians are sometimes faced with patients for whom opioid therapy was initiated without clearly defined endpoints in efforts to achieve analgesia. This may cause a patient to continue experiencing severe pain despite taking relatively high doses of opioids. In efforts to clarify patient and clinician expectations and to make expected treatment outcomes more finite and concrete, the use of some form of GDTA may be useful. As with opioid treatment agreements, a GDTA is not necessarily advocated for all patients or all practices; it is merely suggested in situations where the clinician deems such a measure appropriate.

GDTAs should be tailored to each individual patient, should be clear and concise, should set goals that can reasonably be attained by the patient over a finite period, and optimally should be agreed upon by both patient and clinician. Examples may include increasing daily ambulation by a defined amount, increasing social/recreational activities by a defined amount, and so on. By utilizing GDTAs before instituting opioid therapy, clinicians can establish defined criteria to be met in order for opioid therapy to continue. In this manner, patients may be expected to reach certain reasonably attainable functional goals (which may have to be documented by a physical or behavioral therapist) in order to continue opioid therapy. The specifically defined goals should be clearly stated in the GDTA. It would seem optimal to institute the GDTA prior to instituting opioid therapy. The GDTA is essentially felt to be a contractually agreed-upon, realistic target of translational analgesia (Smith 2005) that should be realized in order maintain opioid treatment.

It is hoped that with the use of GDTAs in certain patients or circumstances, a closer match between the expectations of both patient and clinician can be established (Smith 2005).

Initiating a Trial of Opioid Therapy: Does It Seem Appropriate at This Point in Time?

When considering chronic opioid therapy (COT) for chronic noncancer pain, it has been proposed that it is prudent to contemplate four questions which may be useful and influence medical decision making (Fine and Portenoy 2007).

1. What is the conventional practice?
2. Are there reasonable alternatives to COT?
3. What is the risk of adverse events?
4. Is the patient likely to be a responsible drug-taker?

In an attempt to help primary care prescribers address the first and determine if their opioid prescribing habits were usual/average or a bit out of range of average (beyond 2 standard deviations of the mean opioid dose), Passik and Kirsh published a schematic meant to help primary care physicians with opioid prescribing which they refer to as opioid prescribing "in and out of the box" (Passik and Kirsh 2008). Again, like the first of the four questions discussed above, Passik and Kirsh highlight conventional practice as one of their factors contributing to opioid prescribing in or out of the box. Smith and colleagues (Smith et al. 2009) also noted that pain or painful conditions that are poorly responsive to opioids may predispose to opioid prescribing out of the box (Smith et al. 2009). Smith also noted that there may be many factors which may contribute to variation in opioid responsiveness (Smith 2009; Smith 2008), however, it does appear that certain pains or painful conditions may be better suited for opioid than others. Cancer and perioperative pain were "in the box," and pain syndromes in which opioid use is considered controversial was "out of the box."

Smith developed a schematic (Figure 8.1) in efforts to shed light on which medical conditions may be considered more conventional or traditional to be treated with chronic opioid therapy (prescribing in the box) and for which conditions that COT may be considered less conventional, or prescribing out of the box (Smith 2012a). This schematic is based purely on one factor (e.g., medical condition) and is entirely biased. Obviously many other factors need to be taken into account when considering whether to initiate chronic opioid therapy for a particular patient.

Another factor that may be considered in the pre-opioid period is when the optimal point is in time to initiate a trial of opioid therapy. This is clearly a clinical judgment, however, less experienced clinicians may prefer to have data such as a tool to help them support their judgment. The Readiness for Chronic Opioid Therapy (RCOT) is a brief arbitrary seven item clinician-generated tool in which the prescriber scores each item and then summates the scores to get a total RCOT score (Smith and Kirsh 2009). A high total RCOT score is considered probably ready for COT. If a patient has a low total RCOT score it may be considered uncertain if they are ready for COT and it may be reasonable to wait before initiating COT, or perhaps to send the patient to a pain specialist for an opinion on their suitability for COT at this point in time (Smith and Kirsh 2009) (Figure 8.2).

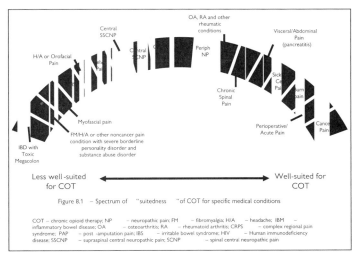

Figure 8.1 – Spectrum of "suitedness" of COT for specific medical conditions

COT – chronic opioid therapy; NP – neuropathic pain; FM – fibromyalgia; H/A – headache; IBM – inflammatory bowel disease; OA – osteoarthritis; RA – rheumatoid arthritis; CRPS – complex regional pain syndrome; PAP – post-amputation pain; IBS – irritable bowel syndrome; HIV – Human immunodeficiency disease; SSCNP – supraspinal central neuropathic pain; SCNP – spinal central neuropathic pain

Figure 8.1 Spectrum of "suitedness" of COT for specific medical conditions

						Points
1.	Age		○ < 40	○ 40-65	○ < 65	
	Point value	*0*	*1*	*2*	*3*	
2.	Prognosis/Life Expectancy	○ Normal	○ < 10 yrs	○ < 5 yrs	○ < 1 yr	
	Point value	*0*	*1*	*2*	*3*	
3.	Certainty of Diagnosis	○ Very Unsure	○ Possible Uncertain	○ Probable	○ Definite with objective	
	Point value	*0*	*1*	*2*	*3*	
4.	Previous Pain Treatments/Management	○ None	○ Little	○ Moderate	○ Extensive	
	Point value	*0*	*2*	*4*	*6*	
5.	Realistic Patient Expectations of COT	○ None	○ Little	○ Intermediate	○ Good	
	Point value	*0*	*1*	*2*	*3*	
6.	Willingness to be actively involved in their treatment or willingness to change aspects of their life/behavior	○ Not at all	○ Little	○ Intermediate	○ Lot	
	Point value	*0*	*1*	*2*	*3*	
7.	Provider/Prescriber/ Patient Relationship	○ None	○ Little	○ Intermediate	○ Good	
	Point value	*0*	*1*	*2*	*3*	
					TOTAL SCORE	

(Smith and Kirsh, 2009)

Figure 8.2 Readiness for Chronic Opioid Therapy (RCOT)

Certain clinicians want to have an idea of how opioid responsive the patient's pain may be before initiating COT. Although definitive evidence does not exist, neuropathic pain tends to be less responsive to opioids than non-neuropathic pain (i.e., nociceptive pain) (Smith 2012b). Also, it is likely that overall, peripheral neuropathic pain is somewhat more responsive to opioids than central neuropathic pain (Smith and Meek 2011). Additionally, within central neuropathic pain it appears likely that supraspinal central neuropathic pain is less responsive to the analgesic effects of opioids than spinal central neuropathic pain (Smith and Meek 2011; Smith 2011b) (see Figure 5f.1 in chapter 5f).

References

Fine PG, Portenoy RK. *A Clinical Guide to Opioid Analgesia*. New York, NY: Vendrome Group, LLC; 2007.

McCleane G, Smith HS. Opioids for persistent noncancer pain. *Med Clin North Am.* 2007;91(2):177–197.

Passik SD, Kirsh KL. The interface between pain and drug abuse and the evolution of strategies to optimize pain management while minimizing drug abuse. *Exp Clin Psychopharmacol.* 2008;16(5):400–404.

Ruta DA, Garratt AM, Leng M, et al. A new approach to the measurement of quality of life. The Patient-Generated Index. *Med Care.* 1994;32(11):1109–1126.

Smith HS. Editorial: Conventional Practice for Medical Conditions for Chronic Opioid Therapy. *Pain Physician.* 2012; 15(3S):ES1–ES7.

Smith HS. Opioids and Neuropathic Pain. *Pain Physician.* 2012; 15(3S):ES93–ES110.

Smith HS, Meek PD. Pain responsiveness to opioids: central versus peripheral neuropathic pain. *J Opioid Manag.* 2011;7(5):391–400.

Smith HS. Opioid Metabolism. *Mayo Clin Proc.* 2009;84(7):613–624.

Smith HS, Kirsh KL. Identifying and managing the risk of opioid misuse. *Therapy.* 2009;6(5):685–693.

Smith HS, Kirsh KL, Passik SD. Chronic opioid therapy issues associated with opioid abuse potential. *J Opioid Manag.* 2009;5(5):287–300.

Smith HS. Variations in opioid responsiveness. *Pain Physician.* 2008;11(2):237–248.

Smith HS. Goal-directed therapy agreements. *J Cancer Pain Symptom Palliat.* 2005;1(3):11–13.

Chapter 9

Identifying Patients at Risk for Pain Medication Misuse

Lynn R. Webster and Howard S. Smith

Chronic pain impairs the lives of millions of people, and this issue must be addressed. Indeed, issues with pain are the number one reason that patients go to see their physicians. However, increased recognition of the problem has been somewhat tempered by the growth of prescription drug abuse and resulting regulatory attention in the form of a risk evaluation mitigation strategy (REMS) to be instituted by the US Food and Drug Administration (FDA). Because of this, some clinicians, particularly nonspecialists, shy away from using high doses of opioids or even from using this modality at all in the treatment of chronic pain. Despite these fears and concerns, practicing pain specialists and research indicate certain patients benefit from the use of opioid therapy to treat chronic pain. In large part, the success of opioid therapy depends on proper patient selection and assessment and ongoing monitoring as therapy progresses.

All clinicians who treat pain with opioids should assess for patient characteristics that may increase a patient's risk of the potential for abuse. To that end, several tools are now available to help clinicians identify patients who may be at risk for prescription drug abuse or misuse.

General Screening Tools

Two brief screening tools for alcohol and drug abuse are the CAGE-AID (Brown and Rounds 1995) and the TICS (Two Item Conjoint Screen) (Brown et al. 1997). Neither of these tools, however, is opioid-specific. Indeed, there is some question as to whether asking patients on opioids whether they take opioids in the morning (some do as part of a prescribed regimen) or feel guilty about opioid use (some do without cause) truly gathers useful information. The CAGE was originally designed as a screening tool for alcoholism but has been adapted to include drugs (CAGE-AID). The CAGE-AID asks patients if they have done any of the following things, with two or more positive responses suggesting a need for further evaluation:

1. Have you tried to cut down or change your pattern of drinking or drug abuse?
2. Have you been annoyed or angry by others' concern about your drinking or drug use?

3. Have you felt guilty about the consequences of your drinking or drug use?
4. Have you had a drink or used a drug in the morning ("eye-opener") to decrease hangover or withdrawal symptoms?

Two affirmative answers constitute a positive screen, but even one affirmative answer suggests a need for caution.

The TICS uses two questions to help clinicians determine the level of risk:

1. In the last year, have you ever drunk or used drugs more than you meant to?
2. Have you felt you wanted or needed to cut down on your drinking or drug abuse in the last year?

A conjoint screening tool like the TICS offers advantages in that it saves time and encourages a patient to answer more honestly than when answering separate questions. However, a disadvantage is that a person who abuses only alcohol may answer negatively, wishing to avoid the appearance of illicit or prescription drug use.

Brief and easy to administer, instruments like the CAGE-AID and TICS may be useful to busy practitioners who otherwise might be tempted to skip the process of substance-abuse assessment. However, it is important to note that in addition to lacking specificity to opioids, these two tools are designed to detect current and lifetime substance abuse, not to assess the risk of future abuse.

Opioid-Specific Screening Tools

Several opioid-specific screening tools have recently been developed for risk assessment in patients with chronic pain. The following tools are endorsed in an opioid treatment guideline from the American Pain Society (APS) and the American Academy of Pain Medicine (AAPM) as having good content, face, and construct validity, although in need of further research to demonstrate clinical utility and predictive validity (Chou et al. 2009a):

- The Screener and Opioid Assessment for Patients with Pain (SOAPP) Version 1
- The revised SOAPP (SOAPP-R)
- The Diagnosis, Intractability, Risk, Efficacy (DIRE) Score
- The Opioid Risk Tool (ORT)

A comparison study found the SOAPP Version 1 to be the most sensitive at detecting high-risk patients, followed by the ORT then the DIRE (Moore et al. 2009). The DIRE is clinician administered, while the others are patient self-report questionnaires. Most tools have been designed to help clinicians decide what level of monitoring would be best for particular patients on chronic opioid therapy (COT). In contrast, the DIRE classifies patients as appropriate or inappropriate candidates for opioid therapy.

More information about those assessments and others follow. These tools are useful as a complement to clinical assessment and as research tools.

Prescription Drug Use Questionnaire (PDUQ)

The PDUQ was created to identify subjects who are likely to be nonaddicted, substance abusing, or substance dependent (Compton et al. 1998). The PDUQ involves a 42-item interview in which data are obtained regarding the patient's pain condition, opioid use, social and family history, and any psychiatric issues. Three items from the PDUQ appear to be especially important in identifying serious concerns of opioid dependency; these include assessing a patient's tendency toward the following:

- Increasing analgesic dose or frequency,
- Having a preferred route of administration, and
- Considering oneself addicted.

Unfavorable features include the fact that the semistructured interview instrument takes significant time to administer, and is geared for use by trained mental health professionals. A 31-item, patient-administered version (PDUQp) was introduced in 2008 (Compton et al. 2008).

Pain Medication Questionnaire (PMQ)

The PMQ is a 26-item self-report questionnaire that uses neutral language to encourage candid responses from patients (Holmes et al. 2006). The tool was designed to identify patients who require more in-depth assessment of risk for opioid misuse. This tool was designed for use in a busy clinic environment.

Diagnosis, Intractability, Risk, Efficacy (DIRE) Score

The DIRE is a seven-item physician-administered tool that is designed to predict which chronic non–cancer pain patients will achieve effective analgesia and be compliant with COT (Belgrade et al. 2006). The total score can range from seven through 21, with a score of ≤13 suggesting an unsuitable candidate and a score of ≥14 suggesting a good candidate for COT.

Screening Instrument for Substance Abuse Potential (SISAP)

The SISAP is a five-item screen that assesses the risk of opioid abuse based on a patient's alcohol consumption, marijuana use, tobacco use, and age (Table 9.1) (Coambs and Jarry 1996). Based on telephone responses in a Canadian epidemiological survey of alcohol and drug use, the SISAP has not been prospectively validated in a chronic pain population; however, it has proven to be useful. This tool is designed to be used when the clinician has sufficient collateral data to confirm the patient's responses.

Screener and Opioid Assessment for Patients with Pain (SOAPP)

The SOAPP is a survey tool used to predict opioid abuse and is available as a 5-, 14-, or 24-item questionnaire (Butler et al. 2004; Akbik et al. 2006). The SOAPP Version 1 contains 14 items found to be most predictive of later aberrant drug-related behaviors and examines predictors that include history of substance misuse, sexual abuse, mood disorders, and legal problems (Butler et

Table 9.1 Screening Instrument for Substance Abuse Potential (SISAP)

Questions

1. If you drink alcohol, how many drinks do you have on a typical day?
2. How many drinks do you have in a typical week?
3. Have you used marijuana or hashish in the past year?
4. Have you ever smoked cigarettes?
5. What is your age?

Interpretation of SISAP results

1. Use caution when prescribing opioids for the following patients:
2. Men who exceed 4 drinks per day or 16 drinks per week.
3. Women who exceed 3 drinks per day or 12 drinks per week.
4. A patient who admits to marijuana or hashish use in the past year.
5. A patient under 40 who smokes.

(Coambs and Jarry, 1996)

Table 9.2 Screener and Opioid Assessment for Patients with Pain (Short Form)

Please answer the question below using the following scale:

0 = never; 1 = seldom; 2 = sometimes; 3 = often; 4 = very often

1. How often do you have mood swings?
2. How often do you smoke a cigarette within an hour after you wake up?
3. How often have you taken medication other than the way it was prescribed?
4. How often have you used illegal drugs (e.g. marijuana, cocaine) in the past 5 years?
5. How often, in your lifetime, have you had legal problems or been arrested?

al. 2004). The cross-validated, 24-item SOAPP-R was created to contain subtler and more socially acceptable questions than the original SOAPP (Butler et al. 2008). Although the 5-item questionnaire (SOAPP V LO-SF [5Q]) is less sensitive and specific than the longer versions, it may suffice for use in primary care settings (Table 9.2). Each version of the SOAPP uses a cut-off score above which the subject may have a potentially increased risk of opioid abuse, thus requiring additional or special precautions and/or monitoring when treated with LTOT (e.g., giving prescriptions at intervals [days or weeks] with limited tablets). While the SOAPP is intended to predict which patients may exhibit drug-related aberrant behaviors in the future, the Current Opioid Misuse Measure (COMM) is designed to help clinicians identify current opioid patients who are exhibiting abuse behaviors (Butler et al. 2007). Information on the SOAPP and the COMM is available at www.painedu.org/index.asp.

The categories include diagnosis, intractability, efficacy, and risk categories (psychological, chemical health, reliability, and social support). Scores for each question are rated from one to three, with higher scores indicating a greater

Table 9.3 SOAPP-R Item (In the Past 30 Days . . .)

1. How often do you have mood swings?
2. How often have you felt a need for higher doses of medication to treat your pain?
3. How often have you felt impatient with your doctors?
4. How often have you felt that things are just too overwhelming that you can't handle them?
5. How often is there tension in the home?
6. How often have you counted pain pills to see how many are remaining?
7. How often have you been concerned that people will judge you for taking pain medication?
8. How often do you feel bored?
9. How often have you taken more pain medication than you were supposed to?
10. How often have you worried about being left alone?
11. How often have you felt a craving for medication?
12. How often have others expressed concern over your use of medication?
13. How often have any of your close friends had a problem with alcohol or drugs?
14. How often have others told you that you had a bad temper?
15. How often have you felt consumed by the need to get pain medication?
16. How often have you run out of pain medication early?
17. How often have others kept you from getting what you deserve?
18. How often, in your lifetime, have you had legal problems or been arrested?
19. How often have you attended an AA or NA meeting?
20. How often have you been in an argument that was so out of control that someone got hurt?
21. How often have you been sexually abused?
22. How often have others suggested that you have a drug or alcohol problem?
23. How often have you had to borrow pain medications from your family or friends?
24. How often have you been treated for an alcohol or drug problem?

Total SOAPP-R Score

(From Butler et al., 2008)

possibility of successful opioid therapy. When the tool was tested on a relatively small sample of 61 patients for nearly 38 months, the results indicated high sensitivity and specificity for predicting both compliance and efficacy (Belgrade et al. 2006). In addition to the relatively small sample, the study was retrospective, and the patients had a variety of pain conditions. To be effective, the physician needs to take a good history and maintain a good relationship with the patient, so this tool might have better utility when used on an ongoing fashion.

Butler and colleagues presented a revised version of the SOAPP-R that is empirically derived with good reliability and validity but less susceptible to overt deception than the original SOAPP version 1 (Butler et al. 2008) (Table 9.3). A score of 18 or higher will identify 80% of those who actually turn out to be at high risk. For this score, the negative predictive value is .87, which means that the vast majority of patients who have a negative SOAPP-R are likely at low risk. Finally, the positive likelihood ratio suggests that a positive SOAPP-R score (at a cutoff of 18) is 2.5 times as likely to come from someone who is actually at high risk (Butler et al. 2008). The SOAPP-R was devised as a self-report measure to predict future misuse behavior based on past behavior and/or cognition (Butler et al. 2008). The SOAPP-R provides clinicians with the ability to help identifying patients who may have greater difficulty modulating their own medical use of opioids and who may require extra monitoring and management, versus patients who are at low risk for addiction or misuse and may require less monitoring (Butler et al. 2008).

Opioid Risk Tool (ORT)

The ORT is a five-question self-administered assessment that can be completed in less than 5 minutes and used on a patient's initial visit (Table 9.4) (Webster and Webster 2005). Personal and family history of substance abuse, age, history of preadolescent sexual abuse, and the presence of depression, attention-deficit disorder (ADD), obsessive-compulsive disorder (OCD), bipolar disorder, and schizophrenia are assessed. The ORT accurately predicted which patients

Table 9.4 **The Opioid Risk Tool (ORT)**			
Item	Mark each box that applies	Item score if female	Item score if male
1. Family History of Substance Abuse			
Alcohol	[ ]	1	3
Illegal Drugs	[ ]	2	3
Prescription Drugs	[ ]	4	4
2. Personal History of Substance Abuse			
Alcohol	[ ]	3	3
Illegal Drugs	[ ]	4	4
Prescription Drugs	[ ]	5	5
3. Age (mark box if 16–45)	[ ]	1	1
4. History of Preadolescent Sexual Abuse	[ ]	3	0
5. Psychological Disease			
Attention Deficit Disorder, Obsessive-Compulsive Disorder, Bipolar, Schizophrenia	[ ]	2	2
Depression	[ ]	1	1
Total ORT Score (sum of 1–5)			
Interpretation of ORT Score			
Low Risk (score of 0–3)			
Moderate Risk (score of 4–7)			
High Risk (score of 8 and above)			

(Webster et al, 2005)

were at the highest and the lowest risk for exhibiting aberrant, drug-related behaviors associated with abuse or addiction (Webster and Webster 2005).

Screening Tool for Addiction Risk (STAR)

The STAR is a 14-item self-administered questionnaire that is designed to identify patients who are at risk for substance abuse (Friedman et al. 2003). This tool is easy to use but, to date, has not been widely validated.

Drug Abuse Screening Test (DAST)

The Drug Abuse Screening Test (DAST) is a 28-item yes-or-no self-report questionnaire (Yudko et al. 2007). Traditionally a cut-off score of six is used to indicate drug abuse or dependence, but this score can be changed to accommodate the needs of different clinical settings. In addition to the full version, which might be too long for some clinics, several abbreviated versions of the DAST can be used, based on either 10 or 20 items. The full-length DAST has face validity and high test-retest reliability, with a correlation coefficient of 0.85, and good internal consistency, with Cronbach's alpha coefficients ranging from 0.92 to 0.94. It exhibits good sensitivity in ranges from 81% to 96%, and its specificity ranges from 71% to 94%. While there are positive aspects to the DAST, it should be noted that the test and retest are only separated by a few weeks, which might make the psychometrics look artificially better than they are. In addition, the tool is susceptible to deception, and it may not identify substance abusers who intentionally give false responses. Also, the measure has yet to undergo a major validation trial in pain patients. Finally, while it predicts substance abuse, it does not specifically explore aberrant behavior during pain treatment.

Other Diagnostic tools

Structured Clinical Interview for DSM Disorders (SCID)

Most screening tools are not designed to diagnose substance-use disorders. If patients demonstrate positive scores on abuse screening tools, they should be considered candidates for an additional step to diagnose whether an actual disorder is present. One such instrument is the SCID (Kranzler et al. 1996), a thorough assessment widely used in research centers and substance-abuse treatment facilities, where staff is specially trained to administer and score it.

Addiction Severity Index (ASI)

Another tool that is especially effective for evaluating the need for substance-abuse treatment is the ASI (McLellan et al. 1992), a 200-item, hour-long assessment of seven potential problem areas designed to be administered by a trained interviewer.

Severity of Opiate Dependence Questionnaire (SODQ)

The SODQ also is not an initial screen, but is meant to be used as an indicator of opiate dependence (Sutherland et al. 1986). It consists of five sections of multiple-choice questions addressing patterns of use, degree of withdrawal symptoms, and other signs of physical and psychological dependence.

More About Risk Factors

Assessments to measure the likelihood of opioid abuse or addiction look at well-supported risk factors already mentioned, including prior and family history of substance abuse, mental-health disorders, legal difficulties, and social environment conducive to drug abuse. Aside from preventing the misuse of pain medications, there is another reason to consistently assess risk in COT: Evidence shows that decedents whose deaths involved prescription drugs had high rates of psychiatric illness, substance abuse, and unemployment (Porucznik et al. 2011). Factors such as major depression, suicidal ideation, personality disorders, impulsivity, catastrophizing, and uncontrolled pain can serve as prelude to problematic opioid usage and can even prove fatal (Cheatle 2011; Passik and Lowery 2011). Screening may help prevent many types of opioid-related harm stemming from improper use.

Ongoing Screening and Risk Management

Passik and Weinreb (Passik and Weinreb 2000) discussed a useful mnemonic device for following the relevant domains of outcome for pain management. The "four As" (analgesia, activities of daily living, adverse events, and aberrant drug-taking behaviors) are clinical domains that reflect progress toward the larger goal of a full and rewarding life. A successful outcome in pain therapy must provide meaningful relief, but it does not end solely with the provision of pain control. Analgesia must make a true difference in the patient's life, and it must be accompanied by stabilization or improvement of psychosocial and physical functioning, manageable side effects (that do not compromise important areas of functioning), and acceptable drug-taking. The Numerical Opioid Side Effect (NOSE) assessment tool was designed specifically for the quantification of opioid-induced adverse effects (Smith 2005). Initially developed as a means for clinicians to monitor and document their patients' progress, the four As are not solely intended for the clinician's benefit. They are also useful for explaining the goals of therapy to patients and for helping them understand the larger goal of being treated in a pain management setting.

Pain Assessment and Documentation Tool

Passik and colleagues (Passik et al. 2004; Passik et al. 2005) introduced the Pain Assessment and Documentation Tool (PADT), which tracks the four As and helps to streamline the assessment of outcomes in the patient with chronic pain. The time for follow-up visits is short, leaving little time to address all the domains of the outcome of treatment, and to discuss how to intervene in and overcome problematic behaviors and build motivation. The principle reason for time limitations is financial; pain physicians often face trading off between financial survival and the desire to "do the right thing" for their patients, such as acting as an agent for positive change. It might take up to 30 minutes to address problematic behavior, but only 30 seconds to write a prescription. Pain clinicians face this dilemma daily and have to learn expedient ways to deal with complex matters or to delegate many of these tasks to other team members. Medication management can often monopolize all of the time the physician and patient spend together, so it was crucial that a tool be developed that could be brief while also comprehensive.

In practice, the PADT is a two-sided chart note that can be readily included in the patient's medical record. It was designed to be intuitive, pragmatic, and adaptable to clinical situations. In the field trial, it took clinicians between 10 and 20 minutes to complete the tool. The finalized PADT is substantially shorter and requires only a few minutes to complete. By addressing the need for documentation, the PADT can assist clinicians in meeting their obligations for ongoing assessment and documentation while maintaining therapies. Although the PADT is not intended to replace a progress note, it is well suited to complement existing documentation with a focused evaluation of outcomes that are clinically relevant and address the need for evidence of appropriate monitoring.

Current Opioid Misuse Measure (COMM)

In addition to the PADT, the Current Opioid Misuse Measure (COMM) was designed for those pain patients already on chronic opioid therapy (Butler et al. 2007). A total of 227 chronic noncancer pain patients were asked to complete a 40-item alpha version of the assessment and the Prescription Drug Use Questionnaire (PDUQ) and were also asked to submit a urine sample for toxicology screening. Physicians were also asked to document any aberrant behavior by patients. A follow-up study among 86 patients with a version that contained the 17 items in the alpha version that were found to adequately measure aberrant behavior indicated that the COMM was promising as an efficient way of assessing current aberrant behavior (Table 9.5). Further study is needed on this tool, but it holds promise as a way to assess current opioid misuse (Smith et al. 2009).

Data suggest that a cutoff score of 9 or higher may be a reasonably conservative choice for the COMM cutoff (Butler et al. 2007). Using a cutoff score of nine or higher, the positive predictive value was .66, while the negative predictive value was .95. The positive likelihood ratio was 3.48, and the negative likelihood ratio was .08 (Butler et al. 2007). These results suggest that the total for the 17 self-report items of the COMM appears to provide a good estimate of whether a patient is currently misusing or abusing their medications (Butler et al. 2007). Each question asks the relative frequency of a thought or behavior over the past 30 days from "0 = Never" to "4 = Very Often." Thus, instead of identifying character and personality traits based on past history, the COMM is mostly interested in current behaviors and cognition (Butler et al. 2007). The goal of the COMM is to identify those patients with chronic pain taking opioids who have indicators of current medication misuse (Butler et al. 2007).

Table 9.5 Assessing Aberrant Drug-Taking Behaviors

The Current Opioid Misuse and Measure (COMM) is a relatively brief, validated, and useful patient self-report instrument recently developed to track and measure the misuse of opioids in chronic pain populations over the course of opioid therapy.

17-Items of Current Opioid Misuse Measure (COMM)

1. How often have you had trouble with thinking clearly or had memory problems?

2. How often do people complain that you are not completing necessary tasks (i.e., doing things that need to be done, such as going to class, work, or appointments)?

3. How often have you had to go to someone other than your prescribing physician to get sufficient pain relief from your medications (i.e. another doctor, the emergency room)?

4. How often have you taken your medications differently from how they are prescribed?

5. How often have you seriously thought about hurting yourself?

6. How much of your time was spent thinking about opioid medications (having enough, taking them, dosing schedule, etc.)?

7. How often have you been in an argument?

8. How often have you had trouble controlling your anger (e.g., road rage, screaming, etc)?

9. How often have you needed to take pain medications belonging to someone else?

10. How often have you been worried about how you're handling your medications?

11. How often have others been worried about how you're handling your medications?

12. How often have you had to make an emergency phone call or show up at the clinic without an appointment?

13. How often have you gotten angry with people?

14. How often have you had to take more of your medication than prescribed?

15. How often have you borrowed pain medication from someone else?

16. How often have you used your pain medicine for symptoms other than for pain (e.g. to help you sleep, improve your mood, or relieve stress)?

17. How often have you had to visit the emergency room?

(Butler et al., 2007)

Addiction Behaviors Checklist (ABC)

Passik and colleagues (Passik et al. 2006) listed behaviors that are less indicative of addiction (e.g., hoarding medications, taking someone else's pain medication, aggressively requesting more drugs from the doctor) and behaviors that are more indicative of addiction (e.g., buying pain medication from a street dealer, stealing money to obtain drugs, selling prescription drugs). Wu and colleagues (Wu et al. 2006) have introduced the Addiction Behaviors Checklist (ABC), a brief (20-item) instrument designed to track behaviors characteristic of addiction related to opioids in chronic pain populations. The ABC items focus on observable behaviors noted during (11 items) and between (eight items) clinic visits, with one item classified as "other" (Wu et al. 2006). These researchers concluded that a cut-off score of three or greater on the ABC shows optimal sensitivity and specificity in helping to determine whether a patient is displaying inappropriate opioid use (Wu et al. 2006). Interrater reliability and concurrent validity data are presented, as well as a cut-off score for use in determining inappropriate medication use. Wu and colleagues concluded that the psychometric findings support the ABC as a viable assessment tool that can increase a provider's confidence in determinations of appropriate vs. inappropriate opioid use (Wu et al. 2006).

Evaluation of Tools to Screen or Monitor for Opioid Abuse Potential

Turk and colleagues performed a MEDLINE database search from 1966 to 2007, exploring the bibliographies from all retrieved articles, as well as articles available in the authors' files, and identified 6 published articles with 16,420 patients addressing clinician-based predictors of substance misuse of opioids. Additionally, they included 9 published studies with 11, 017 patients with chronic noncancer pain evaluating the predictive ability of clinical interviews and self-report measures for aberrant opioid behaviors in patients with chronic noncancer pain (Turk et al. 2008). The screening tools included the Screening Instrument for Substance Abuse Potential (SISAP) (Coambs and Jarry 1996), the Prescription Drug Use Questionnaire (PDUQ) (Compton et al. 1998), the Screening Tool for Addiction Risk (STAR) (Friedman et al. 2003), the Prescription Opioid Therapy Questionnaire (POTQ) (Michna et al. 2004), the Pain Medication Questionnaire (PMQ) (Adams et al. 2004), the Screener and Opioid Assessment for Patients with Pain (SOAPP) (Butler et al. 2004), the Opioid Risk Tool (ORT) (Webster and Webster 2005), the Addiction Behaviors Checklist (ABC) (Wu et al. 2006), and the Current Opioid Misuse Measure (COMM) (Butler et al. 2007). Of the nine instruments reviewed, only the SOAPP (Butler et al. 2004) and the COMM (Butler et al. 2007) assessed all of the psychometric and diagnostic domains outlined (Turk et al. 2008).

Two higher-quality derivation studies found that high scores on the Screener and Opioid Assessment for Patients with Pain (SOAPP) Version 1 and the Revised SOAPP (SOAPP-R) instruments weakly increased the likelihood for future aberrant drug-related behaviors (positive likelihood ratios [PLR], 2.90 [95% CI, 1.91 to 4.39] and 2.50 [95% CI, 1.93 to 3.24], respectively) (Chou et al. 2009b). Low scores on the SOAPP Version 1 moderately decreased the likelihood for aberrant drug-related behaviors (negative likelihood ratio [NLR], 0.13 [95% CI, 0.05 to 0.34]) and low scores on the SOAPP-R weakly decreased the likelihood (NLR, 0.29 [95% CI, 0.18 to 0.46]), but estimates are too imprecise to determine if there is a difference between these instruments (Chou et al. 2009b). One lower-quality study found that categorization as high risk using the Opioid Risk Tool strongly increased the likelihood for future aberrant drug-related behaviors (PLR, 14.3 [95% CI, 5.35 to 38.4]) and classification as low risk strongly decreased the likelihood (PLR, 0.08 [95% CI, 0.01 to 0.62]).

Nine studies evaluated monitoring instruments for identification of aberrant drug-related behaviors in patients on opioid therapy (Chou et al. 2009b). One higher-quality derivation study found higher scores on the Current Opioid Misuse Measure (COMM) weakly increased the likelihood of current aberrant drug-related behaviors (PLR, 2.77 [95% CI, 2.06 to 3.72]) and lower scores weakly decreased the likelihood (NLR, 0.35 [95% CI, 0.24 to 0.52]) (Chou et al. 2009b).

No reliable evidence exists on accuracy of urine drug screening, pill counts, or prescription drug monitoring programs; or clinical outcomes associated with different assessment or monitoring strategies (Chou et al. 2009b). However, these should still be considered useful clinically until definitive empirical evidence becomes available. Recommendations from the clinical guidelines for the use of chronic opioid therapy (COT) in chronic noncancer pain (opioid treatment guidelines) (Chou et al. 2009a) for monitoring included the following suggestions:

Clinicians should reassess patients on COT periodically and as warranted by changing circumstances. Monitoring should include documentation of pain intensity and level of functioning, assessments of progress toward achieving therapeutic goals, presence of adverse events, and adherence to prescribed therapies (strong recommendation, low quality evidence) (Chou et al. 2009a).

In patients on COT who are at high risk or who have engaged in aberrant drug-related behaviors, clinicians should periodically obtain urine drug screens or other information to confirm adherence to the COT plan of care (strong recommendation, low-quality evidence) (Chou et al. 2009a).

In patients on COT not at high risk and not known to have engaged in aberrant drug-related behaviors, clinicians should consider periodically obtaining urine drug screens or other information to confirm adherence to the COT plan of care (weak recommendation, low-quality evidence) (Chou et al. 2009a). Christo et al. have proposed an algorithm for urine drug testing (Christo et al. 2011).

Choice of Assessment

Many factors will determine the choice of assessment tool, including the clinician's expertise or access to specialists and the time available. Predictive tools are useful before treatment begins, and diagnostic tools can help detect a current pattern of abuse. Brief, self-administered instruments are usually best given the typical time limitations of a busy practice (Figure 9.1).

Once an assessment or set of questions is chosen, it should be routinely applied, and patients should be monitored for their response to COT. The purpose behind assessing patients is not to deny high-risk patients pain treatment but to ensure that all patients receive appropriate monitoring and clinical vigilance. The goal is an environment where opioids may be safely prescribed and consumed, resulting in better clinical outcomes and less abuse.

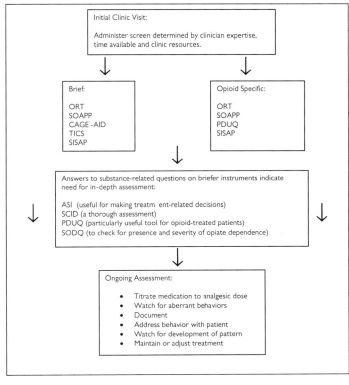

Figure 9.1 Protocol to Assess Patients for Risk of Opioid Abuse:

References

Adams LL, Gatchel RJ, Robinson RC, et al. Development of a self-report screening instrument for assessing potential opioid medication misuse in chronic pain patients. *J Pain Symptom Manage.* 2004;27(5):440–459.

Akbik H, Butler SF, Budman SH, et al. Validation and clinical application of the Screener and Opioid Assessment for Patients with Pain (SOAPP). *J Pain Symptom Manage.* 2006;32(3):287–293.

Belgrade MJ, Schamber CD, Lindgren BR. The DIRE score: predicting outcomes of opioid prescribing for chronic pain. *J Pain.* 2006;7(9):671–681.

Brown RL, Rounds LA. Conjoint screening questionnaires for alcohol and other drug abuse: criterion validity in a primary care practice. *Wisc Med J.* 1995;94(3):135–140.

Brown RL, Leonard T, Saunders LA, et al. A two-item screening test for alcohol and other drug problems. *J Fam Pract.* 1997;44(2):151–160.

Butler SF, Fernandez K, Benoit C, Budman SH, Jamison RN. Validation of the revised Screener and Opioid Assessment for Patients with Pain (SOAPP-R). *J Pain.* 2008;9(4):360–372.

Butler SF, Budman SH, Fernandez K, et al. Development and validation of the Current Opioid Misuse Measure. *Pain.* 2007;130(1–2):144–156.

Butler SF, Budman SH, Fernandez K, et al. Validation of a screener and opioid assessment measure for patients with chronic pain. *Pain.* 2004;112(1–2):65–75.

Cheatle MD. Depression, chronic pain, and suicide by overdose: on the edge. *Pain Med.* 2011;12(Suppl 2):S43–S48.

Chou R, Fanciullo GJ, Fine PG, et al. Clinical guidelines for the use of chronic opioid therapy in chronic noncancer pain. *J Pain.* 2009a;10(2):113–130.

Chou R, Fanciullo GJ, Fine PG, et al. Opioids for Chronic Noncancer Pain: Prediction and Identification of Aberrant Drug-Related Behaviors: A Review of the Evidence for an American Pain Society and American Academy of Pain Medicine Clinical Practice Guideline. *J Pain.* 2009b;10(2):131–146.

Christo PJ, Manchikanti L, Ruan X, et al. Urine drug testing in chronic pain. *Pain Physician.* 2011;14(2):123–143.

Coambs RB, Jarry JL. The SISAP: a new screening instrument for identifying potential opioid abusers in the management of chronic nonmalignant pain in general medical practice. *Pain Res Manage.* 1996;1(3):155–162.

Compton P, Darakjian J, Miotto K. Screening for addiction in patients with chronic pain and "problematic" substance use: evaluation of a pilot assessment tool. *J Pain Symptom Manage.* 1998;16(6):355–363.

Compton PA, Wu SM, Schieffer B, Pham Q, Naliboff BD. Introduction of a self-report version of the Prescription Drug Use Questionnaire and relationship to medication agreement noncompliance. *J Pain Symptom Manage.* 2008;36(4):383–395.

Friedman R, Li V, Mehrotra D. Treating pain patients at risk: evaluation of a screening tool in opioid-treated pain patients with and without addiction. *Pain Med.* 2003;4(2):182–185.

Holmes CP, Gatchel RJ, Adams LL, et al. An opioid screening instrument: long-term evaluation of the utility of the Pain Medication Questionnaire. *Pain Pract.* 2006;6(2):74–88.

Kranzler HR, Kadden RM, Babor TF, Tennen H, Rounsaville BJ. Validity of the SCID in substance abuse patients. *Addiction.* 1996;91(6):859–868.

McLellan AT, Kushner H, Metzger D, et al. The fifth edition of the Addiction Severity Index. *J Subst Abuse Treat.* 1992;9(3):199–213.

Michna E, Ross EL, Hynes WL, et al. Predicting aberrant drug behavior in patients treated for chronic pain: importance of abuse history. *J Pain Symptom Manage.* 2004;28(3):250–258.

Moore TM, Jones T, Browder JH, Daffron S, Passik SD. A comparison of common screening methods for predicting aberrant drug-related behavior among patients receiving opioids for chronic pain management. *Pain Med.* 2009;10(8):1426–1433.

Passik SD, Weinreb HJ. Managing chronic nonmalignant pain: overcoming obstacles to the use of opioids. *Adv Ther.* 2000;17(2):70–83.

Passik SD, Kirsh KL, Whitcomb LA, et al. A new tool to assess and document pain outcomes in chronic pain patients receiving opioid therapy. *Clin Ther.* 2004;26(4):552–561.

Chapter 10

Potential Documentation Tools in Long-Term Opioid Therapy

Howard S. Smith and Kenneth L. Kirsh

When opioids are used for long-term therapy, the clinician must be skilled in opioid prescribing, know the principles of addiction medicine, and be committed to performing and documenting a comprehensive assessment repeatedly over time. Inadequate assessment can lead to under-treatment, compromise the effectiveness of therapy, and prevent an appropriate response when problematic drug-related behaviors occur.

Domains of Interest for Ongoing Assessment

There are several domains of interest in patient assessment during chronic opioid therapy (COT) for those engaged in front-line practice. These include pain relief (i.e., are the medications or treatments leading to pain reduction?), functional outcomes (i.e., is the patient more engaged in life as a result of treatment?), side effects (i.e., how have the medications adversely affected the patient?), and drug-related behaviors (i.e., is the patient acting out in unusual or disturbing ways?). Ongoing assessment of these main domains not only improves pain outcomes for the patient, but protects your practice for those patients on an opioid regimen.

Passik and Weinreb (2000) have described a useful mnemonic for following the relevant domains of outcome in pain management. The so-called four As (analgesia, activities of daily living, adverse events, and aberrant drug-taking behaviors) are the clinical domains that reflect progress toward the larger goal of a full and rewarding life.

Analgesia. Although listed as the first A, analgesia should not necessarily be considered the most important outcome of pain management. An alternate measure is how much relief it takes for patients to feel that their lives are meaningfully changed, enabling them to work toward the attainment of their own goals.

Activities of Daily Living. The second A refers to quality-of-life issues and functionality. It is necessary for patients to understand that they must comply with all of their treatment recommendations in order to be able to return to work, leisure, and social activities in the minimum amount of time.

Adverse Events. Patients must also be made aware of the adverse side effects inherent in the use of opioids and other medications to treat pain. Side effects must be aggressively managed so that sedation and other side effects do not overshadow the potential benefits of drug therapy. The most common side effects of opioid analgesics are constipation, sedation, nausea and vomiting, dry mouth, respiratory depression, confusion, urinary retention, and itching.

Aberrant Drug-Taking Behaviors. Finally, patients must be educated about the parameters of acceptable drug-taking. Even an overall good outcome in every other domain might not constitute satisfactory treatment if the patient is exhibiting worrisome drug-related behaviors (i.e., engaging in unsanctioned dose escalation, visiting multiple providers for controlled substance prescriptions, etc.). Dispensing pain medicine in a highly structured fashion may become necessary for some patients who are in violation, or constantly on the fringes, of appropriate drug taking.

All four domains require vigilant assessment prior to initiation of therapy and throughout COT. Although there is considerable evidence supporting the use of COT for chronic pain, recent studies have suggested that COT in patients with chronic pain can fail to fulfil key outcome opioid-treatment goals in a notable proportion of patients (Eriksen et al. 2006; Ballantyne 2006). One explanation for the failure of COT in some patients may be the failure of clinicians to select the proper patients for this type of therapy. Conversely, there may be issues with patients being nonresponders to the particular opioid molecule chosen (Foster et al. 2007; Samer et al. 2010). Another explanation in some instances may be the failure of a clinician to provide ongoing and vigilant assessment of the four As. Although numerous tools have been developed for assisting with proper patient selection, as described in chapter 9, tools for ongoing assessment, while more limited, are available.

Documentation Tools for Assessing the Efficacy of Chronic Opioid Therapy

A consistent method of documentation can help busy clinicians to remember which of the domains should be assessed on any given visit. Moreover, oversight by regulatory agencies, state medical boards, and various peer-review groups includes examination of appropriate medical care as well as proper documentation. As the old axiom states, "If it isn't written, it didn't happen." In cases of COT for chronic pain, issues beyond typical office-visit charting deserve attention and documentation. Although no explicit requirements are spelled out as to the documentation of issues related to opioid therapy, the use of specific tools and instruments in the chart on some or all visits may boost both adherence to documentation expectations and the consistency of such documentation.

Unidimensional tools such as the numerical rating scale (i.e., "on a scale of 0 to 10, how would you rate your pain?") described in chapter 3 are useful for ongoing assessment of a patient's pain. However, analgesia is only one of the four domains of outcome for pain management, and clinicians must continually assess all four domains. It has been proposed that the use of various tools may provide adjunctive information and help clinicians to create a more complete picture regarding longitudinal trends of overall progress and functioning for their patients with chronic pain (Smith 2005b). Assessing individual outcomes during outpatient multidisciplinary chronic pain treatment is often an extremely challenging task, but fortunately a number of tools are now available to facilitate the ongoing assessment of patients on COT.

The Pain Assessment and Documentation Tool

The Pain Assessment and Documentation Tool (PADT) is a simple charting device based on the four As concept. It is designed to help clinicians focus on key outcomes and consistently document progress in pain management therapy over time (Passik et al. 2004, 2005). The PADT has several advantages in practice:

- It is a brief, two-sided chart note that can be readily included in the patient's medical record.
- It is intuitive, pragmatic, and adaptable to clinical situations.
- It takes between five and ten minutes to complete in its revised version.
- It helps clinicians meet their obligations for ongoing assessment and documentation.
- Although not intended to replace a progress note, it can complement existing documentation with a focused evaluation of outcomes that are clinically relevant, and it addresses the need for evidence of appropriate monitoring.

Numerical Opioid Side Effect Assessment Tool

The Numerical Opioid Side Effect (NOSE) assessment tool was designed specifically for the quantification of adverse effects (Smith 2005a) (see appendix 3). It is not uncommon for patients on COT to ask to discontinue therapy because of adverse effects, even if they have attained reasonable analgesia. Therefore, it is useful to assess opioid adverse effects in such a manner as to be able to follow trends as well as compare the patient's perceived intensity of the adverse effects versus the intensity of pain and/or other symptoms. The NOSE was designed in an effort to provide a tool that facilitates this goal. There are several benefits to the NOSE, including the following:

- It is self-administered and can be completed by the patient in minutes while waiting for an appointment.

- It is easy to interpret and provides clinicians with important information that could potentially affect therapeutic decisions.
- It can be entered into electronic databases or inserted into a hard-copy chart on each patient visit.
- It allows for legible, clear, and concise documentation of such information in outpatient records.

Treatment Outcomes in Pain Survey

The Treatment Outcomes in Pain Survey (TOPS) was specifically designed to assess and follow outcomes in the chronic pain population and has been described as an augmented Medical Outcomes Study Short Form 36-item questionnaire (SF-36) (Ware and Sherbourne 1992). The nine domains of TOPS are pain symptom, family/social disability, functional limitations, total pain experience, objective work disability, life control, solicitous responses, passive coping, and satisfaction with outcomes. Although TOPS is an extremely useful tool, it is time consuming; is based entirely on the patient's subjective responses, and requires that the clinician have access to a means of scoring, whether by a special computer program or by sending forms away. As a result, it may not be an ideal instrument to use in every pain clinic, and may not provide the clinician with an immediate answer as to how the patient is doing relative to previous visits (although it may have that potential with adequate time, scanning equipment, and computer software).

The Translational Analgesic Score

The Translational Analgesia Score (TAS) (see appendix 4) is a patient-generated tool that attempts to quantify the degree of translational analgesia (Smith 2005c), or improvements in physical, social, or emotional function realized by the patient as a result of improved analgesia (Smith 2005c). Improvements may be subtle and can include a range of daily-function activities or other signs (e.g., going out more with friends, doing laundry, showing improved mood, enjoying more rewarding relationships with family members). The TAS is simple, rapid, user-friendly, and suitable for use in busy pain clinics. The patient can complete the tool at each visit while in the waiting room, and the responses are averaged for an overall score, which is recorded in the chart. Patients should be encouraged to write down specific examples of things that they can now do or do frequently that they could not do or did rarely when their pain was less controlled. Alternatively, the patient's responses can be entered into a computerized record (with graphs of trends) if the pain clinic's medical records are electronic. At least one or two specific examples of translational analgesia should be documented on the bottom or reverse side of the TAS score sheet. Treatment decisions regarding escalation or tapering of opioids, changing agents, adding agents, obtaining consultations, and instituting physical or behavioral medicine techniques depend on the medical judgment of practitioners and should be based on a careful reevaluation of the patient, not on numbers. The concept of translational analgesia is not meant to imply that opioids should be tapered, weaned, and/or discontinued. If a patient has a very low TAS that remains essentially unchanged over time, the clinician should reevaluate the patient and consider a change in therapy. This could mean pursuing various therapeutic options including, perhaps, increasing the dose of opioids. The TAS may be helpful as an adjunctive documentation tool and still awaits rigorous validation.

The SAFE score

The SAFE score is a score generated by the health care provider and provides a multidimensional assessment of the outcome of opioid therapy (Smith et al. 2005). The goals of the SAFE score are to demonstrate that the clinician has routinely evaluated the efficacy of the treatment from multiple perspectives, to guide the clinician toward a broader view of treatment options beyond adjusting the medication regimen, and to provide adjunctive data in efforts to document the rationale for continuation, modification, or cessation of opioid therapy. It is a simple, practical tool that may have clinical utility, but it has not yet been rigorously validated. It is not intended to replace more elaborate patient-based assessment tools, but it may be useful as an adjunct to illuminate differences between patients' perceptions of how they are doing on opioid treatment versus the physician's view of the outcome. At each visit, the clinician numerically rates the patient's functioning and pain relief on a scale of one to five in four domains (social functioning, analgesia, physical functioning, and emotional functioning) (see Table 10.1). The ratings in each domain are combined to yield a SAFE score, which can range from four to 20. The green zone is a SAFE score of four to 12 and/or a decrease of two points in total score from baseline. With a score in the green zone, the patient is considered to be doing well, and the plan would be to continue with the current medication regimen or consider reducing the total dose of opioids. The yellow zone is a SAFE score of 13 to 16 and/or a rating of five in any category and/or an increase of two or more from baseline in the total score. With a score in the yellow zone, the patient should be monitored closely and reassessed frequently. The red zone is a SAFE score greater than or equal to 17. With a score in the red zone, a change in treatment would be warranted.

Example A&B illustrates a patient who underwent a treatment in which their pain actually became worse but they improved in various other domains and thus, the patient may potentially be satisfied with their overall status. This does not mean that clinicians would not attempt to further address the patient's pain in attempts to improve analgesia as well. Example C&D illustrates a patient who underwent a treatment in which their pain was improved somewhat, however, they deteriorated in other domains so that overall the patient may be dissatisfied with their overall status.

Table 10-1 Sample SAFE Form

Rating	Criterion				
	1	2	3	4	5
Social Marital, family, friends, leisure, recreational	supportive harmonious socializing engaged				conflictual discord isolated bored
Analgesia Intensity, frequency, duration	comfortable effective controlled				intolerable ineffective uncontrolled
Function Work, ADLs, home management, school, training, physical activity	independent active productive energetic				dependent unmotivated passive deconditioned
Emotional Cognitive, stress, attitude, mood, behavior, neuro-vegetative signs	clear relaxed optimistic upbeat composed				confused tense pessimistic depressed distressed
Total Total Score					

The patient's status in each of the four domains is rated as follows:

1 = Excellent

2 = Good

3 = Fair

4 = Borderline

5 = Poor

Tracking a Change in Status Using the SAFE Scoring Tool

Example A		Example B	
Social	5	Social	3
Analgesia	3	Analgesia	4
Function	5	Function	3
Emotional	5	Emotional	3
Red Zone "SAFE" score	18	Green Zone "SAFE" score	13
Example C		Example D	
Social	3	Social	4
Analgesia	3	Analgesia	2
Function	3	Function	4
Emotional	3	Emotional	5
Green Zone "SAFE" score	12	Yellow Zone "SAFE" score	15

Conclusion

Assessment and documentation are cornerstones for both protecting your practice and obtaining optimal patient outcomes in opioid therapy. There are a growing number of assessment tools designed to guide clinicians in the evaluation of important outcomes during opioid therapy and to provide a simple means of documenting patient care. They all may prove helpful in clinical management and offer mechanisms for documenting the types of practice standards that those in the regulatory and law enforcement communities seek to insure.

References

Ballantyne JC. Opioids for chronic nonterminal pain. *South Med J.* 2006; 99(11):1245–1255.

Butler SF, Budman SH, Fernandez K, et al. Validation of a screener and opioid assessment measure for patients with chronic pain. *Pain.* 2004;112(1–2):65–75.

Eriksen J, Sjogren P, Bruera E, et al. Critical issues on opioids in chronic non-cancer pain: an epidemiological study. *Pain.* 2006;125(1–2):172–179.

Foster A, Mobley E, Wang Z. Complicated pain management in a CYP450 2D6 poor metabolizer. *Pain Pract.* 2007;7(4):352–356.

Passik SD, Kirsh KL, Whitcomb LA, et al. A new tool to assess and document pain outcomes in chronic pain patients receiving opioid therapy. *Clin Ther.* 2004;26(4):552–561.

Passik SD, Kirsh KL, Whitcomb LA, et al. Monitoring outcomes during long-term opioid therapy for non-cancer pain: results with the pain assessment and documentation tool. *J Opioid Manag.* 2005;1(5):257–266.

Passik SD, Weinreb HJ. Managing chronic nonmalignant pain: overcoming obstacles to the use of opioids. *Adv Ther.* 2000;17(2):70–80.

Samer CF, Daali Y, Wagner M, et al. Genetic polymorphisms and drug interactions modulating CYP2D6 and CYP3A activities have a major effect on oxycodone –analgesic efficacy and safety. *Br J Pharmacol.* 2010;160(4):919–930.

Smith HS. The numerical opioid side effect (NOSE) assessment tool. *Journal of Cancer Pain & Symptom Palliation.* 2005a;1(3):75–79.

Smith HS. Perspectives in long-term therapy for persistent noncancer pain. *Journal of Cancer Pain & Symptom Palliation.* 2005b;1(4):31–32.

Smith HS. Translational analgesia and the Translational Analgesia Score (TAS). *Journal of Cancer Pain & Symptom Palliation.* 2005c;1(3):15–19.

Smith HS, Audette J, Witkower A. Playing it "SAFE." *Journal of Cancer Pain & Symptom Palliation.* 2005;1(1):3–10.

Ware JE Jr, Sherbourne CD. The MOS 36-item short-form health survey (SF-36). I. Conceptual framework and item selection. *Med Care.* 1992;30(6):473–483.

Chapter 11

Managing the Risk of Abuse, Addiction, and Diversion

Howard S. Smith

There is no single behavior that is pathognomonic of a substance use disorder, thus there is no foolproof instrument that can reliably assess the risk of opioid addiction (Gourlay and Heit 2006). As the prevalence of addiction in the general population is not insignificant, it seems prudent to utilize the 10 steps of universal precautions in patients receiving chronic opioid therapy (COT) (Gourlay et al. 2005). These are (1) reasonable attempts to make a diagnosis with an appropriate differential; (2) comprehensive patient assessment, including risk of addictive disorders; (3) informed consent; (4) treatment agreement; (5) pre- and postintervention assessment of pain level and function; (6) appropriate trial of opioid therapy "adjunctive" medications; (7) reassessment of pain score and level of function; (8) regular assessment of the four As of pain medicine (see chapter 10); (9) periodic review of pain diagnosis and comorbid conditions, including addictive disorders; and (10) documentation. Application of the universal precautions is intended to help the clinician identify and interpret aberrant behavior and, where they exist, diagnose underlying substance misuse disorders.

In the interest of balance as well as documentation, many have advocated utilizing a risk-management plan in prescribing COT. Currently, no specific elements are required as part of such a plan; however, popular risk-management elements include obtaining informed consent for chronic opioid therapy, using opioid treatment agreements, performing urine drug tests, and implementing specific policies to manage aberrant behaviors. Controlled substance agreements, regular urine drug screens, and interventions such as motivational counselling have been shown to help improve patient compliance with opioids and to minimize aberrant drug-related behaviour (Jamison et al. 2011).

Informed Consent

The prescriber must discuss the opioid treatment plan clearly with the patient and answer any questions the patient may have. The patient must be informed of the anticipated benefits of COT as well as the foreseeable risks, including the issues of addiction, physical dependence, and tolerance (Gourlay et al. 2005). The American Academy of Pain Medicine has a sample informed consent form titled "Consent for Chronic Opioid Therapy," available in both English and Spanish on their website at www.painmed.org/productpub/statements.

Opioid Treatment Agreements

It may also be reasonable to use an opioid treatment agreement when prescribing COT for patients with persistent noncancer pain. However, such a treatment agreement may not be necessary for all patients in all settings. Therefore the use of opioid contracts is left to the clinician's judgment and/or policies (see appendices 1 and 2). Elements of opioid treatment agreements may include the following:

- Only one physician prescribing opioids while the patient is being treated at a pain clinic;
- Use of only one pharmacy for medications;
- Random drug (blood or urine) screens and/or pill counts allowed;
- Refill requests must be made according to pain clinic policy and not on nights or weekends;
- Selling, trading, or sharing opioids with anyone constitutes grounds for discontinuation of opioids and possible dismissal;
- Forged or abused prescriptions constitute grounds for discontinuation of opioids and possible dismissal;
- Use of any illegal controlled substances (e.g., marijuana, cocaine) constitutes grounds for discontinuation of opioids and possible dismissal;
- Opioids must be safeguarded from loss or theft (lost or stolen opioids will not be replaced);
- The patient agrees to take medication exactly as prescribed; and
- All unused opioid medication must be brought to the pain clinic at every visit.

An extension of the traditional opioid treatment agreement is the use of a trilateral opioid treatment agreement, which is seen, agreed upon, and signed by the pain specialist, patient, and patient's primary care physician (Fishman et al. 2002).

Urine Drug Testing

Urine drug testing (UDT) is considered one of the mainstays of adherence monitoring in conjunction with prescription monitoring programs and other screening tools, however, UDT is associated with multiple limitations secondary to potential pitfalls related to drug metabolism, reliability of the tests, and the knowledge of the pain physician (Christo et al. 2011). The practice of UDT is more common in a noncancer pain setting than in an oncology or primary care setting; however, it sometimes seems to be incorrectly utilized in a punitive manner to "catch" the patient with an inappropriate positive or negative test. Unfortunately, this often results in dismissal of the patient from the practice. While drug testing can be used in a variety of ways, it is most commonly used for two quite different purposes: to identify substances that should not be present in the urine (i.e., forensic testing) and to detect the presence of prescribed medications (compliance testing).

The use of UDT in efforts to monitor patients on COT treated in a pain clinic is reasonable. This type of testing is not mandatory for all patients on COT in all settings. UDT should be utilized based on the clinical judgment of the prescribing clinician; however, some clinicians and/or clinics test all patients on COT sporadically based on policy. Katz and Fanciullo (2002) have proposed that although further research is needed, it may be easier and more uniform to conduct routine urine toxicology testing in patients with chronic pain treated with opioids. By adopting a uniform policy of testing, stigma is reduced while ensuring that those persons dually diagnosed with pain and substance use disorders receive optimal care. With careful explanation of the purpose of testing, any patient concerns can be easily addressed (Gourlay et al. 2002; Heit 2003). Caveats to the use of UDT include the following:

1. Ensuring the proper collection, handling, and documentation of the urine specimen;
2. Being knowledgeable regarding interpretation of UDT results;
3. Knowing exactly what your patient consumed and when it was consumed prior to the urine collection; and
4. Knowing what you are looking for and what you will do when various results come back.

One of the most common urinary drug screens involves fluorescence polarization immunoassay, which detects the "federal five" of marijuana metabolite (delta-9-THC), cocaine metabolite (Benzoylecgonime), opiates, phencyclidine (PCP), and amphetamines/methamphetamines. This test has a relatively low sensitivity for semisynthetic and synthetic opioids (e.g., hydrocodone, oxycodone, fentanyl). Therefore, if the test on the patient's urine is negative for the presence of one of these drugs, it does not exclude use. Furthermore, even if the test is positive for a specific drug, a confirmatory test should follow. The confirmatory UDT is based on principles of gas chromatography and mass spectrometry (GC/MS) or high-performance liquid chromatography (HPLC). GC/MS is considered to be the gold standard. The expanded "federal ten" also tests for methadone, propoxyphene (no longer available), methaqualone, benzodiazepines, and barbiturates.

Manchikanti et al. (2011) prospectively studied the diagnostic accuracy of POC testing with immunoassay, comparing it with laboratory testing with chromatography in 1,000 patients. Compared with laboratory testing for opioids and illicit drugs, immunoassay in-office testing at high specificity and agreement but variable sensitivity demonstrates the value of immunoassay drug testing, but a cautious approach is advocated. Agreement for prescribed opioids was high with the index test (80.4%). The reference test of opioids improved the accuracy by 8.9% from 80.4% to 89.3%.

Fishbain and colleagues gathered urine toxicology results among 122 patients who were prescribed opioids for noncancer pain and found abnormal results in 43% of this sample (Fishbain et al. 1999). Michna and colleagues published a report on 226 patients primarily with chronic back pain and found 46.5% of the sample to have abnormal urine toxicology screens (Michna et al. 2007). In a retrospective study of 470 patients, four of 10 patients prescribed opioids also had abnormal urine toxicology screens (Katz and Fanciullo 2002). In 2003, Katz and colleagues reported that roughly 20% of patients with persistent pain on chronic opioid therapy who seem compliant will test positive for an illicit drug and/or another non-prescribed opioid (Katz et al. 2003). Cone et al. analyzed a large number (n = 10,922) of urine samples from patients with persistent pain on chronic opioid therapy and found that the overall prevalence of illicit drug use was 10.9% (Cone et al. 2008). The illicit drugs found in the urine of these patients most often were marijuana, cocaine, and ecstasy-related drugs (Cone et al. 2008). Couto and colleagues reported that they found over 30% of urine drug testing results in chronic pain patients contained at least one other controlled substance in addition to the prescribed opioid (Couto et al. 2009). These studies underscore the importance of urine toxicology screens along with behavioral observation and self-report measures to help identify aberrant drug-related behaviour (Jamison et al. 2011).

It is becoming more and more frequent that many physicians, specifically in pain management settings, believe that UDT may be helpful routinely to establish baseline information regardless of how much information is available from physicians, prescription monitoring programs, and other sources.

The health care professional must know which drugs to test for and by what methods, as well as the expected use of the results. It is critical that the clinician be knowledgeable regarding the limitations of the tests (i.e., low sensitivity of immunoassay for semisynthetic and synthetic opioids). Confirmatory tests should be specifically requested. If the purpose of testing is to find unprescribed or illicit drug use, combination techniques such as GC/MS or HPLC are the most specific for identifying individual drugs or their metabolites (Vandevenne et al. 2000).

Starrels and colleagues performed a systematic review of treatment agreements and urine drug testing in efforts to reduce opioid misuse in patients with chronic pain, and found that the evidence was relatively weak in supporting the effectiveness of opioid treatment agreements and urine drug testing in reducing opioid misuse by patients with chronic pain (Starrels et al. 2010). Although there does not exist robust/rigorous evidence that urine drug testing positively affects outcomes, multiple authors (Michna et al. 2007; Fishbain et al. 1999, Cone et al. 2008; Kahan et al. 2006; Heit and Gourlay 2004; Passik and Kirsh 2004; Macario and Pergolizzi 2005) believe that urine drug testing provides valuable information when making clinical decisions and caring for patients with persistent pain on chronic opioid therapy. It appears that opioid misuse occurring in patients with persistent pain on chronic opioid therapy may have a variable and wide-ranging prevalence of 3–40% (Fishbain et al. 2008; Hoffmann et al. 1995; Trescot et al. 2006). Manchikanti et al. reported that there may be fair evidence that urine drug testing: (a) has good diagnostic accuracy; (b) is helpful in identifying non-compliance, opioid misuse, and/or use of illicit drugs; and (c) may decrease prescription drug abuse or illicit drug use for patients with persistent pain on chronic opioid therapy (Manchikanti et al. 2012).

Gupta and colleagues retrospectively reviewed physician opioids prescribing practices in patients with aberrant behaviors for patients at an academic center's chronic pain outpatient clinic and assessed what occurred after they interpreted the patient's urine drug test results (Gupta et al. 2011). The urines were categorized as having urine screens that were "normal" (expected findings based on their prescribed drugs) or abnormal. Abnormal findings were those with either (1) the absence of a prescribed opioid, (2) the presence of an additional nonprescribed controlled substance, (3) detection of an illicit substance, or (4) an adulterated urine sample.

When an aberrance occurred, it was most likely in the form of an abnormal UDT, followed by the presence of an illicit drug, and then self-escalating doses, with other types of aberrance comprising a small fraction of the total (Gupta et al. 2011). Provider responses to this aberrance generally took the form of five basic types, with a smaller percentage of patients not returning to the clinic and therefore effectively discharging themselves. Of note, the preferred response to the discovery of aberrant behavior was actually to continue to prescribe opioids. This occurred approximately 55% of the time (Gupta et al. 2011). Discontinuation of opioid therapy was a distant second at roughly 20% of the responses (Figure 11-1) (even with instances in which the same patient had aberrant behavior on multiple occasions). Thus, it appeared that despite their interpreting urine drug testing as abnormal with the presence of an illicit drug, the majority of physicians continued chronic opioid therapy without significant changes to treatment.

Barth and colleagues retrospectively reviewed medical records of patients on chronic opioids for more than 22 months in a primary care clinic and found patients on chronic opioids who have a UDT positive for an illicit opioid or unprescribed opioids alone are more likely to respond to monitored opioid pharmacotherapy (Barth et al. 2010). Patients with a UDT positive for cocaine,

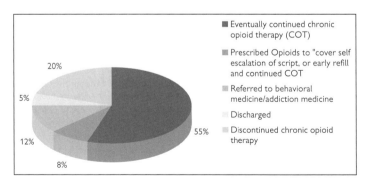

Figure 11.1 Rough estimates of provider action breakdown by percent (adapted from Gupta et al. 2011)

alone or in combination, are less likely to resolve aberrant behavior within the structure of a monitored opioid pharmacotherapy program and are more likely to be discharged electively or administratively from the program without significant transition to addiction treatment (Barth et al. 2010).

There exists a growing appreciation that many physicians, specifically in pain management settings, believe that UDT may be helpful when utilized routinely to establish baseline information regardless of how much information is available from physicians, prescription monitoring programs, and other sources. In 2008, the Biomedical Research and Education Foundation (BREF) (Miami Beach, FL, USA) conducted a study based on a questionnaire distributed to 250 attendees of the American Congress of Pain Medicine in New York City (Pegolizzi et al. 2010). Forty-nine attendees completed it ($n = 49$) mostly being anesthesiologists, primary care physicians or physiatrists. When selecting patients for urine testing, some respondents tested all patients who were being prescribed a controlled substance, while others tested a subset of that group. Seven respondents (14%) did not use UDT, 34 (69%) tested only patients who displayed aberrant behavior/drug-taking, and 25 (51%) tested any patient that they were considering prescribing a controlled substance for.

The patient population subjected to urine drug testing varied from 0% to 25% of patients (testing practice of 38.8% of respondents) to testing 76% to 100% of patients (22.4% of respondents). The frequency of testing in the survey appears to be most frequently random ("other" as opposed to a more calendar-oriented schedule—23 respondents [47%]), but some respondents reported testing monthly (16%)[27]or quarterly (10%) (CMS Manual System 2004). Five respondents performed biannual testing and six (12%) said they tested annually. Testing was sometimes scheduled, but might also be driven by a specific patient action or change in treatment (Pegolizzi et al. 2010).

Caution must be exercised in interpreting UDT results in a pain practice. True negative urine results for prescribed medication may indicate a pattern of bingeing rather than drug diversion. Time of last use of the drugs can be helpful in interpreting the results.

However, clinicians need to be careful not to immediately jump to the "final" conclusion that just because the laboratory reports a negative result for the opioid that the patient is being prescribed, does not automatically mean that the patient is not taking the opioid. There may be many possible scenarios to explain this including that the patient is an ultra-rapid metabolizer of this opioid, bacterial contamination lead to a lower opioid level in the specimen, or perhaps a random urine sample with a slightly lower specific gravity (e.g. If the concentration of the opioid is just sub-threshold such as 199 ng/ml with a cutoff of 200 ng/ml; the test will be reported as negative for that particular opioid.) If the concentration of the opioid is roughly half that of the expected value, then potential scenarios may be that the patient is a rapid metabolizer of the opioid or perhaps the patient is taking a lower dose of opioid because of miscommunication, or be the patient is doing well with less pain and decreased their dose but did not let their pain specialist know yet, or maybe the patient is taking half their dose and selling the rest. Time of last use of the drug(s) and/or the use of serum drug testing for the opioid that the patient is being prescribed, may be helpful in interpreting the results (Smith 2012).

Care must be taken in the collection of the urine specimen and in ensuring that the handling chain or chain of custody process to the lab is executed and documented properly. The collection facility should be a private area with no sink basin or access of water or liquids, and the toilet should have pigmented toilet water (e.g., blue). Measurements of urinary creatinine, pH, specific gravity, and temperature should also be ordered and recorded to assist with results interpretation and to increase specimen reliability. To confirm reliability and authenticity of the urine sample, values for each of these variables should be within the following limits:

- Temperature (within 4 minutes of voiding): 90°F to 100°F
- Urinary pH: 4.5 to 8.0
- Urinary creatinine: 20mg/dL
- Additionally, specimen validity testing (SVT) to determine if adulterants or foreign substances were added to urine or if specimen was substituted should occur (e.g., testing for nitrite, pyridine, glutaraldehyde, bleach, and soap). Adulterated specimens may be suspected if nitrate is ^{3}500 mcg/ml, or pH is ^{3}11, or exogenous substances are present, or substances are present at significantly higher concentrations than normal physiologic concentration (e.g., Chromium+6 in significant supraphysiologic concentrations).

Multiple variables affecting the results of urine testing include cutoff selection; pharmacokinetics, pharmacodynamics, and pharmacogenetics; laboratory technology used in the urine drug test; and subversion and adulteration of the urine specimen (Table 11.1) (Christo et al. 2011).

In certain cases, UDT may detect traces of unexplained opioids secondary to drug metabolism. For example, a patient taking codeine may show trace quantities of hydrocodone (up to 11%) that is unrelated to hydrocodone use (Oyler et al. 2000). Detection of minor amounts of hydrocodone in urine containing a high concentration of codeine should not be interpreted as evidence of hydrocodone misuse. In the case of a patient who is prescribed hydrocodone, quantities of hydromorphone may also be detected due to hydrocodone metabolism (Gourlay et al. 2002). Morphine may be metabolized to produce small amounts of hydromorphone (up to 10%) through a minor metabolic pathway (Cone et al. 2006). It appears that quetiapine (Seroquel) may produce false methadone-positive urine drug screens (Cherwinski et al. 2007).

Normetabolites such as norcodeine, norhydrocodone, and noroxycodone are unique metabolites that are not available commercially (Table 11.2). Consequently, detection of normetabolite in specimens not containing parent drug, provides conclusive evidence that the parent drug was consumed (Cone et al. 2010). Cone and colleagues analyzed 2654 urine specimens of pain patients in a chronic pain clinic treated with COT. For specimens containing normetabolite, the prevalence of norcodeine, norhydrocodone and noroxycodone in the absence of parent drug was 8.6%, 7.8%, and 9.4%, respectively. From one-third to two-thirds of these specimens also did not contain other metabolites that could have originated from the parent drug. The authors

Table 11.1 Urine Drug Testing: Typical Screening and Confirmation Cut-Off Concentrations and Detection Times for Drugs of Abuse

Drug	Screening cut-off oncentrations ng/mL urine	Confirmation cut-off concentrations g/Ml (non-regulated)	Confirmation cutoff concentrations g/mL (federally egulated)	Urine detection time
Opioids	300	50	2,000	3–4 days
Morphine	300	50	2,000	1–3 days
Codeine Hydrocodone	300	50	2,000	1–2 days
Oxycodone	100	50	2,000	1–3 days
Methadone	300	100	2,000	2–4 days
Benzodiazepines	200	20–50	NA	Up to 30 days
Cocaine	300	50	150	1–3 days
Marijuana	50	15	15	1–3 days for casual use; up to 30 days for chronic use
Amphetamine	1,000	100	500	2–4 days
Methamphetamine	1,000	100	500	2–4 days
Heroin*	10	10	NA	1–3 days
Phencyclidine	25	10	25	2–7 days for casual use; up to 30 days for chronic use

*6-MAM, the specific metabolite is detected only for 6 hours
(Christo et al., 2011)

concluded that inclusion of norcodeine, norhydrocodone, and noroxycodone may be useful in interpretation of opiate drug source and may reduce potential false negatives that would occur without tests for these unique metabolites (Cone et al. 2010).

UDT may also have the potential to be useful for identifying potential patients who may be "poor metabolizers" or "ultra-fast metabolizers." Yee et al. evaluated the metabolism of oxycodone to oxymorphone in a pain patient population using a quantitative liquid chromatography-tandem mass spectrometry analysis of 32,656 urine specimens obtained from pain patients between March 2008 and February 2010 (Yee et al. 2012). Urine samples containing oxycodone without oxymorphone allowed an estimation of the proportion of poor metabolizers (2.4 ± 2.1%) in the population. A similar analysis of samples containing oxymorphone without oxycodone gave an estimate of the proportion of ultra-rapid metabolizers (1.8 ± 1.1%) in the population; and showed that

Table 11.2 Major Opioid Metabolites			
Opioid	Major Metabolites	Bioactive Metabolite	Major Metabolic Enzymes
Morphine	Morphine-3-glucuronide	I	UGT2B7
Morphine	Morphine-6-glucuronide	A	UGT2B7
Hydromorphone	Hydromorphone-3-glucuronide	I	UGT2B7
	Hydromorphone-6-glucuronide	A	UGT1A3
Oxycodone	Noroxycodone	A	CYP3A4
Oxycodone	Oxymorphone	A	CYP2D6
Codeine	Codeine-6-glucuronide	A	UGT2B7
Codeine	Morphine	A	CYP2D6
	Norcodeine	A	CYP3A4
Hydrocodone	Norhydrocodone	A	CYP3A4
	Hydromorphone	A	CYP2D6
Oxymorphone	Oxymorphone-3-glucuronide	I	UGT2B7
Oxymorphone	6-hyroxy-oxymorphone	A	U.C.
Propoxyphene	Norpropoxyphene	A	CYP3A4
Meperidine	Normeperidine	A	CYP3A4, CYP2B6, CYP2C19
Fentanyl	Norfentanyl	I	CYP3A4
Buprenorphine	Norbuprenorphine	A	CYP3A4
Methadone	EDDP	I	CYP2B6
Tramadol	O-desmethyl tramadol (M1)	A	CYP2D6
Tapentadol	Tapentadol-O-glucuronide	I	UGT1A9 UGT2B7
I = inactive for analgesia; A = active for analgesia; U.C.= uncertain			

it may be possible to identify fast or slow metabolizers who may be at risk for adverse events (Yee et al. 2012).

If urine drug testing is utilized, it is crucial to avoid inappropriate interpretation of results, which may adversely affect clinical decision making. Health care providers should not jump to conclusions of noncompliance or appropriate opioid use versus opioid misuse based on positive or negative detection of opioid in the urine. Clinicians should use the results of the drug test in conjunction with other clinical information when deciding whether to alter the treatment plan.

There is no specific uniform strategy to deal with specific abnormal results of urine drug testing. Each practice should be comfortable dealing with abnormal results in a specific way but it should be consistent for each practice. Algorithms for UDT have been published that may help certain clinicians/practices (Christo et al. 2011; Koyyalagunta et al. 2011). Furthermore, the various options of what to do with different abnormal results should be known in advance, and preferably patients should be informed of these plans ahead of time when they first become part of the practice (as long as the clinicians stick to what they state).

Aberrant Drug-Taking Behaviors

Ongoing assessment of drug-taking behavior (one of the four As) is clearly a part of risk management. Keeping track of opioid analgesics (e.g., unscheduled pill counts) may constitute one particular aspect of a risk-management plan. However, the presence of aberrant drug-taking behaviors is not always indicative of addiction and should not automatically lead clinicians to suspect addiction. As discussed more fully in other chapters, several reasons other than addiction may account for aberrant drug-taking behaviors, including pseudoaddiction or psychiatric complications. A recent study (Passik et al. 2006) lists behaviors that are less indicative of addiction (e.g., hoarding medications, taking someone else's pain medication, aggressively requesting more drugs from the doctor) and behaviors that are more indicative of addiction (e.g., buying pain medication from a street dealer, stealing money to obtain drugs, selling prescription drugs). Wu et al. (2006) have introduced the Addiction Behaviors Checklist (ABC), a brief (20-item) instrument designed to track behaviors characteristic of addiction related to opioids in chronic pain populations. The ABC items focus on observable behaviors noted during (11 items) and between (eight items) clinic visits, with 1 item classified as "other."

Several strategies can be adopted at the initiation of or during opioid therapy based on the perceived level of risk for the patient. These strategies include the following:

- Adopting a structured, strict prescription policy with no early refills and no replacement of lost prescriptions (without a police report documenting the loss);
- Requiring the patient to attend frequent visits, with small quantities of opioids being prescribed;
- Requiring that the patient use only one pharmacy;
- Requiring the patient to bring the pill bottle to each appointment for a pill count;
- Requiring unscheduled, spontaneous calls for the patient to bring the bottle in for a pill count between regular appointments;
- Performing UDT at screening and informing the patient that occasional tests will be required in the future (with proper monitoring of the collection to ensure that the urine is fresh and real, not imitation or another person's urine sample);
- Requiring the use of nonpharmacologic/nonopioid therapies; and
- Requiring that the patient see an addiction medicine specialist.

Based on the level of the problematic behavior and a reassessment of the four As, the clinician must make the decision as to whether COT should be continued, whether the patient should be referred to a pain specialist and/or an addiction specialist, and whether the patient should be released from the practice.

References

Barth KS, Becker WC, Wiedemer NL, et al. Association between urine drug test results and treatment outcome in high-risk chronic pain patients on opioids. *J Addict Med.* 2010;4(3):167–173.

Cherwinski K, Petti TA, Jekelis A. False methadone-positive urine drug screens in patients treated with quetiapine. *J Am Acad Child Adolesc Psychiatry.* 2007;46(4):435–436.

Christo PJ, Manchikanti L, Ruan X, et al. Urine Drug Testing in Chronic Pain. *Pain Physician.* 2011;14(2):123–143.

CMS Manual System. (2004) Pub 100-04 medicare claims processing, transmittal 1884. [WWW document]. URL http://www.cms.hhs.gov/transmittals/downloads/ R1884CP.pdf. Accessed on June 4, 2012.

Cone EJ, Caplan YH, Black DL, Robert T, Moser F. Urine drug testing of chronic pain patients: licit and illicit drug patterns. *J Anal Toxicol.* 2008;32(8):530–543.

Cone EJ, Heit HA, Caplan YH, et al. Evidence of morphine metabolism to hydromorphone in pain patients chronically treated with morphine. *J Anal Toxicol.* 2006;30(1):1–5.

Cone EJ, Zichterman A, Heltsley R, Black DL, Cawthon B, Robert T, Moser F, Caplan YH. Urine testing for norcodeine, norhydrocodone, and noroxycodone facilitates interpretation and reduces false negatives. *Forensic Sci Int.* 2010;198(1–3):58–61.

Couto JE, Rommey MC, Leider HL, Sharma S, Goldfarb NI. High rates of inappropriate drug use in the chronic pain population. *Popul Health Manag.* 2009;12(4):185–190.

Fishbain DA, Cole B, Lewis J, Rosomoff HL, Rosomoff RS. What percentage of chronic nonmalignant pain patients exposed to chronic opioid analgesic therapy develop abuse/addiction and/or aberrant drug-related behaviors? A structured evidence-based review. *Pain Med.* 2008;9(4):444–459.

Fishbain DA, Curlter RB, Rosomoff HL, Rosomoff RS. Validity of self-reported drug use in chronic pain patients. *Clin J Pain.* 1999;15(3):184–191.

Fishman SM, Mahajan G, Jung SW, et al. The trilateral opioid contract. Bridging the pain clinic and the primary care physician through the opioid contract. *J Pain Symptom Manage.* 2002;24(3):335–344.

Gourlay D, Heit HA. Universal precautions: a matter of mutual trust and responsibility. *Pain Med.* 2006;7(2):210–211.

Gourlay DL, Heit HA Almahrezi A. Universal precautions in pain medicine: a rational approach to the treatment of chronic pain. *Pain Med.* 2005;6(2):107–112.

Gourlay DL, Heit HA, Caplan YH. *Urine Drug Testing in Primary Care: Dispelling the Myths & Designing Strategies.* Pharmacom Group, 2002. California Academy of Family Physicians Web site. www.familydocs.org/assets/Professional_ Development/CME/UDT.pdf. Accessed March 7, 2006.

Gupta A, Patton C, Diskina D, Cheatle M. Retrospective review of physician opioid prescribing practices in patients with aberrant behaviors. *Pain Physician.* 2011;14(4):383–389.

Heit HA. *Use of Urine Toxicology Tests in a Chronic Pain Practice.* 3rd ed. Chevy Chase, MD: American Society of Addiction Medicine, 2003.

Heit HA, Gourlay DL. Urine drug testing in pain medicine. *J Pain Symptom Manage.* 2004; 27(3): 260–267.

Hoffmann NG, Olofsson O, Salen B, Wickstrom L. Prevalence of abuse and dependency in chronic pain patients. *Int J Addict.* 1995;30(8):919–927.

Jamison RN, Serraillier J, Michna E. Assessment and treatment of abuse risk in opioid prescribing for chronic pain. *Pain Res Treat.* 2011. DOI: 10.1155/2011/941808.

Kahan M, Srivastava A, Wilson L, Gourlay D, Midmer D. Misuse of and dependence on opioids. *Can Fam Physician.* 2006;52(9):1081–1087.

Katz N, Fanciullo G. Role of urine toxicology testing in the management of chronic opioid therapy. *Clin J Pain.* 2002;18(4 Suppl):S76–82.

Katz N, Sherburne S, Beach M, et al. Behavioral monitoring and urine toxicology testing in patients receiving long-term opioid therapy. *Anesth Analg.* 2003;97(4):1097–1102.

Koyyalagunta D, Burton AW, Toro MP, Driver L, Novy DM. Opioid abuse in cancer pain: report of two cases and presentation of an algorithm of multidisciplinary care. *Pain Physician.* 2011;14(4):E361–371.

Macario A, Pergolizzi JV Jr. Urine drug testing in chronic pain patients taking opioids: a clinical practice update. *Int J Pain Med Palliat Care.* 2005;4:133–139.

Manchikanti L, Abdi S, Arluri S, et al. American Society of Interventional Pain Physicians (ASIPP) Guidelines for Responsible Opioid Prescribing in Chronic Non-cancer Pain: Part I – Evidence Assessment. *Pain Physician.* 2012;In Press.

Manchikanti L, Malla Y, Wargo BW, Fellows B. Comparative evaluation of the accuracy of immunoassay with liquid chromatography tandem mass spectrometry (LC/MS/MS) of urine drug testing (UDT) Opioids and illicit drugs in chronic pain patients. *Pain Physician.* 2011;14(2):175–188.

Michna E, Jamison RN, Pham LD, et al. Urine toxicology screening among chronic pain patients on opioid therapy: frequency and predictability of abnormal findings. *Clin J Pain.* 2007;23(2):173–179.

Oyler JM, Cone EJ, Joseph RE Jr, et al. Identification of hydrocodone in human urine following controlled codeine administration. *J Anal Toxicol.* 2000;24(7):530–535.

Passik SD, Kirsh KL. Opioid therapy in patients with a history of substance abuse. *CNS Drugs.* 2004;18(1):13–25.

Passik SD, Kirsh KL, Donaghy KB, et al. Pain and aberrant drug-related behaviors in medically ill patients with and without histories of substance abuse. *Clin J Pain.* 2006;22(2):173–181.

Pegolizzi J, Pappagallo M, Stauffer J, et al. The Integrated Drug Compliance Study Group. The Role of Urine Drug testing for patients on Opioid Therapy. *Pain Pract.* 2010;10(6):497–507.

Smith HS. Urine Drug Testing. In Bajwa ZH, Wootton J, Warfield CA, eds. *Principles and Practice of Pain Medicine.* 3rd ed. New York: McGraw-Hill, 2012.In Press.

Starrels JL, Becker WC, Alford DP, et al. Systematic review: Treatment agreements and urine drug testing to reduce opioid misuse in patients with chronic pain. *Ann Intern Med.* 2010;152(11):712–720.

Trescot AM, Boswell MV, Arluri SL, et al. Opioid guidelines in the management of chronic non-cancer pain. *Pain Physician.* 2006;9(1):1–39.

Vandevenne M, Vandenbussche H, Verstraete A. Detection time of drugs of abuse in urine. *Acta Clin Belg.* 2000;55(6):323–333.

Wu SM, Compton P, Bolus R, et al. The Addiction Behaviors Checklist: validation of a new clinician-based measure of inappropriate opioid use in chronic pain. *J Pain Symptom Manage.* 2006;32(4):342–351.

Yee DA, Best BM, Atayee RS, Pesce AJ. Observations on the urine metabolic ratio of oxymorphone to oxycodone in pain patients. *J Anal Toxicol.* 2012;36(4):232–238.

Chapter 12a

Special Populations: Pediatric

Amy L. Mitchell and Howard S. Smith

Transition into the twenty-first century still finds the pediatrician searching for guidance with the management of pain. Few practices have implemented clinical guidelines. This lack of direction is one of the many challenges that face practitioners treating children (Greco and Berde 2005; Anand et al. 2006). Early maturation of the anatomic, neurophysiologic, and hormonal components necessary for pain perception leaves practitioners struggling to provide comfort to even the smallest of the micropremies in their care (Anand and Carr 1989; Fitzgerald et al. 1989; Giannakoulopoulos et al. 1994; Perreault et al. 1997; Berde and Sethna 2002; Berde et al. 2012). This chapter provides some suggestions and strategies for overcoming challenges in the use of opioids for treating pain in children.

Assessment of Pain

The first significant challenge is the identification of pain in children. The belief that physicians cannot accurately assess pain in children is incorrect. Accurate pain assessment can be achieved through physiologic indicators, systematic observation of behavior, and reports by the children themselves. The key to successful pain assessment is finding the scale that simplifies the means by which even the smallest child can communicate his or her pain (Walco et al. 1994). Since one common pain scale is not practical for the widely varying population in a children's hospital, pain scales have been developed with various subpopulations in mind, such as neonates and preverbal children. Pain scales used within an institution should correspond to a common numerical scale of one to 10, so that single definitions of moderate and severe pain may be used. Refer to Table 12a.1 for suggested pain scales referenced by age.

Expressions of pain reflect the individual's physical and emotional state, coping style, and family and cultural expectations, and can easily be misinterpreted by the practitioner. Barriers to communication can also limit the assessment of pain, making it imperative that the practitioner refrain from imposing his or her own interpretation onto the situation (AAP 2001). Although children five years of age and older are very reliable self-reporters of pain, circumstances do not always afford the ability to speak, particularly in the critical care setting. In these situations, inadequate analgesia is a significant risk (Herr et al. 2006). Several scales have been developed that augment the objectivity necessary for pain

Table 12a.1 Pain Assessment Scales*	
Premature infants and term infants (neonates)	N-PASS (critical care setting) CRIES
Preverbal toddlers and non-verbal children through age 7 years	FLACC
Any verbal child over 4 years old	FACES scales, Self-report (1-10)
Non verbal Adolescents	APPT
Intellectually Disabled Children	PICIC, NCCPC-PV, PPP, CPB, rFLACC, INRS

*This only a selection of the pain scales available. Take care to choose the scale that best works for your population and has been properly validated by the literature.

assessment in the nonverbal patient at the various developmental stages: the Neonatal Pain, Agitation, and Sedation Scale (N-PASS) for critically ill infants (Hummel and Puchalski n.d.); CRIES [**C**ry, **R**equires oxygen, **I**ncreased vital signs, **E**xpression, **S**leeplessness] for postoperative infants (Krechel and Bildner 1995); FLACC (**F**ace, **L**egs, **A**ctivity, **C**ry, **C**onsolability) for children up to age seven (Merkel et al. 1997; Willis et al. 2003; Manworren and Hynan 2003) and the Adolescent Pediatric Pain Tool (APPT) (Savedra et al. 1993).

A growing area of interest in the field of pain management is pain assessment in the intellectually disabled child. Developmental disabilities including intellectual disability (also known as mental retardation) are prevalent and affect nearly one out of six children in the United States according to data collected from 2006 to 2008. (Boyle et al. 2011). Intellectual disability is characterized by significant limitations both in intellectual functioning and in adaptive behavior. Depending upon the level or degree of disability, children with intellectual disability might have a hard time letting others know their wants and needs. While self-report is the gold standard for pain assessment, this may not be a viable option for these children. Validated observational pain assessment scales for intellectually disabled children are available and should be applied as necessary (Valkenburg et al. 2010).

Prescribing Opioids

As previously mentioned in this text, opioids are the drugs of choice for moderate to severe pain associated with surgery or invasive procedures, cancer, sickle cell disease, and various other disease states where there is a chronic pain component (Berde and Sethna 2002). Specific selection of an opioid depends upon practitioner preference, patient comorbidities, patient tolerability, and the dosage forms available. Table 12a.2 reviews the opioid choices for pediatric patients and considerations that should be taken into account in prescribing. Table 12a.3 describes best initial dosing of some opioids.

Table 12a.2 Opioid Selection for Pediatric Patients (online.lexi.com)W

Opioid	Dose forms available	Recommended Dosing	Comments
Codeine	15 mg/ml and 30 mg/ml injection 30 mg and 60 mg tabs (phosphate salt) 15 mg, 30 mg and 60 mg tabs (sulfate salt) acetaminophen 120 mg and codeine 12 mg per 5 ml elixir acetaminophen 300 mg and codeine 15 mg (or 30 mg or 60 mg) tabs	0.5–1 mg codeine/kg/dose (max of 60 mg/dose) po q4–6 h Alternatively, for acetaminophen/codeine: 3–6 years: 5 ml 3–4 times per day as needed of elixir 7–12 years: 10 ml 3–4 times per day as needed of elixir >12 years: 15 ml 3–4 times per day as needed of elixir	Associated with >10% incidence of vomiting Combination product has lower maximum daily dose due to limitations of daily acetaminophen dosage Variable response due to genotype; slow metabolizers have limited effect and fast metabolizers have potentially-life threatening apnea
Fentanyl	0.05 mg/ml injection	Intermittent: 1–4 mcg/kg/dose (max of 50 mcg/dose) IV every 2–4 hours as needed Continuous: (1–2 mcg/kg load) 1–5 mcg/kg/h Patient Controlled Analgesia/Authorized Agent Analgesia: Hourly limit as above; divide between basal and on-demand dose according to patient situation	Other dose forms such as the lozenge, buccal tabs, and iontophoretic transdermal system are not practical, nor approved for use in children Refer to table 3 for partially occluded patch administration procedure Must be used with caution outside of the critical care setting due to ability to cause chest wall rigidity if administered too quickly (in less than 5 minutes)
	12.5 mcg/h, 25 mcg/h, 50 mcg/h, 75 mcg/h, 100 mcg/h transdermal patch	(Requires conversion to fentanyl equivalents) Partially occluded patch: Determine mcg/kg/day in fentanyl equivalents Round to nearest portion of patch (¼, ½, ¾)	

(continued)

Table 12a.2 Continued

Opioid	Dose forms available	Recommended Dosing	Comments
Buprenorphine	5 mcg/h, 10 mcg/h, 20 mcg/h transdermal patch	Limited information—until established, use adult dosing: <30 mg morphine equivalents = 5 mcg/h 30–80 mg morphine requivalents = 10 mcg/h	Dosing not well established for partial patches Serious concern for respiratory depression: 30–50 times more potent than morphine
Hydrocodone (only in combination with acetaminophen)	Hydrocodone 7.5 mg and acetaminophen 500 mg per 15 ml elixir Hydrocodone 7.5 mg and acetaminophen 325 mg per 15 ml oral solution Hydrocodone (2.5 mg, 5 mg, 7.5 mg, 10 mg) and acetaminophen (325 mg, 500 mg, 650 mg) tabs – varies by brand	0.2 mg/kg/dose (max of 10 mg/dose) po every 3–4 hours as needed	Combination product has lower maximum daily dose due to limitations of daily acetaminophen dosage; unfortunately not available as single agent dose form Likely to have same genotype impact on metabolism as codeine
Hydromorphone	1 mg/ml, 2 mg/ml, 4 mg/ml, 10 mg/ml injection 1 mg/ml oral liquid 3 mg suppository 2 mg, 4 mg, 8 mg tabs	Oral: Younger children: 0.03–0.08 mg/kg/dose (max of 5 mg/dose) po every 3–4 hours as needed Adolescents: 1–4 mg/dose po every 3–4 hours as needed; doses up to 8 mg have been used Intravenous: 0.015 mg/kg/dose (max dose of 0.6 mg) IV every 3–6 hours as needed Rectal: 3 mg (1 suppository) PR every 6–8 hours as needed	Patient Controlled analgesia/authorized agent analgesia using hydromorphone not usually recommended for children due to tolerance and limited information on dosing Difficult to obtain dose from single strength suppository

Methadone	5 mg/5 ml, 10 mg/5 ml oral solution	0.1 mg/kg/dose every 4 hours for 2–3 doses, then every 6–12 hours as needed or 0.7 mg/kg/24 hours divided every 4–6 hours as needed; maximum dose: 10 mg/dose	Must be individualized to patient if used to manage opioid withdrawal
	5 mg, 10 mg tabs		Concentrated oral solution available; caution should be used to avoid confusion with diluted concentration
	40 mg dispersible tabs		Even using dilute concentration of oral solution, difficult to measure doses needed by neonates
Morphine	0.5 mg/ml, 1 mg/ml, 25 mg/ml injection	Oral: 0.2–0.5 mg/kg/dose (max of 30 mg/dose) po every 3–4 hours as needed **ONLY USE IMMEDIATE-RELEASE TABS OR ORAL SOLUTION**	Drug of choice for some NICUs due to higher incidence of adverse events during the weaning of fentanyl
	10 mg/5 ml, 20 mg/5 ml, 20 mg/ml oral solution		Only immediate-release tabs can be broken and given as partial tabs
	5 mg, 10 mg, 20 mg, 30 mg suppository	Intravenous: Intermittent:	Controlled-release, extended-release and sustained-release tabs are inappropriate for younger children
	10 mg, 15 mg, 30 mg immediate-release tabs	0.05–0.1 mg/kg/dose (max dose of 15 mg/dose) IV every 2–4 hours as needed	
	15 mg, 30 mg, 60 mg, 100 mg, 200 mg controlled-release and extended-release tabs	Continuous: 0.01–0.04 mg/kg/h IV	
	15 mg, 30 mg, 60 mg, 100 mg sustained-release tabs	Patient Controlled Analgesia/Authorized Agent Analgesia: Hourly limit as above; divide between basal and on-demand dose according to patient situation	

(continued)

Table 12a.2 Continued

Opioid	Dose forms available	Recommended Dosing	Comments
Oxycodone	Oxycodone 5 mg and acetaminophen 500 mg capsule or caplet (capsule also available this strength without acetaminophen)	0.05–0.3 mg/kg/dose (max of 30 mg/dose) po every 4–6 hours as needed	Concentrated elixir available—caution should be used to avoid confusion with diluted elixir
	Oxycodone 5 mg and acetaminophen 325 mg per 5 ml oral solution (also available without acetaminophen)		Note that brand names are very similar and easily confused (Roxicodone® and Roxicet®)
	Oxycodone (2.5 mg, 5 mg, 7.5 mg, 10 mg) and acetaminophen (325 mg, 500 mg, 650 mg) tabs—varies by brand		Only immediate-release tabs can be broken and given as partial tabs
	Oxycodone 5 mg, 15 mg, 30 mg tabs		Controlled-release, extended-release and sustained –release tabs are inappropriate for younger children
	Oxycodone 10 mg, 20 mg, 40 mg, 80 mg Extended-release tabs		Combination product has lower maximum daily dose due to limitations of daily acetaminophen dosage
	Oxycodone 10 mg, 20 mg, 40 mg, 60 mg, 80 mg, 160 mg Controlled-release tabs		

Table 12a.3 Initial Dosage Guidelines for Onoid Analgesics*							
Drug	Equianalgesic Doses		Usual Starting Intravenous or Subcutaneous Doses and Intervals		Parenteral:Oral Dose Ratio	Usual Starting Oral Doses and Intervals	
	Parenteral	Oral	Child < 50 kg	Child > 50 kg		Child < 50 kg	Child > 50 kg
Codeine	120 mg	200 mg	NR	NR	1:2	0.5–1.0 mg/kg every 3–4 hr	30–60 mg every 3–4 hr
Morphine	10 mg	SO mg (long-term) 60 mg (single dose)	Bolus: 0.1 mg/ kg every 2–4 hr Infusion: 0.03 mg/ kg/hr	Bolus: 5–8 mg every 2–4 hr Infusion: 1.5 mg/hr	1:3 (long-term) 1:6 (single dose)	Immediate release: 0.3 mg/kg every 3–4 hr Sustained release: 20–35 kg: 10–15 mg every 8–12 hr 35–50 kg: IS-30 mg every 8- 12 hr	Immediate release: 15–20 mg every 3–4 hr Sustained release: 30–45 mg every 8–12 hr
Oxycodone	NA	15–20 mg	NA	NA	NA	0.1–0.2 mg/kg every 3–4 hr	5–10 mg every 3–4 hr
Methadone†	10 mg	10- 20 mg	0.1 mg/kg every 4–8 hr	5–8 mg every 4–8 hr	1:2	0.1–0.2 mg/kg every 4–8 hr	5–10 mg every 4–8 hr
Fentanyl	100 μg (0.1 mg)	NA	Bolus: 0.5–1.0 μg/ kg every 1–2 hr Infusion: 0.5–2.0 μg/kg/hr	Bolus: 25–50 μg every 1–2 hr Infusion. 25–100 μg/hr	NA	NA	NA

(continued)

Table 12a.3 Continued

Drug	Equianalgesic Doses		Usual Starting Intravenous or Subcutaneous Doses and Intervals	Parenteral:Oral Dose Ratio	Usual Starting Oral Doses and Intervals	
Hydromorphone	1.5–2 mg	6–8 mg	Bolus: 0.02 mg every 2–4 hr Infusion: 0.006 mg/kg/hr	Bonis: 1 mg every 2–4 hr Infusion: 0.3 mg/hr	1:4	0.04–0.08 mg/kg every 3–4 hr	2–4 mg every 3–4 hr
Meperidine (pethiline)‡	75–100 mg	300 mg	Bolus: 0.8–1.0 mg/kg every 2–3 hr	Bolus: 50–75 mg every 2–3 hr	1:4	2–3 mg/kg every 3–4 hr	100–150 mg every 3–4 hr

* Doses are for patients over six months of age. In infants under six months of age, initial per-kilogram doses should begin at roughly 25 percent of the per-kilogram doses recommended here. Higher doses are often required for patients receiving mechanical ventilation. All doses are approximate and should be adjusted according to clinical circumstances. Recommendations are adapted from previous summary tables, including those of a consensus statement from the World Health Organization and the International Association for the Study of Pain.49 NA denotes not applicable, and NR not recommended.

† Methadone requires additional vigilance because it can accumulate and produce delayed sedation. If sedation occurs, doses should be withheld until sedation resolves. Thereafter, doses should be substantially reduced, the interval between doses should be extended to 8 to 12 hours, or both.

‡ The use of meperidine should generally be avoided if other opioids are available, especially with long-term use, because its metabolite can cause seizures.

Continuous opioids are recommended for the management of acute post-operative pain or severe chronic pain (AAP 2001; Morton 2007). Morphine and fentanyl are readily provided continuously as patient-controlled analgesia/authorized-agent-controlled analgesia or continuous infusions. In pediatric hematology and oncology, long-acting morphine for analgesia has proved to be safe and effective even in very young patients (Zernikow and Lindena 2001). Zernikow and Lindena (2001) report that children under the age of seven years requiring opioid therapy for malignancies generally received an average of 2.6mg/kg/day of morphine equivalents, while patients over age 12 received 1.4mg/kg/day. Use of continuous opioids in the critically ill child requires a careful balance between undersedation (vulnerability of the child if paralyzed, ineffective ventilation, accidental extubation, or loss of invasive access or monitors) and oversedation (delayed recovery, tolerance or dependence, or distressing withdrawal symptoms such as agitation, seizures, hallucinations, psychosis, fever, or tachycardia). Neonates are more vulnerable to opioid adverse events and are likely to have ineffective pain control due to reduced opioid doses. Older infants and young children may require large doses in combination with other sedative agents to maintain comfort and relatively quiescent state. (Wolf 2011). Regardless of age, other factors such as reduced cardiac output, cardiovascular instability, the need for ECMO or cooling therapies, prolonged respiratory failure, or high fever will complicate the opioid dosing, requiring each patient situation to be individualized.

Intermittent opioid dosing (e.g., every four to six hours) is recommended for the treatment of moderate pain or acute post-procedural pain. Early weaning of a patient from continuous opioids directly to intermittent intravenous/oral doses rarely addresses pain adequately, causing the caregiver to respond to pain rather than to anticipate it. Anticipation of pain leads to a lower daily opioid requirement and a more comfortable patient (AAP 2001). Consequently, a step-down approach to weaning opioids in acute pain management works best, in which continuous intravenous administration is transitioned to scheduled intermittent intravenous/oral doses, and then to as-needed oral intermittent doses. As-needed intermittent opioids should be used for breakthrough pain when the pain is mild or moderate and/or episodic. The use of adjunctive nonopioid analgesics is another opioid-sparing strategy. Table 12a.4 provides some examples of dosing for several nonsteroidal anti-inflammatory agents.

Children can receive opioids from all of the same routes as adults, but the route must take into account the specific situational and emotional factors that play into the child's perception of pain. Injections should be avoided whenever possible because of the fear and pain they can cause (Kart et al. 1997). Oral opioids are an attractive alternative to needles, particularly if the pain is mild to moderate in intensity and is expected to be of short duration. Acetaminophen in combination with either codeine or hydrocodone is commonly prescribed to pediatric patients. A growing controversy surrounding codeine use in children and breastfeeding mothers has led prescribers to consider whether this opioid

Table 12a.4 Oral Dosage Guidelines for Commonly Used Nonopioid Analgesics

Drug	Dose for Patients <60 kg	Dose for Patients >60 kg	Interval	Maximal Daily Dose for Patients <60 kg	Maximal Daily Dose for Patients >60 kg
	mg/kg	mg	hr	mg/kg	mg
Acetaminophen	10–15	650–1000	4	100*	4000
Ibuprofen	6–10	400–600†	6	40‡	2400†
Naproxen	5–6‡	250–375†	12	24††	1000†
Aspirin§	10–15†§	650–1000†	4	80††§	

* The maximal daily doses of acetaminophen for infants and neonates are a subject of current controversy. Provisional recommendation are that daily dosing should not exceed 75 mg per kilogram per day infants, 60 mg per kilogram per day for term neonates and preterm neonates of more than 32 weeks of postconceptional age, and 40 mg per kilogram per day for perterm neonates 28 to 32 weeks of postconceptional age. Fever, dehydration, hepatic disease and lack of oral intake may all increase the risk of hepatotoxicity.

† Higher doses may be used in selected cases for treatment of rheumatologic conditions in children.

‡ Dosage guidelines for neonates and infants have not been established.

§ Aspirin carries a risk of provoking Reye's syndrome in infants and children. If other analgesics are available, aspirin should be restricted to indications for which an antiplatelet or antiinflammatory effect is required, rather than being used as a routine analgesic or antipyretic in neonates, infants, or children. Dosage guidelines for asprin in neoenates have not been established.

has an ongoing role in pediatric pain management (Koren et al. 2006; Voronov et al. 2007; Ciszkowski 2009; Madadi et al. 2009; Tremlett et al. 2010; Madadi et al. 2011). At the center of this controversy are the highly variable unpredictable effects of codeine that range from lack of effect to life-threatening complications. Codeine is converted to morphine by an enzyme showing substantial genetic polymorphism. Without the ability to determine the genotype of the child, we will not know if the usual dose will be too little, too much or just right for that patient (Tremlett et al. 2010). Research looking at the effectiveness of codeine in tonsillectomy (Sutters et al. 2004) and musculoskeletal pain (Clark et al. 2007) did not find this opioid to be helpful in treating pain. Active trials are now ongoing to access the impact of patient genotype on the effectiveness of codeine in sickle cell patients. Hydrocodone is an effective alternative to codeine for tonsillectomy (Sutters et al. 2004), but may have toxicity issues similar to codeine. Hydrocodone is metabolized to hydromorphone also using the same enzyme pathway as codeine (Madadi et al. 2010).

Although transdermal fentanyl patches have not been approved by the FDA for pediatric patients, the use of these patches may be medically appropriate for certain patients with persistent severe pain (e.g., intractable cancer pain). These patches may provide an option for children with a stable pain pattern who are treated with regularly scheduled daily oral morphine equivalent to $\geq$30mg/day. Because it is not possible to titrate the opioid dose precisely in real time, transdermal fentanyl patches should not be used in opioid-naïve patients or those suffering from acute pain (e.g., postoperative or procedural pain).

The time to reach steady-state serum drug concentrations seems to be longer, clearance (expressed as liters per kilogram per hour) is higher, and elimination half-life is shorter for the fentanyl transdermal therapeutic system (TTS) in children than in adults (Zernikow et al. 2007). The side-effect profile of the low-dose fentanyl TTS in children appears to be similar to that in adults (with less constipation than caused by morphine). A rough conservative conversion of 45mg/day oral morphine to 12.5µg/h fentanyl TTS is used for initial therapy dose estimation in children receiving long-term morphine therapy (Zernikow et al. 2007). Partially occluded transdermal patches have been considered in some circumstances as cutting of the patch is contraindicated and may lead to fentanyl leakage with inadvertent overdose (Mitchell and Smith 2010).

Buprenorphine is another opioid that has recently become of interest in the management of pediatric pain. At low doses it may be 25 to 40 times more potent than morphine and has the advantage of a long duration of action with a metabolism largely independent of renal function. An extended release delivery system is available that delivers five, 10, or 20 mcg/h over seven days. Similar to the fentanyl transdermal patches, these are based upon matrix technology and the delivery rate is proportional to the application surface area (Michel et al. 2011). The same safety considerations concerning avoiding cutting of the patch apply. Also, exposure to direct external heat sources should be avoided, since buprenorphine release from the patch is temperature-dependent and this may result in overdose. Although the package insert states that the safety and effectiveness of Butrans® have not been established in patients below 18 years, clinicians have anecdotally used Butrans® in select pediatric patients without significant issues. Considerable caution should be used in relation to risk for respiratory depression as buprenorphine, if it occurs, since it is much more difficult to reverse than morphine induced respiratory depression. High doses of naloxone may be required for reversal and may not even provide effective reversal due to relative inability of nalaxone to displace bound buprenorphine (Michel et al. 2011).

Pain management is rarely a "cookbook" enterprise. Although the general concepts can be applied to any patient, customization of the pain-management plan to the patient is essential. Some of strategies that may be used to optimize opioid use are discussed in Table 12a.5.

Table 12a.5 Strategies For Optimize Opioids In Children

1. *Anticipate need for pain management* – by proactively giving doses around-the-clock following a painful experience, less pain is experienced and less opioid is necessary to control pain.

2. *Continuous infusion affords more steady pain control than intermittent doses* – if the child "can't wait" for the next dose of opioid and pain scores remain above 5/10, consider changing to continuous infusion or adding a basal rate to the patient controlled analgesia

3. *Stage the wean of opioids* – begin with continuous infusion for severe pain and as pain becomes stable and controlled, reduce dose of infusion (not more than 25-50% daily), when at minimum hourly dose, change to around-the-clock intermittent dosing and then change to as needed dosing; this will shorten the duration of opioid use.

4. *Overlap continuous opioid use with around-the-clock acetaminophen or ibuprofen* – this establishes a steady state level of adjunctive pain medication before the child has to begin to rely on the drug for pain management and contributes to a shorter course of opioid, perhaps eliminating the need for outpatient opioid prescriptions.

5. *Match the delivery mode for continuous opioid to circumstance to allow optimal flexibility to control pain* – patient controlled analgesia/authorized agent controlled analgesia is ideal for pain that waxes and wanes such as that seen with cancer or sickle cell disease by allowing for continuous drug throughout the 24 hours but the ability to administer more when needed immediately upon demand; whereas epidural works best for controlling post-operative pain localized to the lower extremities. Non-parenteral formulations such as Transdermal fentanyl or sustained release oral opioids should be reserved to circumstances where the pain is severe and persistent such as with cancer pain.

6. *Do not be afraid to separate combination products and administer opioid and acetaminophen independently* – loss of convenience from a combination tablet/liquid is more than made up for with the added flexibility to schedule the acetaminophen throughout the 24 hours and titrate the opioid as needed; unnecessary periods of time when drug can't be given due to exceeded 24 hour acetaminophen dose are avoided as are acetaminophen overdoses.

7. *Persistent pain may be a sign of something not being right – look for its cause* – before dismissing pain as a lack of patient "tolerance" consider that an unanticipated source of pain may be recognizable and possibly eliminated.

8. *Opt for the least painful route of administration* – if a child perceives the pain medication is more painful than just suffering, they will refuse the medication and minimize their report of pain; avoid IM injections whenever possible.

Challenges of Opioid Use

Getting the drug into the child is the single biggest challenge of opioid use, with issues ranging from taste to ability to measure prescribed dose volume. The limitations posed by the solid oral dosage forms often preclude their use in younger patients as younger children have difficulty swallowing pills and will insist on a liquid formulation. Although oral liquids are available for most opioids, the taste or "yummy factor" may still make it difficult to ensure that the whole dose is retained. Table 12a.6 describes strategies to make oral drug administration to a child more successful. Intravenous doses are not immune to the difficulties in measuring appropriate dose volumes. This often results in further dilution of intravenous doses prior to administration, particularly in the neonates.

Developmental pharmacokinetics is an area that has been well studied (Kearns and Read 1989; Olkkola et al. 1995; Kearns et al. 2003) and should be taken into account in optimizing the pain-management plan. Although dosing recommendations have compensated for much pharmacokinetic variability, the practitioner may wish to apply age-specific monitoring. For example, time to peak concentration varies by age; hence one may wish to observe one age group more closely for sedation within the hour of administration, versus two to three hours after administration for another age group. Table 12a.7 details other examples of how developmental-pharmacokinetics principles can affect the pain-management plan. Adverse effects may also be different between the age groups due to the differences in pharmacodynamics or the maturity/presence of drug receptor sites.

Table12a.6 Strategies For More Successful Drug Administration

General Principles	Making oral liquids "yummier"
Be firm and consistent	Follow medicine with spoonful of sugar or chocolate
Avoid forcing the child to swallow	Mix in juice or chocolate milk (use caution as altered taste of these foods may lead to future food avoidance)
Avoid references to candy or treats	Hide in jello or peanut butter
Let them do it themselves	Stagger the dose (offer brief breaks)
Set the mood	Mix in pudding, ice cream or applesauce
Explain why it is necessary	Chill it
Make it a game of song	Have child suck on a popsicle or ice cube before and after dose to numb tongue
Be consistent about when and where	"Rinse" afterwards (but not with water)
Offer choices (e.g. apple or orange juice)	
Bribes and negotiation are permissible	

Table 12a.7 Developmental Pharmacokinetics Impact on Pain Management in Children

Developmental Pharmacokinetics Principles	Impact on Opioid Prescribing
1. Neonates have increased percutaneous absorption due to thinner stratum corneum layers of the skin, increased water content within the dermis and a higher ratio of surface area to body weight	Use of transdermal opioid patches is not first line practice for neonates and young infants.
2. Neonates have enhanced permeability into the blood brain barrier which will persist until nearly a year of age	Neonates and young infants are prone to increased sedation and other neurological adverse events with opioids and need to be monitored closely.
3. Neonates have reduced plasma protein binding due to reduced amount of protein, fewer binding sites on the available proteins and reduced binding affinity	Neonates and young infants are prone to increased sedation and other neurological adverse events with opioids and need to be monitored closely.
4. Adipose tissue composition and mass of tissue available for binding varies with age – neonates are 75% water composition compared to adults who are 60%	Most opioids are not strongly lipophilic with the exception of fentanyl. Fentanyl is more likely to accumulate within the body as the child matures and becomes larger – leaving them vulnerable for drug accumulation and prolonged adverse effects.
4 All enzymes are present at birth. Specific enzymes will mature at variable rates that are unique to each patient. It is generally believed that between 2-6 months of age the rate of activity jumps to 2-6 times the rate of adults until 2-3 years of age when they start to gradually decline, reaching adult levels of function around 8-10 years of age	Young children will require more drug per kilogram of weight compared to adolescents or adults, as opioids are predominately metabolized. Genotype will determine if child is slow or fast metabolizer of codeine/hydrocodone – children are more vulnerable to higher levels of morphine/hydromorphone if fast metabolizer.
5. Renal elimination is reduced in the first year as proximal tubules are small relative to corresponding glomeruli at birth; the extremely premature at birth may take two years to mature kidneys to adult functionality	A small portion of opioids are eliminated unchanged in the urine – with reduce kidney function, the clearance of these drugs is reduced. Considering the increased complimentary liver function, this should have little impact on how the practitioner cares for the patient.

Monitoring

Morphine side effects have been known to include sedation, pruritus, urinary retention, nausea and vomiting, respiratory depression, constipation, myoclonic movements, and dependence (both physical and psychological). Prescribing of opioids coupled with a bowel regimen may go far in preventing constipation. Nausea and vomiting may be minimized by administration of the oral opioid with food and optimization of adjunctive analgesics to allow for opioid dose reduction.

Severe respiratory depression needing treatment is rarely described, even after intrathecal administration, but respiratory depression can persist for several hours and its onset may be delayed for hours after administration (Kart et al. 1997). Despite the barrier of nursing workload, a monitoring guideline for intravenous morphine will improve early detection of respiratory depression and oversedation. A study conducted in the Children's Hospital of Eastern Ontario (Ellis et al. 2011) demonstrated that a monitoring protocol for intravenous morphine will identify incidents otherwise undetected, even with suboptimal adherence to the protocol. The consideration of continuous cardiopulmonary monitoring or perhaps end tidal CO_2 of the young child receiving opioids (continuous or high dose oral) is as yet difficult to implement due to resource limitations.

Conclusion

Despite it being nearly a decade into the twenty-first century, practitioners still fail to provide adequate pain management to children (Walco et al. 1994; Morton 2007). The reasons for this are multifactorial, but often lead back to the inexperience of the practitioner. Implementation of standardized pain-management guidelines at your institution or in your practice can have the most significant impact on improving pain management for the child in your care (Mackenzie 2006).

As is often stated, more clinical studies need to be conducted to address the numerous unresolved issues relating to pediatric pain management. Fortunately, consensus on aspects of pediatric analgesic trial design was reached at a recent US Food and Drug Administration sponsored scientific workshop. Specifics relating to outcome measures for acute and chronic pain, patient population selection and study design concepts were put forth as provisional recommendations for future study design. Pediatric analgesic trials are challenging and necessitate a delicate balance between scientific, ethical and practical concerns. As established clinical trials consortia evolve much sought after information relating to pediatric analgesia should emerge (Berde et al. 2012).

References

American Academy of Pediatrics (AAP). Committee on Psychosocial Aspects of Child and Family Health; Task Force on Pain in Infants, Children, and Adolescents. The assessment and management of acute pain in infants, children and adolescents. *Pediatrics.* 2001;108(3):793–797.

Anand KJ, Carr DB. The neuroanatomy, neurophysiology and neurochemistry of pain, stress and analgesia in newborns and children. *Pediatr Clin North Am.* 1989;36(4):795–822.

Anand KJ, Aranda JV, Berde CB, et al. Summary proceedings from the neonatal pain-control group. *Pediatrics.* 2006;117(3 Pt 2):S9–S22.

Berde CB, Sethna NF. Analgesics for the treatment of pain in children. *NEJM.* 2002;347(14):1094–1103.

Berde CB, Walco GA, Krane EJ, et al. Pediatric analgesic clinical trial designs, measures, and extrapolation: report of an FDA scientific workshop. *Pediatrics.* 2012;129(2):354–364.

Boyle CA, Boulet S, Schieve LA, et al. Trends in the prevalence of developmental disabilities in US children, 1997–2008. *Pediatrics.* 2011;27(6):1034–1042.

Ciszkowski C. Codeine, Ultrarapid-Metabolism Genotype, and Postopreative Death. *NEJM.* 2009;361(8):827.

Clark E, Plint AC, Correll R, Gaboury I, Passi B. A randomized, controlled trial of acetaminophen, ibuprofen, and codeine for acute pain relief in children with musculoskeletal trauma. *Pediatrics.* 2007;119(3): 460–467.

Ellis J, Martelli B, Lamontagne, et al. Improved practices for safe administration of intravenous bolus morphine in a pediatric setting. *Pain Manag Nurs.* 2011;12(3):146–153.

Fitzgerald M, Millard C, McIntosh N. Cutaneous hypersensitivity following peripheral tissue damage in newborn infants and its reversal with topical anesthesia. *Pain.* 1989;39(1):31–36.

Giannakoulopoulos X, Sepulveda W, Kourtis P, et al. Fetal plasma cortisol and beta-endorphin response to intrauterine needling. *Lancet.* 1994;344(8915):77–81.

Greco C, Berde C. Pain management for the hospitalized pediatric patient. *Pediatr Clin North Am.* 2005;52(4):995–1027.

Herr K, Coyne PJ, Key T, et al. Pain assessment in the nonverbal patient: position statement with clinical practice recommendations. *Pain Manage Nurs.* 2006;7(2):44–52.

Hummel P, Puchalski M. N-PASS: *Neonatal Pain, Agitation, & Sedation Scale—Scoring Criteria.* N-PASS website. www.n-pass.com/scoring_criteria.html. n.d. Accessed July 3, 2007.

Kart T, Christrup Lona L, Rasmussen M. Recommended use of morphine in neonates, infants and children based on a literature review: Part 2—Clinical use. *Paediatr Anesth.* 1997;7(2):93–101.

Kearns GL, Reed MD. Clinical pharmacokinetics in infants and children. A reappraisal. *Clin Pharmacokinet.* 1989;17(1):29–67.

Kearns GL, Bel-Rahman SM, Alander SW, et al. Developmental pharmacology—drug disposition, action and therapy in infants and children. *NEJM.* 2003;349(12):1157–1167.

Koren G, Cairns J, Chitayat D, Gaedigk A, Leeder S. Pharmacogenetics of morphine poisoning in a breastfed neonate of a codeine-prescribed mother. *Lancet.* 2006;368(9536):704.

Krechel SW, Bildner J. CRIES: A new neonatal postoperative pain measurement score. Initial testing of validity and reliability. *Paediatr Anesth.* 1995;5(1):53–61.

Mackenzie A. Guideline statements on the management of procedure-related pain in neonates, children and adolescents. *J Pediatr Child Health.* 2006;(42):14–15.

Madadi P, Ross CJ, Hayden MR, et al. Pharmacogenetics of neonatal opioid toxicity following maternal use of codeine during breastfeeding: a case-control study. *Clin Pharm Ther.* 2009;85(1):31–35.

Madadi P, Hildebrandt D, Gong IY, et al. Fatal hydrocodone overdose in a child: pharmacogenetics and drug interations. *Pediatrics.* 2010;126(4):e986–e989.

Madadi P, Ciszkowski C, Gaedigk A, et al. Genetic transmission of cytochrome P450 2D6 (CYP2D6) ultrrapid metabolism: implications for breastfeeding women taking codeine. *Curr Drug Saf.* 2011;6(1):36–39.

Manworren RC, Hynan LS. Clinical validation of FLACC: preverbal patient pain scale. *Pediatr Nurs.* 2003;29(2):140–146.

Merkel SI, Voepel-Lewis T, Shayevitz JR, et al. The FLACC: a behavioral scale for scoring postoperative pain in young children. *Pediatr Nurs.* 1997;23(3):293–297.

Michel E, Anderson BJ, Zernikow B. Buprenorphine TTS for children – a review of the drug's clinical pharmacology. *Paediatr Anesth.* 2011;21(3):280–290.

Mitchell AL, Smith HS. Applying partially occluded fentanyl transdermal patches to manage pain in pediatric patients. *J Opioid Manag.* 2010;6(4):290–294.

Morton NS. Management of postoperative pain in children. *Arch Dis Child Educ Pract.* 2007;92(1):ep14–ep19.

Olkkola KT, Hamunen K, Maunuksela E-L. Clinical pharmacokinetics and pharmacodynamics of opioid analgesics in infants and children. *Clin Pharmacokinet.* 1995;28(5):385–404.

Perreault T, Fraser-Askin D, Liston R, et al. Pain in the neonate. *Paediatr Child Health.* 1997;2(3):201–209.

Savedra MC, Holzemer WL, Tesler MD, et al. Assessment of postoperation pain in children and adolescents using the Adolescent Pediatric Pain Tool. *Nurs Res.* 1993;42(1):5–9.

Sutters KA, Miaskowski C, Holdridge-Zeuner D, et al. A randomized clinical trial of the effectiveness of a scheduled oral analgesic dosing regimen for the management of postoperative pain in children following tonsillectomy. *Pain.* 2004;110(1–2):49–55.

Tremlett M, Anderson BJ. Pro-con debate: is codeine a drug that still has a useful role in pediatric practice? *Paediatr Anesth.* 2010;20(2):183–194.

Valkenburg AJ, van Dijk M, de Klein A, vander Anker VN, Tibboel D. Pain management in intellectually disabled children: assessment, treatment and translational research. *Dev Disabil Res Rev.* 2010;16(3):248–257.

Voronov P, Przybylo HJ, Jagannathan N. Case Report Apnea in a child after oral codeine: a genetic variant – an ultra-rapid metabolizer. *Paediatr Anesth.* 2007;17(7):684–687

Walco GA, Cassidy RC, Schechter NL. Pain, hurt, and harm: the ethics of pain control in infants and children. *NEJM* 1994;331(8):541–544.

Willis MH, Merkel SI, Voepel-Lewis T, Malviya S. FLACC Behavioral Pain Assessment Scale: a comparison with the child's self-report. *Pediatr Nurs.* 2003;29(3):195–198.

Wolf AR, Jackman L. Analgesia and sedation after pediatric cardiac surgery. *Paediatr Anesth.* 2011:21(5):567–576.

Zernikow B, Lindena G. Long-acting morphine for pain control in paediatric oncology. *Med Pediatr Oncol.* 2001;36(4):451–458.

Zernikow B, Michel E, Anderson B. Transdermal fentanyl in childhood and adolescence: a comprehensive literature review. *J Pain* 2007;8(3):187–207.

Chapter 12b

Special Populations: Geriatric

Gary McCleane

Opioids and the Elderly Patient

In the year 2000 there were more than 400 million people aged 65 or over in the world (roughly 37 million in the United States, comprising 13% of the population); this number is expected to increase to 1.5 billion by the year 2050. This represents a fourfold increase, compared to a 50% increase in the world population as a whole. By 2030, it is expected that one in five Americans will be over the age of 66. Of these people, around 25% will be above age 80 (Lunenfeld 2002). Unfortunately, many of the studies providing evidence-based approaches have been based on studies conducted in younger populations (less than 80 years). Therefore, age-specific evidence-based guidelines on how to treat those persons 80 years and older are not based on a high number of large well-designed robust age-specific (over 80 years) studies. It is currently accepted that the incidence of acute pain is broadly similar throughout all age groups, while pain of a more chronic nature increases in incidence up to the seventh decade (Corran et al. 1997; Helme and Gibson 2001). This, along with the increased incidence of malignancy with advancing age, increases the likelihood that these elderly patients may require pain relief, and that in many instances consideration may need to be given to the use of opioids. The issue, therefore, is whether we can prescribe opioid analgesics to the elderly patient in the same fashion as we would utilize this class of drug in patients of less advanced years, or whether special considerations exist.

Effect of Age on Animal Pain Models

In aged animals there is a loss of myelinated and unmyelinated fibers, with at least some of this decrease in myelin being a result of decreased expression of the major myelin proteins. In addition, axonal atrophy is more commonly observed with advancing age and decreases in endoneural blood flow. When regeneration of damaged neurons occurs, these regenerated fibers have a smaller number of terminal and collateral synapses (Khalil et al. 1984; Verdu et al. 2000).

In addition to these changes, other observations in aged animals include the following:

- Increased mRNA content of tyrosine and galanin in dorsal root ganglia neurons (Bergman et al. 1996);
- Decreased cellular content of calcitonin-gene-related peptide and substance P (Cruce et al. 2001);
- Decreased encoding for high-affinity tyrosine receptors (TrkA, TrkB, and TrkC) in dorsal root ganglia neurons;
- A progressive loss of serotonergic and noradrenergic neurons in the superficial lamina of the spinal dorsal horn;
- Decreased neurotransmitter content at the supraspinal level (Laporte et al. 1996; Iwata et al. 2002);
- Decreased metabolic turnover in cerebral cortex, midbrain, and brainstem (Barili et al. 1998);
- Increased size of receptive-field area of wide-dynamic-range neurons; and
- Decreased receptive field of low-threshold neurons.

When peripheral nerve injury is induced in rats, aged rats develop hyperalgesia and tactile allodynia more slowly than younger rats. Younger rats appear to recover from the mechanical allodynia produced by paw incision more quickly than older rats (Jourdan et al. 2000). It has also been observed that paw-withdrawal latency is significantly shorter in aged as compared to adult rats when heat stimulation is applied (Gagliese and Melzack 2000; Ririe et al. 2003). It is likely, therefore, that advancing age will be accompanied by alterations in the perception and modulation of pain and that pharmacologic interventions will produce different results in older versus younger subjects.

Effect of Age on Human Experimental Pain

The two major issues to be considered in terms of human experimental pain are pain threshold and tolerance. When all available evidence is considered, there appears to be definite evidence that pain threshold increases with advances in age, while pain tolerance decreases (Gibson et al. 1994; Harkins 1996; Harkins et al. 1996; Heft et al. 1996; Gibson and Helme 2001).

When, for example, an intraesophageal balloon is dilated in healthy young and healthy older adults and the volume required to produce pain is measured, that volume is significantly higher in older subjects. Indeed, some fail to report pain even on maximal dilation (Lasch et al. 1997). Clinically, this failure to appreciate distension in a hollow internal space may mean that warning signs of a constrictive and obstructing lesion could be absent and time to clinical presentation much delayed.

Pharmacologic Differences in the Elderly Patient

A number of factors may affect drug absorption in elderly patients, including the following:

- Decreased gastrointestinal blood flow,
- Slowed intestinal transit (a function of age and concomitant medications),
- Dermal thinning,
- Decreased saliva production, and
- Muscle and fat atrophy.

Drug distribution may be influenced by a relative increase in fat mass and a decrease in muscle mass, when body water may also be reduced (Bressler and Bahl 2003). Water-soluble drugs such as morphine are less efficiently distributed, and higher plasma concentrations are obtained, in older than in younger subjects. With the relative increase in body fat—and hence volume of distribution—with increased age, lipophilic drugs such as fentanyl may be sequestered in the fat, thus prolonging the drug's duration of action (Noble 2003).

In terms of drug elimination, liver and kidney function decreases with age; therefore, drugs are less efficiently cleared from the body in older persons.

Opioid analgesics undergo significant first-pass metabolism during passage from the gastrointestinal tract into the liver. In the elderly hepatic function may be decreased, along with cardiac output; therefore, drug metabolism may be slowed, leading to higher peak plasma concentrations. Renal blood flow decreases by approximately 1% per annum after the age of 50, so all elderly patients should be considered to have reduced renal function. Morphine is metabolized to morphine-6-glucuronide, a renally excreted compound derived from phase II conjugation of morphine that is responsible for a significant proportion of the analgesic effect of morphine. Therefore, renal impairment will prolong the effect of morphine and may produce toxicity.

From a pharmacodynamic perspective, opioid action may differ between adults and the elderly. Studies in rats have shown that elderly animals have fewer μ and k opioid receptors, while the number of d opioid receptors remains unchanged. In terms of pharmacokinetics and pharmacodynamics, then, elderly patients may handle opioid analgesics differently from younger subjects, and these influences should be borne in mind when consideration is given to opioid use in those of advanced years (Turnheim 2003).

Assessment of Pain in Older Persons

Proper assessment of pain in older persons is key to appropriate clinical decision making, optimal care, and the determination of treatment outcomes. The American Geriatrics Society Panel on Persistent Pain in Older Persons (American Geriatrics Society 2002), the American Medical Director Association (AMDA 2003), and, more recently, an interdisciplinary expert consensus (Hadjistavropoulos et al. 2007) have addressed issues surrounding the assessment of pain in older persons. A comprehensive assessment of pain

Table 12b-1 Selected Measures to Assess Pain in Older Persons
Self-report Assessment of Pain Intensity
Numeric Rating Scale (NRS)
Verbal Descriptors Scale (VDS) or Verbal Rating Scale (VRS)
21-point Box Scale
Observational Assessment Tools for People with Severe Dementia
Pain Assessment Checklist for Seniors with Limited Ability to Communicate (PACSLAC)
The DOLOPLUS-2
Functional Assessment
Functional Status Index (FSI)
Human Activity Profile (HAP)
Physical Performance Test
Emotional Function
Depression
Geriatric Depression Scale (GDS)
Anxiety
Beck Anxiety Inventory (BAI)
Pain Related Anxiety
Pain Anxiety Symptom Scale (PASS)
Modified from Hadjistravopoulos, 2007

entails identification of physical, emotional, cognitive, and communicative disturbances, including the assessment of functional limitations (e.g., impairment in the performance of activities of daily living, as well as reduced mobility, sleep, and appetite), psychosocial function (e.g., mood, interpersonal interactions, beliefs about pain and its meaning, fear of pain-related activity), and cognitive function (e.g., dementia, delirium) (Hadjistavropoulos et al. 2007).

It does seem that both the estimation of pain and the amount of opioids used in its treatment may be less in older patients than younger patients, at least in an emergency department situation (Hwang et al. 2010).

Hadjistavropoulos et al. (2007) have recommended a brief assessment battery consisting of the administration of two instruments: the Brief Pain Inventory (Cleeland and Ryan 1994) and the short-form McGill Pain Questionnaire (Melzack 1987). When time permits or clinical needs dictate a more comprehensive evaluation of specific domains (e.g., mood, functional ability), Hadjistavropoulos et al. have suggested an additional menu of instruments that can be utilized in various domains and circumstances (Table 12b.1).

Opioid Use in Older Persons

Regardless of issues that may influence opioid use in elderly patients, these agents are extensively used. A study of 10,372 nursing home residents who had persistent pain found that 18.9% were taking short-acting opioids, while 3.3%

were taking long-acting opioids. Interestingly, there was an increased association between opioid use and depression and a decreased association with opioid use and the risk of falls (Won et al. 2006). In contrast, a large study undertaken in Denmark found that when 124,655 patients who had suffered a fracture were compared with 373,962 controls from the background population, morphine and other opiates were taken by 8.0% of the fracture subjects and by only 3.2% of the control population. The odds ratios for sustaining a fracture were 1.47 with morphine, 2.23 with fentanyl, 1.39 with methadone, 1.36 with oxycodone, 1.54 with tramadol, 1.16 with codeine, and 0.86 with buprenorphine.

The risk may be maximal in the first two weeks after initiation of the opioids with short acting opioids being a greater risk factor than longer acting opioids (Miller et al 2011). Buckeridge and colleagues (2010) report that of 403,339 subjects over the age of 65, opioids increased the risk of injury and that this risk was greatest in those using codeine combinations.

When analgesia is required in an elderly patient, a number of factors must influence the choice of pain relief, including the following:

- With advancing age, general health often declines; therefore, the opioid chosen may be absorbed, metabolized, and/or excreted in a different manner than in younger subjects.
- There is an increased likelihood of concomitant drug use in older persons, and thus the risks of drug–drug interactions are also increased.
- There is a greater likelihood that the older patient will be living alone; therefore, institution of any new drug may cause side effects that the patient may have to cope with alone and unobserved. (It may be prudent to suggest that the older person starting on opioids stay with another person during the initial titration period.)
- The chances that the older patient will have cognitive impairment are increased; therefore, he or she may misunderstand dosing instructions and take a prescribed drug inappropriately (Manfredi et al. 2003). Furthermore, an older person may forget having taken an opioid dose and thus take more than one. Opioids should be used in elderly patients at risk of delirium with caution because of the risk of it being initiated or exacerbated (Clegg and Young 2011).
- Sensory loss may mean that written or verbal instructions about use are not picked up, leading to the drug being taken inappropriately.
- The incidence of painless cardiac ischemia (or, for example, painless peritonitis) increases with age, and may be further increased and compounded by an opioid prescription.
- The risk of side effects associated with analgesic use is increased in the elderly.

When a decision to employ analgesia is made, the aim of treatment must be to improve quality of life. This does not necessarily equate with total pain relief. Many patients are more content with partial pain relief in the absence of side effects than they are with total pain relief with troublesome side effects. Furthermore, there may be a difference between what is proven to be of value in terms of pain relief in scientific studies and what is in the patient's best interest. For example, it is accepted that opioids for severe pain can reduce the pain of postherpetic neuralgia. That does not mean that they are the best initial choice for a particular patient, as the opioid for severe pain may cause or worsen cognitive impairment, constipation, nausea, or unsteadiness.

Institution of Opioid Therapy

A variety of opioid analgesics can be chosen from to treat persistent pain in older persons (Table 12b.2). Rational selection of a particular opioid for a particular older person is dependent on multiple factors, including the pattern and intensity of the patient's pain, previous responses to opioid therapy, adherence to dosing regimens, routes of administration, associated comorbidities, associated symptoms, preexisting organ impairment, convenience (for both patient and caregiver), and cost (Hanks and Cherny 1998; Fine 2004).

As with any pharmacologic treatment, the aim and possible consequences of opioid therapy must be considered prior to its initiation. These consequences may be positive in that the patient gets pain relief or, more importantly, experiences an improvement in quality of life; or they may be negative, in that

Table 12b-2 Opioids for the Treatment of Persistent Pain in Older Persons

Opioid	Starting Dose
Short-Acting	
Tramadol	25 mg q6h
Tramadol (37.5 mg)/APAP (325 mg)	37.5 mg q6h
Hydrocodone (5 mg)/APAP (325 mg)	5 mg q6h
Oxycodone IR	5 mg q6h
Morphine sulfate IR oral liquid	2.5 mg–10 mg q4h
Oxymorphone IR	5 mg q6h
Hydromorphone IR	2 mg q6h
Tapentadol IR	50 mg q8h
Long-Acting	
Oxycodone sustained release	10 mg q12h
Morphine sustained release	15 mg–20 mg q12h
Transdermal Fentanyl	12 mcg/h–25 mcg/h q72h
Methadone	2.5–5 mg q12h
Oxymorphone ER	5 mg q12h
Transdermal Buprenorphine	5 mcg/h q7d
Tramadol ER (Ultram® ER, Ryzolt™)	100 mg once daily
Tapentadol ER	50 mg once daily
Hydromorphone ER (Exalgo™)	8 mg once daily

Modified from Hadjistravopoulos, 2007

unwanted side effects result. When relief is produced but is complicated by side effects, the clinician must consider whether, on balance, the therapy is of sufficient value to justify its continued use.

In 2009, the American Geriatrics Society (AGS) Panel on the Pharmacological Management of Persistent Pain in Older Persons updated their original 1998 and 2002 guidelines and noted that since therapy with NSAIDs and COX-2 inhibitors may result in serious and life-threatening gastrointestinal and cardiovascular adverse events or gastrointestinal bleeding, clinicians choosing analgesic therapy for persistent pain have shifted attention to opioids, especially for older patients who may be at particular risk for NSAID-related adverse effects (Singh et al. 2006; American Geriatrics Society 2009; Antman et al. 2007). They stated that nonselective NSAIDs and COX-2 selective inhibitors may be considered rarely, and with extreme caution, in highly selected individuals (high quality of evidence, strong recommendation) (American Geriatrics Society 2009). Controlled trials have established the efficacy of various opioids in the treatment of persistent pain associated with musculoskeletal conditions, including osteoarthritis (Caldwell et al. 1999) and low back pain (Hale et al. 1999; Rauck et al. 2006), and in the management of several neuropathic pain conditions, such as diabetic peripheral neuropathy and postherpetic neuralgia (Dworkin et al. 2007). The AGS panel stated that "all patients with moderate to severe pain, pain-related functional impairment, or diminished quality of life due to pain should be considered for opioid therapy" (low quality of evidence, strong recommendation) (American Geriatrics Society 2009). If chronic opioid therapy is initiated in older persons, it should be done cautiously and monitored closely (Figure 12b-1).

There is no doubt that opioids are useful pain relievers in patients of all ages. Unfortunately, it is also without doubt that their use may be complicated by adverse effects (Gloth 2000). Some of the complications of opioids are obvious and predictable: nausea and constipation are not uncommon, and prophylactic measures should be taken to minimize the risk of their occurrence; somnolence can be a short-term issue when the dose is increased. But other more insidious side effects can also occur. For example, paradoxical pain—that is, pain produced by and consequent to sustained opioid use—has been described (Heger et al. 1990; De Cono et al. 1991; Sjogren et al. 1994; Ossipov et al. 2003), and hormonal and endocrine upset can also occur with prolonged opioid use (Abs et al. 2000). The features of these last two complications will not necessarily be attributed by either patient or physician to opioid consumption.

Overall, there is a responsibility for the physician initiating treatment in the elderly patient to be absolutely clear regarding the goals of therapy, to be sure that the benefits of therapy are actively considered after initiation of treatment, and to discontinue the opioid if the goals of therapy are not achieved.

The following checklist may be helpful prior to and during opioid use:

1. Is an opioid for severe pain the best form of treatment available for the presenting pain?
2. Will the opioid interact in a negative fashion with any concomitantly administered medication?

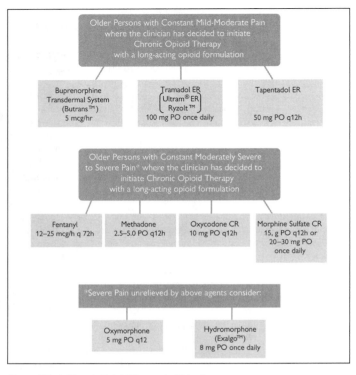

Figure 12b-1 Chronic Opioid Therapy in Older Persons

3. Can other therapeutic agents be added to minimize the dose of opioid required to achieve analgesia?
4. Can other agents be added to minimize the risk of analgesic tolerance?
5. Will other therapeutic agents (e.g., laxatives, antiemetics) be given to reduce the risk of side effects?
6. Which route of administration is most appropriate?
7. At what dose will the opioid be initiated?
8. What is the expected duration of treatment?
9. Will rules be imposed that limit the rate of dose escalation?
10. Will there be a limit to the dose of the opioid used?
11. How will the effect of treatment be measured?
12. After what period of time will the effect of treatment be assessed?
13. Will the therapy be kept under long-term review?

Conclusion

There can be no doubt that opioids, both for mild to moderate pain and for severe pain, are efficacious in the treatment of a broad range of pain conditions. It is also certain that they are not universally effective; therefore, it is most important that opioid therapy not be seen as the only option for pain control in any patient, but rather as one of a number of options whose merits and weaknesses are all assessed prior to the construction of a treatment plan.

A number of factors should influence the choice of opioid treatment in elderly patients. Because of pharmacokinetic and pharmacodynamic differences, the elderly patient may not handle an opioid in the same way as an individual of less advanced age. An older person may be taking a number of other medications, and may have other health problems. Furthermore, older people may live alone or have sensory impairments that could hinder their understanding of and compliance with treatment protocols. For these reasons, if opioid therapy is to be considered, careful thought should be given to the potential positive and negative consequences of treatment and, on an intermittent basis, to the wisdom of continued treatment. However, although caution should be used, there is certainly a place in the pain practitioner's armamentarium for the use of opioids in treating severe, persistent pain in older persons.

References

Abs R, Verhelst J, Maeyaert J, et al. Endocrine consequences of long-term intrathecal administration of opioids. *J Clin Endocrinol Metab.* 2000;85(6):2215–2222.

American Medical Directors Association (AMDA). *Pain Management in the Long Term Care Setting: Clinical Practice Guideline.* Rev. ed. Columbia, MD: AMDA, 2003.

American Geriatrics Society. Panel on Persistent Pain in Older Persons. Clinical practice guidelines: the management of persistent pain in older persons. *J Am Geriatr Soc.* 2002;50:S205–S224.

American Geriatrics SocietyPanel on Pharmacological Management of Persistent Pain in Older Persons. Pharmacological management of persistent pain in older persons. *J Am Geriatr Soc.* 2009;57(8):1331–1346.

Antman EM, Bennett JS, Daugherty A, et al. Use of nonsteroidal anti-inflammatory drugs: an update for clinicians: a scientific statement from the American Heart Association. *Circulation.* 2007;115(12):1634–1642.

Barili P, De Carolis G, Zaccheo D, et al. Sensitivity to ageing of the limbic dopaminergic system: a review. *Mech Ageing Dev.* 1998;106(1–2):57–92.

Bergman E, Johnson H, Zhang X, et al. Neuropeptides and neurotrophin receptor mRNAs in primary sensory neurons of aged rats. *J Comp Neurol.* 1996; 375(2)303–319.

Bressler R, Bahl JJ. Principles of drug therapy for the elderly patient. *Mayo Clin Proc.* 2003;78(12):1564–1577.

Buckeridge D, Huang A, Hanley J et al. Risk of injury associated with opioids use in older adults. *J Am Geriatr Soc* 2010;58(9):1664–1670.

Caldwell JR, Hale ME, Boyd RE, et al. Treatment of osteoarthritis pain with controlled release oxycodone or fixed combination oxycodone plus acetaminophen added to nonsteroidal antiinflammatory drugs: A double blind, randomized, multicenter, placebo controlled trial. *J Rheumatol.* 1999;26(4):862–869.

Chipnail JT, Tait RC. Pain assessment in cognitively impaired and unimpaired older adults: a comparison of four scales. *Pain.* 2001;92(1–2):173–186.

Cleeland CS, Ryan KM. Pain assessment: global use of the Brief Pain Inventory. *Ann Acad Med Singapore.* 1994;23(2):129–138.

Clegg A, Young J. Which medications to avoid in people at risk of delirium: a systematic review. *Age Ageing* 2011;40(1): 23–29.

Corran TM, Farrell MJ, Helme RD, et al. The classification of patients with chronic pain: age as a contributing factor. *Clin J Pain.* 1997;13(3):207–214.

Cruce WL, Lovell JA, Crisp T, et al. Effect of aging on the substance P receptor, NK-1, in the spinal cord in rats with peripheral nerve injury. Somatosens Mot Res. 2001;18(1):66–75.

De Cono F, Caraceni A, Martini C, et al. Hyperalgesia and myoclonus with intrathecal infusion of high-dose morphine. *Pain.* 1991;47(3):337–339.

Dworkin RH, O'Connor AB, Backonja M, et al. Pharmacologic management of neuropathic pain: Evidence-based recommendations. *Pain.* 2007;132(3):237–251.

Fine PG. Pharmacological management of persistent pain in older patients. *Clin J Pain.* 2004;20(4):220–226.

Gagliese L, Melzack R. Age differences in nociception and pain behaviour in the rat. *Neurosci Biobehav Rev.* 2000;24(8):843–854.

Gibson SJ, Helme RD. Age related differences in pain perception and report. *Clin Geriatr Med.* 2001;17(3):433–456.

Gibson SJ, Katz B, Corran TM, et al. Pain in older persons. *Disabil Rehabil.* 1994;16(3):127–139.

Gloth FM. Geriatric pain: factors that limit pain relief and increase complications. *Geriatrics.* 2000;55(10):51–54.

Hadjistavropoulos T, Heer K, Turk D, et al. An interdisciplinary expert consensus statement on assessment of pain in older persons. *Clin J Pain.* 2007;23(Suppl 1):S1–S43.

Hale ME, Fleischmann R, Salzman R, et al. Efficacy and safety of controlled release versus immediate-release oxycodone: Randomized, double-blind evaluation in patients with chronic back pain. *Clin J Pain.* 1999;15(3):179–183.

Hanks G, Cherny N. Opioid analgesic therapy. In Doyle D, Hanks G, McDonald N, eds. *Oxford Textbook of Palliative Medicine.* 2nd ed. Oxford: Oxford University Press, 1998; 331–355.

Harkins SW, Davis MD, Bush FM, et al. Suppression of first pain and slow temporal summation of second pain related to age. *J Gerontol A Biol Sci Med Sci.* 1996;51(5):260–265.

Harkins SW. Geriatric pain: pain perceptions in the old. Clin Geriatr Med. 1996;12(3):435–459.

Heft MW, Cooper BY, O'Brien KK, et al. Aging effects on the perception of noxious and non-noxious thermal stimuli applied to the face. *Aging.* 1996;8(1):35–41.

Heger S, Maier C, Otter K, et al. Morphine induced allodynia in a child with brain tumor. *Br Med J.* 1990;319(7210):627–629.

Helme RD, Gibson SJ. The epidemiology of pain in elderly people. *Clin Geriatr Med.* 2001;17(3):417–431.

Hwang U, Richardson LD, Harris B, Morrison R. The quality of emergency department pain are for older adult patients. *J Am Geriatr Soc* 2010;58(11):212–218

Iwata K, Fukuoka T, Kondo E, et al. Plastic changes in nociceptive transmission of the rat spinal cord with advancing age. *J Neurophysiol.* 2002;87(2)1086–1093.

Jourdan D, Boghossian S, Alloui A, et al. Age related changes in nociception and the effect of morphine in the Lou rat. *Eur J Pain.* 2000;4(3):291–300.

Khalil Z, Ralevic V, Bassirat M, et al. Effects of ageing on sensory nerve function in rat skin. *Brain Res.* 1984;641(2):265–272.

Laporte AM, Doyen C, Nevo IT. Autoradiographic mapping of serotonin 5HT1A, 5HT1D, 5HT2A and 5HT3 receptors in the aged human spinal cord. *J Chem Neuroanat.* 1996;11(1):67–75.

Lasch H, Castell DO, Castell JA. Evidence for diminished visceral pain with aging: studies using graded intraesophageal balloon distension. *Am J Physiol.* 1997;272(1 Pt 1):G1–G3.

Lunenfeld B. The ageing male: demographics and challenges. World J Urol. 2002;20(1):11–16.

Manfredi PL, Breuer B, Meier DE, et al. Pain assessment in elderly patients with severe dementia. *J Pain Symptom Manage.* 2003;25(1):48–52.

Melzack R. The short-form McGill Pain Questionnaire. *Pain.* 1987;30(2):191–197.

Miller M, Stürmer T, Azrael D, Levin R, Solomon D. Opioid analgesics and the risk of fractures in older adults with arthritis. *J Am Geriatr Soc* 2011;59(3):430–438.

Noble RE. Drug therapy in the elderly. *Metabolism.* 2003;52(10 Suppl 2):27–30.

Ossipov MH, Lai J, Vanderah TW, et al. Induction of pain facilitation by sustained opioid exposure: relationship to opioid antinociceptive tolerance. *Life Sci.* 2003;73(6):783–800.

Rauck RL, Bookbinder SA, Bunker TR, et al. The ACTION study: A randomized, open-label, multicenter trial comparing once-a-day extended-release morphine sulfate capsules (AVINZA) to twice-a-day controlled-release oxycodone hydrochloride tablets (OxyContin) for the treatment of chronic, moderate to severe low back pain. *J Opioid Manage.* 2006;2(3):155–166.

Ririe DG, Vernon TL, Tobin JR, et al. Age-dependent responses to thermal hyperalgesia and mechanical allodynia in a rat model of acute postoperative pain. *Anesthesiology.* 2003;99(2):443–448.

Singh G, Wu O, Langhorne P, et al. Risk of acute myocardial infarction with nonselective non-steroidal anti-inflammatory drugs: A meta-analysis. *Arthritis Res Ther.* 2006;8(5):R153.

Sjogren P, Jensen N-K, Jensen TS. Disappearance of morphine induced hyperalgesia after discontinuing or substituting morphine with other opioid analgesics. *Pain.* 1994;59(2):313–316.

Turnheim K. When drug therapy gets old: pharmacokinetics and pharmacodynamics in the elderly. *Exp Gerontol.* 2003;38(8):843–853.

Verdú E, Ceballos D, Vilches JJ, et al. Influence of aging on peripheral nerve function and regeneration. *J Peripher Nerv Syst.* 2000;5(4):191–208.

Won A, Lapane KL, Vallow S. Long-term effects of analgesics in a population of elderly nursing home residents with persistent non-malignant pain. *J Gerontol A Biol Sci Med Sci.* 2006;61(2):165–169.

Yesavage JA, Brink TL, Rose TL, et al. Development and validation of a geriatric depression screening scale: a preliminary report. *J Psychiatr Res.* 1983;17(1):37–49.

Special Populations: Palliative Care

Lida Nabati and Janet L. Abrahm

Dame Cicely Saunders, who founded the modern hospice movement in the 1960s, coined the term "total pain," which embodies the notion that pain endured by those facing a life-limiting illness is multifaceted and can include psychological, physical, spiritual, and social elements (Saunders 1981). From this concept, a new subspecialty, palliative medicine, emerged. Pain poses a tremendous burden of suffering for those with serious illness and at the end of life, and relief of pain is an important goal for palliative care clinicians. Opioids are part of the standard of care for patients with cancer-related pain, pain at the end of life, and dyspnea at the end of life. In this chapter we will review unique issues related to opioids and pain management in palliative care patients.

Overview of Palliative Medicine

The Institute of Medicine reported in 1997 that the quality of end-of-life care in the United States suffered because of inadequate attention to it in medical school curricula and postgraduate medical training, as well as lack of adequate research funding (Field and Cassel 1997). Hospice and Palliative Medicine, an established and burgeoning subspecialty recognized in 2006 by the American Board of Medical Specialties, seeks to reverse these findings.

Palliative medicine includes clinical palliative care, education, and research. The National Consensus Project for Quality Palliative Care defines palliative care as "medical care provided by an interdisciplinary team, including the professions of medicine, nursing, social work, chaplaincy, counselling, nursing assistants and other health care professionals, focused on the relief of suffering and support for the best possible quality of life for patients facing serious life-threatening illness, and their families. It aims to identify and address the physical, psychological, spiritual and practical burdens of illness" (National Consensus Project 2009), and singled out communication skills, along with symptom assessment and management, as core components of the delivery of palliative care (National Consensus Project 2009; Tulsky 2005).

Palliative care supports patients' goals, whether focused on comfort or life-prolongation. Palliative care and hospice programs serve patients with cancer, congestive heart failure, chronic obstructive pulmonary disease, progressive neurodegenerative disease, and HIV/AIDS, as well as advanced renal and liver disease and other life-limiting illnesses. Palliative care services are available to patients at all stages of a life-limiting illness and can be delivered concurrently with disease-modifying therapy. A recent randomized trial showed improved survival for patients with advanced lung cancer who received palliative care services early in their diagnosis (Temel et al. 2010). In the United States, the population with potential to benefit from and eligible for hospice and/or palliative care is growing, owing to aging and increasing rates of chronic illness (Morrison and Meier 2004). Palliative care can continue to offer relief from suffering when disease-modifying or life-prolonging therapy can no longer be pursued.

Prevalence of Pain in the Palliative Care Population

While palliative care tends to a broad array of symptom management needs, expert management of pain is an important skill for palliative care providers across settings, especially for patients with cancer. On average, patients with advanced cancer report a median of six symptoms, with pain being the most common (Coyle et al. 1990). It is estimated that 60% to 90% of patients with advanced cancer experience pain (Coyle et al. 1990; Curtis et al. 1991; Levy 1996), and an investigation of prescribing practices in an outpatient palliative care team showed that morphine was the most commonly prescribed medication (Curtis and Walsh 1993). A qualitative study identified adequate pain and symptom control (comfort) as one of five domains of end-of-life care most valued by patients (Singer et al. 1999). It has been clearly shown, however, that pain is often undertreated in patients with cancer (Cleeland et al. 1994). For instance, the Institute of Medicine report on end-of-life care in the United States, which included data on patients with and without a cancer diagnosis, documented that undertreated pain causes needless suffering (Field and Cassel 1997).

Pain Management in Palliative Care

Management of pain in a palliative care patient begins with a thorough history and physical, with special attention given to assessing coping, psychosocial state, and the patient's goals of care. A thorough assessment of pain includes identifying nullifying or aggravating factors, a detailed description of the characteristics of the patient's pain, and reviews of any prior workup or previous therapeutic modalities used. Assessments in these patients must be individualized to the individual's goals of care. The burdens of any diagnostic workup or invasive treatment for a pain complaint must be weighed against the potential benefit to the patient. If the burden is too great, the initiation of empiric symptomatic treatment may be more appropriate. If possible, imaging studies should be obtained when they are likely to reveal a specific, reversible etiology for the pain; provide important prognostic information; or prevent an outcome that would severely diminish the patient's quality of life (e.g., an MRI to evaluate for spinal cord compression in a cancer patient with back pain).

While the etiology is being sought or if empiric therapy is chosen, the World Health Organization's analgesic ladder outlines a basic approach to cancer pain management including both opioid and nonopioid medications. Patients are also encouraged to use nonpharmacologic techniques such as heat, massage, relaxation, and meditation (Abrahm 2005). Interventional approaches such percutaneous injections of neurolytic substances and continuous infusion of spinal analgesics can also improve the quality of life of patients with pain refractory to more conventional therapies, though they are needed only in 5% or fewer patients (Sloan 2004). Radiation therapy offered as a single fraction can be very effective for managing painful bone metastases (Dy et al. 2008; Dy 2010). Back pain in a cancer patient can indicate spinal cord compression, and prompt evaluation and treatment is indicated to preserve neurologic function. Treatment should include corticosteroids and radiation therapy, though some patients may benefit from surgery to prolong their ambulatory status (Loblaw et al. 2005).

Common concerns related to managing pain at the end of life include fears that opioids hasten death. Opioids are used to treat dyspnea at the end of life as well as pain. While morphine is most commonly associated with treating patients at the end of life, the effect on relieving air hunger is felt to be an opioid class effect. While opioids do carry risk of respiratory depression, it is generally held that when opioid titrations are managed by skilled providers and target symptoms of pain or dyspnea, death is not in fact hastened (Morita et al. 2001). Respiratory depression from opioids is typically preceded by sedation, though patients with cardiorespiratory comorbidity or compromise may be more susceptible to experiencing respiratory depression in the absence of preceding sedation.

A common yet problematic practice for hospitalized patients at the end of life is to initiate a morphine infusion in a patient who has not previously reported pain. Orders are typically written for a broad range of doses (e.g., 0–10 or 1–100 mg morphine), with vague instructions to "titrate to comfort." This practice may worsen the patient's distress at the end of life. For example, a patient who is experiencing agitation due to delirium may be perceived to be in pain. Treating with opioids may worsen delirium and agitation when in fact the patient would benefit from treatment of any reversible etiologies and from neuroleptics.

Not all patients require continuous opioid infusions for control of pain or dyspnea. Many patients are able to achieve effective symptom control with intermittent dosing. For patients who need a continuous infusion, the top of the dose range should be no more than three times the lowest dose in the range (e.g., 2–6 mg), and any acute escalation of symptoms is best managed with opioid boluses for rapid relief. Increasing the rate of continuous opioid infusion will increase the opioid plasma level in several hours, but there is both the risk of overshooting the analgesic dose as well as failing to control escalating symptoms in a timely manner. Generally, titration of the continuous infusion rate need not occur more frequently than every eight hours, as this interval is sufficient to achieve steady state between titrations.

Tasks of Patients at the End of Life

Clinicians caring for patients with pain can help them and their families with spiritual or existential concerns that arise as their lives end. These concerns include deriving meaning from their lives, wondering whether they are loved by family and friends, asking for or giving forgiveness, and wondering how to say goodbye or thank you (Byock 1997). For some patients and families, discussing "the five things" ("forgive me; I forgive you; thank you; I love you; and goodbye") together will bring healing and closure (Byock 1997). When patients are unable to speak or are spending a great deal of time sleeping, clinicians can encourage their family members to tell one another what they remember about the patient. For many patients and families this difficult time can become a time of growth and healing, resolution, remembrance of good times together, and transmission of a legacy (Block 2001).

While patients are still able to do so, physicians can urge them to talk more about their lives. Through the telling patients prioritize, order, celebrate, and mourn. Clinicians can help patients find solace and closure at the end of life by exploring religious and spiritual beliefs and by listening empathetically (Lev et al. 1998; Block 2001).

Through these discussions, patients begin to understand that they are cared for as people, not just as patients. Some may reveal fears that their clinicians can dispel, such as a fear of dying in uncontrolled pain, of suffocating, or of being abandoned. Some want to reconnect with religious traditions and carry out the rituals that surround dying in their culture or religion (Bigby 2003). Chaplains, social workers, and psychiatrists can address many of these problems well, and the clinician can make appropriate referrals.

Hospice Programs

Hospice is a system for providing specialist palliative care for patients with a life expectancy of six months or less, if the disease takes its expected course. Unfortunately, in the United States, the current reimbursement system, which is driven by the Medicare hospice benefit, leads many hospice programs to exclude patients who are receiving costly life-prolonging or palliative therapies.

Hospice programs provide a continuum of care, from home to the inpatient setting. While by law 80% of days of patient care must take place in the home, all Medicare-certified hospices are required to provide four levels of care: routine home care, continuous home care, respite care in nursing homes, and inpatient care (Medicare Hospice Regulations 1993) (Table 12c.1).

For a patient to be eligible to enroll in a hospice program, both the attending physician and the hospice medical director must certify that the patient is terminally ill with a prognosis of six months or less if the disease follows its usual course (Saunders 1981; Medicare Hospice Regulations 1993). There are

Table 12c-1. Routine Clinical Care Provided by Hospice Programs

SERVICE	FREQUENCY
"on call"	24 hours/day
HHA	≤ 2hr/day
RN visits	≤ 3 / wk +prn
SW visits	q 2 wks
Chaplain visits	q 2–4wks
Volunteer	2–4 hrs/wk
MD	prn
Occuptional/physical/recreation therapist	prn

Additional mandated services:

(1) *Continuous home care.* Patients with, for example, refractory cough, dyspnea, pain, or delirium can receive 24 hour/day nursing and home health aide services.

(2) *Inpatient care.* Rarely utilized. For refractory symptoms that cannot be controlled at home, even with continuous care. The referring physician admits the patient and may bill for his/her services under Medicare Part B (Medicare Hospice Regulations. 1983).

(3) *Respite care.* The goal of the respite (in a community skilled or intermediate nursing facility) is either to provide a rest for the caregiver, or to remove the patient to an adequate facility when the home is temporarily inadequate to meet the patient care needs. Respite care is offered for 5 days for every month the patient is enrolled in hospice.

Table 12c-2 Common Misconceptions about Hospice Care

- **Misconception:** *Patients enrolling in hospice must choose not to be resuscitated.*

- **Misconception:** *Patients enrolled in hospice lose their primary physicians.* The referring primary care physician or oncologist continues to direct and approve all of the patient's care. If the patient requires either inpatient hospice admission for symptom control or routine admission for a diagnosis unrelated to the terminal illness, the physician may bill Medicare under Part B for any visits.

- **Misconception:** *Hospice patients cannot be hospitalized and remain enrolled in hospice.*

- **Misconception:** *Hospice patients cannot participate in research projects while enrolled in hospice.* Yes they can, so long as the project is consistent with the mission of hospice.

- **Misconception:** *Hospice nursing personnel do not provide sophisticated care.* The palliative care delivered by hospice nurses requires astute assessment and expert intervention tailored to the patient and family goals. Tube feedings, intravenous hydration or nutrition, or intravenous medications to control symptoms may be included in the hospice plan of care.

- **Misconception:** *Patients can "use up" their hospice eligibility.* Patients who live longer than six months will continue to receive services, so long as they continue to meet eligibility criteria for hospice care. And patients who chose to revoke the hospice benefit to seek life-prolonging therapies may chose to re-enroll if their goals change.

- **Misconception:** *Patients must have a live-in caregiver to enroll in hospice.* Hospices that care for "live-alone' patients have special protocols to enhance their safety.

a number of misconceptions, however, that can delay or prevent referrals to hospice (Table 12c.2).

The services provided by hospice are listed in Table 12c.3. Hospice covers 95% of the cost of prescription drugs related to the terminal diagnosis and

Table 12c-3 Hospice Services
Personnel:
Medical director, nurses, social workers, home health aides, chaplains, volunteers, administrative personnel, medical consultations, occupational therapy, physical therapy, speech therapy, bereavement counseling
Items Needed for Palliation of Terminal Illness:
Prescription medications
Durable Medical equipment and supplies
Oxygen
Radiation and chemotherapy
Laboratory and diagnostic procedures
Other:
Transportation when medically necessary for changes in level of care
When needed, continuous care at home or in a skilled nursing facility or inpatient setting
Respite care (care in a nursing facility that provides a "respite" for the caregivers)

necessary for the patient's palliative treatment (and many waive the other 5% if there is no insurance coverage). Hospice programs provide all durable medical equipment, supplies, and oxygen for needs related to the terminal diagnosis, laboratory and diagnostic procedures related to the terminal diagnosis, and transportation when medically necessary for changes in the patient's level of care.

Relief of Suffering in the Last Weeks

Patients report that the components of a "good death" include (1) optimizing physical comfort, (2) maintaining a sense of continuity with oneself, (3) maintaining and enhancing relationships, (4) finding meaning in one's life and death, (5) achieving a sense of control, and (6) confronting and preparing for death (Block 2001). Control of physical and psychological suffering is a prerequisite for allowing both patients and caregivers to address these social and spiritual/ existential dimensions of their lives and for minimizing the suffering of bereaved survivors.

Even in patients on stable drug regimens, physiologic changes at the end of life make it necessary to monitor carefully for the appearance of opioid-related side effects such as myoclonus or delirium. With decreasing renal function, for example, patients taking sustained-release preparations of morphine or oxycodone may develop these side effects as a result of decreased clearance of the drugs and their metabolites. If the respiratory rate declines to fewer than six breaths per minute and opioids are thought to be the cause, opioid doses should be decreased 25% and the patient should be monitored carefully for increasing discomfort. Naloxone is almost never indicated. If a sedated patient demonstrates a dangerous reduction in respiratory rate that is thought to be

Table 12c-4 Common Disorder at the End of Life		
Source	Medication(s)	Dose and route (PO/SL/IV/SC/PR*)
Fatigue	Methylphenidate	2.5–5 mg PO 8am/noon; can increase as needed
Insomnia	Temazepam	7.5–30 PO hs (lower dose in elderly)
	Zoldipem	5–10 mg PO hs
	Trazadone	25–100 mg PO hs
Pain (continuous)	Opioid (morphine, oxycodone)	Oral concentrates or IV or SQ infusion
	Fentanyl	Transdermal
Pain (intermittent)	Morphine, oxycodone	SL oral concentrates
	Hydromorphone	PR
Depression	Methylphenidate	2.5–5 mg PO qam or qam and noon
Anxiety	Lorazepam	0.5–2 mg SL q2h
	Clonazepam	0.5–2 mg PO bid
Delirium	Haloperidol	1–5 mg PO, SQ, IV, PR q2-12h
	Chlorpromazine	12.5–50 mg PO, IV, PR q4-8h
	Olanzapine wafer	5 mg SL qhs or bid; 5 mg SL prn q4h
Agitated Delirium	Midazolam	1–2.5 mg IV/SC load; 0.5–1.5 mg/hr IV/ SC or 25% of loading dose; increase as needed
Dyspnea (anxiety)	Lorazepam	1 mg PO, SL q2h
Dyspnea (other)	Opioid	For example, morphine 5-10 mg PO, IV
	Chlorpromazine	25–50 mg PO, PR q4–12h
Cough	Opioid	Nebulized with dexamethasone, e.g. morphine 5–10 mg PO, IV or by nebulizer q2h
	Lidocaine	2 ml of 2% lidocaine in 1 ml of NL saline for 10"
	Albuterol/terbutaline	Nebulized
Hiccups	Baclofen	10–20 mg PO tid
	Metoclopramide	10–20 mg PO/IV/SC/PR qid
	Nifedipine	10–20 mg PO tid
	Haloperidol	1–4 mg PO/SC/PR tid
	Chlorpromazine	25–50 mg PO/IV qd-qid
"Death rattle"	Scopolamine	Trans-derm Scop patch 1-3 q3d
	Hyoscyamine	0.125–0.25 SL tid–qid
	Glycopyrrolate	0.2–0.6 mg PO/SC/IV tid
Nausea	Olanzapine	2.5 to 5 mg SL hs to bid

(continued)

247

Table 12c-4 Continued		
Source	Medication(s)	Dose and route (PO/SL/IV/SC/PR*)
	Lorazepam, metoclopramide, dexamethasone, or haloperidol	IV or compounded suppositories with desired agents (depending on presumed cause of nausea) q6 PR
Palliative Sedation for Refractory Symptoms	Midazolam	1–2.5 mg IV/SC load; 0.4 mg/hr IV/SC drip; increase as needed
	Pentobarbital	2–3 mg/kg IV load; 1–2 mg/kg/hr IV drip
	Lorazepam	0.5–1 mg/hour IV
	Propofol	2.5–5 ug/kg/minute IV
* PO = oral; SL = sublingual; IV= intravenous; SQ = subcutaneous; PR = per rectum		

caused by opioids, 1mL (0.4mg) of naloxone can be diluted to 10mL and given as 1 or 2mL (0.04mg–0.08mg) at a time until the respiratory rate recovers to more than six breaths per minute. If the naloxone is given undiluted, the patient is likely to experience severe opioid withdrawal.

If the patient becomes unable to take pills, liquid opioid concentrates or other forms—for example, transmucosal (Payne et al. 2001), rectal (Kaiko et al. 1992; Davis et al. 2002), transdermal, or pelleted opioids—can be used. A nasal preparation of fentanyl shows promise for treating breakthough pain (Kress et al. 2009). Kadian and Avinza contain morphine sustained-release pellets packaged into capsules that can be opened. The pellets can be sprinkled on food or suspended in liquid and either swallowed or placed into feeding tubes every 12 to 24 hours. Patients whose opioid dose is too large to be delivered by sublingual, transdermal, or rectal routes will need subcutaneous or intravenous continuous opioid infusions. Parenteral opioid administration is also needed for patients who would benefit from patient-controlled analgesia.

The xerostomia that is common in this population is usually due to opioids, not dehydration (Ellershaw et al. 1995). There is no correlation between reports of thirst or dry mouth and hydration status (Ellershaw et al. 1995), and no controlled studies have shown that rehydration is effective. Moistening the mouth with swabs or offering sips of water, ice chips, or fruit-flavored ice usually ameliorates the xerostomia.

Not all patients who exhibit distress are in pain. Delirium may mimic pain. Patients who moan without any apparent provocation or in response to non-painful stimuli, such as having their lips moistened, may be delirious. Delirium is especially likely in patients exhibiting such behaviors who did not report pain before they became nonverbal. Therapy to prevent and treat constipation in dying patients should be continued because constipation can cause delirium in this population. Delirious patients may appear agitated or hypoactive or may vacillate between these states (Abrahm 2005). Symptoms of delirium include insomnia and daytime somnolence, nightmares, restlessness or agitation (which mimics uncontrolled pain), irritability, distractibility, hypersensitivity to light and sound, anxiety, difficulty in concentrating or marshaling thoughts, and fleeting illusions. Table 12c.4 lists the effective treatments for delirium in patients at the end of life.

Anxiety

Anxiety in this population is often situational, involving concerns related to the terminal illness. Fear of death, impairment, or pain and concerns about the past all contribute (Stark 2002). Hospitalization can add a sense of isolation, loneliness, a sense of uselessness, and concerns about lack of information or misinformation about what is happening. Other causes include drugs (corticosteroids, metoclopramide, opioid neurotoxicity, withdrawal from benzodiazepines or alcohol), uncontrolled pain, hypoxia, dyspnea, metabolic abnormalities (sepsis, hypoglycemia), insomnia, and preexisting psychiatric disorders (Storey et al. 2003).

The Final Days

If the patient is not enrolled in hospice, the treatment team needs to explain to the family what to expect as the patient dies and how to recognize when the patient's last days are approaching. Many relatives have limited support from someone who can care for the rest of the family while they support the dying patient, and vacation, sick, and family leave days are often limited. Signs that the patient is entering the last 10 to 14 days include the following:

- Dehydration, tachycardia, followed by decrease in heart rate and blood pressure;
- Perspiration, clammy skin, cool extremities, and just before death, mottling;
- Diminished breath sounds, irregular breathing pattern with periods of apnea or full Cheyne-Stokes respiration, grunting or moaning with exhalation;
- Mouth droop, difficulty swallowing, loss of gag reflex, with pooling of secretions causing "death rattle";
- Incontinence of bladder or rectum; and
- Agitation and/or hallucinations, stillness, being difficult to arouse (Pitorak 2003).

For patients in a hospital or nursing home, discussions should be held with the family to learn whether their religious or cultural tradition has any specific requirements for the days immediately preceding or immediately following the death. The family can then begin to assemble the group who will perform the rituals and begin to explain to the unit staff what they will need.

Table 12c.4 lists the common causes of disorders in the last days of life and medications that can ease these problems.

Aberrant Drug-Related Behaviors and Substance Use in the Palliative Care Patient

As patients with cancer and other life-limiting illnesses are living longer with improved therapies and as palliative care referrals occur earlier in the disease trajectory, the challenges of opiod misuse seen in patients with chronic pain may become more prevalent in palliative care populations (Starr et al. 2010). Substance use and misuse and aberrant drug related behaviors are seen in the palliative care population, though incidence and prevalence is not well understood. Even in patients whose prognosis is very limited, eliciting a prior history of substance use or active substance use can be very useful information. Additionally, identifying patients at risk for misuse of prescribed medications or at risk of withdrawal syndromes can prevent adverse outcomes if appropriate measures are taken. Tools used to screen for risk of opioid misuse in the chronic pain setting may be used to screen cancer pain patients at risk of opioid misuse. In a patient with a life-limiting illness, the differential diagnosis of apparently aberrant drug-related behaviors accompanying a complaint of pain must be thoroughly explored in order to ensure appropriate clinical management. The differential diagnosis includes undertreated pain or pseudoaddiction, chemical coping, psychiatric disorders, and other alternatives, including, in a distinct minority of cases, substance abuse disorders.

Pseudoaddiction likely arises when the treating clinician has an inadequate understanding of appropriate pain assessment or of the pharmacology of opioids used for pain management, or excessive fear of addiction in patients managed with opioids (Weissman and Haddox 1989). Regressive behavior (moaning or crying out in pain) or failure to cooperate with the health care team may develop if the patient's attempts to obtain more analgesics are unsuccessful. This pattern will continue to escalate until a crisis of mistrust arises, leading to feelings of anger and isolation on the part of the patient. Only after a patient trusts that his health care team believes his or her pain and that analgesia will be a priority of care will the aberrant behaviors cease. Given the fact that pain is typically undertreated in patients who are at the end of life, pseudoaddiction is an important cause of suffering in this population.

Chemical coping describes a patient who uses pain medicines to alleviate symptoms other than pain, such as anxiety or depression. Careful assessment of psychiatric symptoms and availability of psychiatric consultation are important components of a comprehensive, multidisciplinary approach to serving these patients (Passik and Kirsh 2003). The prevalence of anxiety disorders in patients with advanced cancer is 22% (Smith et al. 2003); although panic disorder at the end of life has not yet been studied, clinical experience has shown this to be a commonly encountered phenomenon (Periyakoil et al. 2005) (see discussion on anxiety, above). Depression at the end of life is also quite common. Clinicians must be alert to the presence of depression in the palliative care patient manifesting guilt, hopelessness, or anhedonia; it is not advisable to rely on somatic or neurovegetative criteria such as fatigue or anorexia, as these symptoms are often present in nondepressed patients with advanced medical illness (Block 2000). Counseling, psychotherapy, or psychopharmacologic treatment with benzodiazepines, other anxiolytics, or antidepressants may be indicated in these circumstances. If the guilt is associated with spiritual or existential concerns, further questioning and counseling in these areas by the primary or palliative care team or by the chaplain should be pursued (Lo et al. 2002).

Delirium is experienced by 28% to 83% of patients near the end of life (Casarett et al. 2001; Nowels et al. 2002); it can explain aberrant drug-taking behaviors in patients who are responsible for taking their own medications but are not closely monitored to make sure that they are taking the correct amounts at the correct times. Delirium manifests as an alteration of cognition, consciousness, and perception, and it may wax and wane. Recognition and treatment of the delirium can eliminate the aberrant drug-taking behaviour (see the section on relief of sufferring in the last weeks, above).

Personality disorders can also cause patients to seem to be taking their medications strangely. If the patient's goal is contact with or attention from the health care team, a patient with a personality disorder may engage in impulsive or attention-seeking drug-related behaviors.

In the palliative care patient with substance abuse, a pain complaint may manifest or be intensified by spiritual suffering, social isolation, and guilt for past behaviors. Spiritual well-being actually protects against despair at the end of life (McClain et al. 2003). But patients with a history of substance abuse or a prior criminal history may be isolated from family and friends and feel guilty about past or ongoing betrayals. They may also fear punishment or be estranged from their religious tradition. They may even resist taking medication so that they can atone before they die (e.g., "I'd rather burn here than burn there").

Managing Patients on Opioid Replacement

Patients on methadone maintenance can also be successfully treated for pain. It is incorrect to assume, however, that the methadone used in the maintenance program will provide adequate analgesia for those with acute or chronic pain (Alford et al. 2005). Alternative opioids can and often should be used for analgesia, as patients on methadone likely have significant tolerance to opioids and may need higher doses. Nonetheless, methadone itself can be used to treat the patient's pain. For patients on active methadone maintenance, receiving the methadone for maintenance from their program allows them to benefit from the additional support and structure that the program offers. Collaboration, therefore, between the team at the facility and the palliative care or primary physician managing the patient's pain would seem ideal.

Summary

The approach to palliative care patients with pain and other symptoms is not unique; it comprises careful communication, compassionate delivery of care, and multidisciplinary management. Skillful use of opioids is an important tool in providing expert palliative care. Coordinated efforts of palliative care teams, primary treating physicians, and hospice teams can allow for personal and spiritual growth, legacy leaving, and closure.

References

Abrahm JL. *A Physician's Guide to Pain and Symptom Management in Cancer Patients.* Baltimore, MD: Johns Hopkins University Press, 2005.

Alford DP, Compton P, Samet JH. Acute pain management for patients receiving maintenance methadone or buprenorphine therapy. *Ann Intern Med.* 2005;144(2):127–134.

Bigby JA, ed. *Cross-Cultural Medicine.* Philadelphia: American College of Physicians, 2003.

Block SD. Assessing and managing depression in the terminally ill patient. *Ann Intern Med.* 2000;132(3):209–218.

Block SD. Perspectives on care at the close of life. Psychological considerations, growth, and transcendence at the end of life: the art of the possible. *JAMA.* 2001;285:2898–2905.

Byock I. *Dying Well: The Prospect of Growth at the End of Life.* New York: Riverhead Books, 1997.

Casarett DJ, Inouye SK. Diagnosis and management of delirium near the end of life. *Ann Intern Med.* 2001;135(1):32–40.

Cleeland CS, Gonin R, Hatfield AK, et al. Pain and its treatment in outpatients with metastatic cancer. *N Engl J Med.* 1994;330(9):592–596.

Coyle N, Adelhardt J, Foley KM, et al. Character of terminal illness in the advanced cancer patient: pain and other symptoms during the last four weeks of life. *J Pain Symptom Manage.* 1990;5(2):83–93.

Curtis EB, Krech R, Walsh TD. Common symptoms in patients with advanced cancer. *J Palliat Care.* 1991;7(2):25–29.

Curtis EB, Walsh TD. Prescribing practices of a palliative care service. *J Pain Symptom Manage.* 1993;8(5):312–316.

Davis MP, Walsh D, LeGrand SB, et al. Symptom control in cancer patients: the clinical pharmacology and therapeutic role of suppositories and rectal suspensions. *Support Care Cancer.* 2002;10(2):117–138.

Dy SM. Evidence-based approaches to pain in advanced cancer. *Cancer J.* 2010;16(5):500–506.

Dy SM, Asch SM, Naeim A, et al. Evidence-based standards for cancer pain management. *J Clin Oncol.* 2008;26(23):3879–3885.

Ellershaw JE, Sutcliffe JM, Saunders CM. Dehydration and the dying patient. *J Pain Symptom Manage.* 1995;10(3):192–197.

Field MJ, Cassel CK, eds. *Approaching Death: Improving Care at the End of Life.* Washington, DC: National Academies Press, 1997.

Kaiko RF, Fitzmartin RD, Thomas GB, et al. The bioavailabilty of morphine in controlled-release 30mg tablets. *Pharmacotherapy.* 1992;12(2):107–134.

Kress HG, Oronska A, Kaczmarek G, et al. Efficacy and tolerability of intranasal fentanyl spray 50 to 200 µg for breakthrough pain in patients with cancer: A phase III, multinational, randomized, double-blind, placebo-controlled, crossover trial with a 10-month, open-label extension treatment period. *Clin Therap.* 2009;31(6):1177–1191.

Lev EL, McCorkle R. Loss, grief, and bereavement in family members of cancer patients. *Semin Oncol Nurs.* 1998;14(2):145–151.

Levy MH. Pharmacological treatment of cancer pain. *N Engl J Med.* 1996; 335(15):1124–1132.

Lo B, Ruston D, Kates LW, et al. Discussing religious and spiritual issues at the end of life; a practical guide for physicians. *JAMA.* 2002;287(6):749–754.

Loblaw DA, Perry J, Chambers A, Laperriere NJ. Systematic review of the diagnosis and management of malignant extradural spinal cord compression: the Cancer Care Ontario practice guidelines intiative's nuero-oncology disease site group. *J Clin Oncol* 2005;23(9):2028–2037.

McClain CS, Rosenfeld B, Breitbart W. Effect of spiritual well-being on end-of-life despair in terminally-ill cancer patients. *Lancet.* 2003;361(9369):1603–1607.

Medicare Hospice Regulations. Title 42 Code of Federal Regulations, Pt. 418. 1983 ed.

Morita T, Tsunoda J, Inoue S, Chihara S. Effects of high dose opioids and sedatives on survival in terminally ill cancer patients. *J Pain Symptom Manage* 2001;21(4):282–289.

Morrison RS, Meier DE. Clinical Practice. Palliative care. *N Engl J Med.* 2004;350(25):2582–2590.

National Consensus Project for Quality Palliative Care. *Clinical Practice Guidelines for Quality Palliative Care.* Pittsburgh: National Consensus Project, 2009.

Nowels DE, Bublitz C, Kassner CT, et al. Estimation of confusion prevalence in hospice patients. *J Palliat Med.* 2002;5(5):687–695.

Passik SD, Kirsh KL. The need to identify predictors of aberrant drug-related behavior and addiction in patients being treated with opioids for pain. *Pain Med.* 2003;4(2):186–189.

Payne R, Coluzzi P, Hart L, et al. Long-term safety of oral transmucosal fentanyl citrate for breakthrough cancer pain. *J Pain Symptom Manage.* 2001;22(1):575–583.

Periyakoil VS, Skultety K, Sheikh J. Pain, anxiety, and chronic dyspnea. *J Palliat Med.* 2005;8(2):453–459.

Pitorak EF. Care at the time of death. *Am J Nurs.* 2003;103(7):42–52.

Saunders C. The founding philosophy. In Saunders C, Summers DH, Teller N, eds. *Hospice: The Living Idea.* Philadelphia: W. B. Saunders, 1981.

Schuman ZD, Abrahm JL. Implementing institutional change: an institutional case study of palliative sedation. *J Palliat Med.* 2005;8(3):666–676.

Singer PA, Martin DK, Kelner M. Quality end-of-life care: patients' perspectives. *JAMA.* 1999;281(2):163–168.

Sloan PA. The evolving role of interventional pain management in oncology. *J Support Oncol.* 2004;2(6):491–500.

Smith EM, Gomm SA, Dickens CM. Assessing the independent contribution to quality of life from anxiety and depression in patients with advanced cancer. *Palliat Med.* 2003;17(6):509–513.

Stark D, Kiely M, Smith A, et al. Anxiety disorders in cancer patients: their nature, associations, and relation to quality of life. *J Clin Oncol.* 2002;20(14):3137–3148.

Starr TD, Rogak LJ, Passik SD. Substance abuse in cancer pain. Curr Pain Headache Rep. 2010;14(4):268–275.

Storey P, Knight CF, Schonwetter RS. *Pocket Guide to Hospice/Palliative Medicine.* Glenview, IL: American Academy of Hospice and Palliative Medicine, 2003. Temel JS, Greer JA, Muzikansky A, et al. Early palliative care for patients with metastatic non–small-cell lung cancer. *NEJM.* 2010;363(8):733–742.

Tulsky JA. Beyond advance directives: importance of communication skills at the end of life. *JAMA.* 2005;294(3):359–365.

Weissman DE, Haddox JD. Opioid pseudoaddiction—an iatrogenic syndrome. *Pain.* 1989;36(3):363–366.

Chapter 13

Patients with a History of Substance Abuse

Kenneth L. Kirsh and Steven D. Passik

Addiction and drug abuse are common in the US population: some 6% to 12% have abused illicit drugs, 15% have abused alcohol, 25% are addicted to nicotine, and 33% have sampled illicit drugs at least once (Colliver and Kopstein 1991; Groerer and Brodsky 1992; Lopez-Quintero et al. 2011; Spiller et al. 2009). Given that substance abuse of one form or another is a risk for some chronic pain patients, it is inevitable that these problems will be seen in a sizable, often labor-intensive subset of patients with chronic pain. There is no reason to think that abuse rates would be any lower among these patients than in the general population.

Given this, there is an interesting phenomenon concerning the perception of opioid medications both in our society and within the health care system. Some sectors of the medical community consider these drugs to be a major cause of abuse, associated with dire consequences for the individual and society at large, whereas others view them as essential medications, capable of bringing about one of the highest goals of medicine—the relief of pain and suffering. Generally, addiction specialists focus on the former characterization, and pain specialists project the latter (Portenoy et al. 2005). Given the antithetical nature of these perspectives, it is not surprising that historically, there has been little communication between these two groups.

In diverse patient populations with chronic pain issues, a remote or current history of drug abuse presents a constellation of stigmatizing physical and psychosocial issues that can both complicate the management of the underlying disease and undermine therapies. The interface between the therapeutic use of potentially abusable drugs and the abuse of these drugs is complex and must be understood if pain management is to be optimized. Additional studies are needed to clarify the epidemiology of substance abuse and addiction in patients with chronic pain. These patients can be adequately and successfully treated only when the addiction problems are noted by staff and these patients' special needs are addressed (Bruera et al. 1995; Savage et al. 2008).

Defining Addiction in Chronic Pain Patients

In order to intervene with these difficult patients, it is first necessary to have a common set of terms that can be used to identify them. The traditional definitions of addiction, which include phenomena related to physical dependence or tolerance, cannot be the model terminology for medically ill populations who receive potentially abusable drugs for legitimate medical purposes. Instead, a more appropriate definition of addiction notes that it is a chronic disorder characterized by "the compulsive use of a substance resulting in physical, psychological or social harm to the user and continued use despite that harm" (Rinaldi 1988). Therefore, any appropriate definition of addiction must include the concepts of loss of control over drug use, compulsive drug use, and continued use despite harm (ASAM 2011). The concept of aberrant drug-taking behavior is a useful first step in operationalizing the definitions of abuse and addiction, and it recognizes the broad range of behaviors that may be considered problematic by prescribers. If drug-taking behavior in a medical patient can be characterized as aberrant, a differential diagnosis for this behavior can be explored. The following points highlight potential differential diagnoses to consider:

- Addiction, meeting the criteria for continued use despite harm, as discussed above;
- Pseudoaddiction, or the concept that the analgesic regimen is subtherapeutic, which causes patients to engage in desperate behaviors to achieve adequate analgesia (Passik et al. 2011);
- Presentations complicated by psychiatric diagnoses such as encephalopathy, borderline personality disorder, depression, or anxiety; and
- Criminal intent by those with an eye toward diversion.

Psychiatric Complications Expanded

Building on one of the differential diagnoses listed above, it is important to assess whether a psychiatric disorder is complicating the patient's presentation. Impulsive drug use may indicate the existence of another psychiatric disorder, the diagnosis of which may have therapeutic implications. The following list expounds on the potential complications that might be encountered by specific psychiatric diagnoses:

- Patients with borderline personality disorder can express fear and rage through aberrant drug taking and behave impulsively and self-destructively during pain therapy. Hay and Passik (2000) reported a case in which one of the more worrisome aberrant drug-related behaviors, forging of a prescription for a controlled substance, was an impulsive expression of fears of abandonment having little to do with true substance abuse in a borderline patient.
- Patients who self-medicate anxiety, panic, depression, or even periodic dysphoria and loneliness can present as aberrant drug takers.
- Careful diagnosis and treatment of psychiatric problems can sometimes obviate the need for such self-medication with opioids.

Exploring the Level of Aberrancy of Behaviors

In assessing the differential diagnosis for drug-related behavior, it is useful to consider the degree of aberrancy (see Table 13.1). Less aberrant behaviors (such as aggressively complaining about the need for medications) are more

Table 13.1 Aberrant Behaviors and Their Proposed Levels of Aberrancy

Behaviors *LESS* Indicative of Aberrancy:	Behaviors *MORE* Indicative of Aberrancy:
Drug hoarding during periods of reduced symptoms	Prescription forgery
Acquisition of similar drugs from other medical sources	Concurrent abuse of related illicit drugs
Aggressive complaining about the need for higher doses	Recurrent prescription losses
Unapproved use of the drug to treat another symptom	Selling prescription drugs
Unsanctioned dose escalation one or two times	Multiple unsanctioned dose escalations
Reporting psychic effects not intended by the clinician	Stealing or borrowing another patient's drugs
Requesting specific drugs	Obtaining prescription drugs from nonmedical sources

likely to reflect untreated distress of some type than true addiction-related concerns. Conversely, the more aberrant behaviors (such as injection of an oral formulation) are more likely to reflect true addiction. Although empirical studies are needed to validate this conceptualization, it may be a useful model in evaluating aberrant behaviors.

Tailoring the Approach

The differential between patients with no histories of substance abuse and those who are prior addicts, as well as all the gradations between, has created a need to tailor chronic pain management to the individual patient. To this end, we offer an oversimplified three-level conceptualization of prototypical patients and the amount of follow-up necessary for each. Although these are caricatures, they can be used to create mental prototypes as we see and assess our chronic pain patients.

The Uncomplicated Patient

- Minimal structure required owing to lack of comorbid psychiatric problems and lack of connection to a drug subculture;
- Routine medical management is generally sufficient;
- Suggested practice includes 30-day supply of medications with liberal rescue-dose policy; and
- Monthly follow-ups.

The Chemical Coper

- Behavior resembles that of an addict, with a central focus on obtaining drugs (Kirsh et al. 2007);

- Needs structure, psychiatric input, and drug treatments that decentralize the pain medication from coping strategies;
- Decentralize meaning: reduce the meaning of medications, undo conditioning, and undo the socialization around the drug; and
- Best accomplished via use of pain-related psychotherapy.

The Addicted Patient

- Includes the active abuser, the patient in drug-free recovery, and the patient on methadone maintenance;
- Requires the most structure, including frequent visits;
- Patient should be given a limited supply of medications;
- Drug choices should be tailored to include long-acting opioids with little street value;
- Rescues should be offered judiciously;
- Implement use of urine toxicology screening and follow up on results; and
- Patient should be required to be in active recovery program or psychotherapy.

Optimizing Therapy for Abusers with Pain

The treatment of pain in those with a history of substance abuse should not be taken lightly. Optimal drug therapy for substance abusers with pain, first and foremost, employs the basic principles of good pain treatment with consideration of the unique pharmacologic needs of addicts, and then adds the psychosocial, recovery, and additional structures necessary to maximize the likelihood of a good outcome. These are truly complex patients who have, in essence, two distinct diseases. Treatment of one with the assumption that it is most important and that resolving it will take care of the other is a common mistake that frequently results in additional suffering for the patient from either or both illnesses.

Good opioid pain treatment in any patient follows two key rules. First, the clinician must maintain an accepting and thoughtful attitude directed toward self-reports of pain. Second, prudent drug selection that leads to the decision to use an opioid must be followed by skilled titration that focuses on maintaining a balance of analgesia and side effects. The following are recommendations that build upon these principles:

- Connecting with the patient and forming a therapeutic bond can often lead to more reliable self-reporting if trust can be maintained by both parties.
- Pain reports should be followed by a nonjudgmental, interested, and concerned assessment that recognizes the patient's cry of distress and helps the patient to articulate what it is that he or she most needs help with.
- Drug addicts have often been described as alexithymic, and many are unable to label distress other than globally "good" or "bad"; it is often this trait that leads to global distress in the face of the negative emotions associated with pain and chronic illness (Handelsman 2000).

- Drug selection in such patients is often limited to sustained-release delivery to avoid feeding into compulsive pill popping and/or the use of opioids in service of chemical coping (Bruera et al. 1995; Kirsh et al. 2007).
- Use of a drug with a relatively low street value is recommended for patients who are battling for their recovery but who still maintain contact with the addiction subculture, which can be unavoidable for some patients.
- Titration is aimed at and continued until effect or toxicity, bearing in mind that addicts will often be highly tolerant and may require very large doses of opioids for pain control.

Use of Urine Toxicology Screening

Urine toxicology screening has the potential to be a very useful tool for diagnosing potential abuse problems and monitoring patients with an established history of abuse. Unfortunately, recent work suggests that urine toxicology screens are employed infrequently, as seen in the case of tertiary care centers (Passik et al. 2000). When such screens are ordered, documentation tends to be inconsistent regarding the reasons for ordering as well as any follow-up recommendations based on the results. The aforementioned survey found that nearly 40% of the charts surveyed listed no reason for obtaining the urine toxicology screen and that the ordering physician could not be identified nearly 30% of the time (Passik et al. 2000). Therefore, while useful, toxicology screens do need to be employed in a consistent and rational manner.

Managing Patients on an Outpatient Basis

Managing patients in a primary care or other outpatient setting presents challenges. A written contract between the treating physician and the patient helps to provide structure to the treatment plan, establishes clear expectations of the roles played by both parties, and outlines the consequences of aberrant drug taking. The following are useful guidelines for engaging in outpatient management:

- The inclusion of spot urine toxicology screens in the contract can be useful in maximizing treatment compliance. Expectations regarding attendance of clinic visits and the management of the patient's supply of medications should also be stated.
- Limit the amount of drug dispensed per prescription, and make refills contingent upon clinic attendance.
- Consider requiring the patient to attend a 12-step program and having the patient document such attendance as a condition for ongoing prescribing.
- Involve family members and friends in the treatment to help bolster social support and functioning. Becoming familiar with the family may help the team to identify family members who are themselves drug abusers and who may, as facilitators of the patient's noncompliance, potentially divert the patient's medications.

Managing Patients in the Inpatient Setting

Inpatient management of patients with active substance abuse problems both includes and expands upon the guidelines discussed above for outpatient settings. The first point of order is to discuss the patient's drug use in an open manner. In addition, it is necessary to reassure the patient that steps will be taken to avoid adverse events such as drug withdrawal. For certain specific situations, such as with preoperative patients, patients should be admitted several days in advance, when possible, to stabilize the drug regimen. In addition, the following may be helpful:

- It is important to provide the patient with a private room near the nurses' station to aid in monitoring the patient and to discourage attempts to leave the hospital for the purchase of illicit drugs.
- The team should require visitors to check in with nursing staff prior to visitation.
- Daily urine specimens for random toxicology analysis should be collected and pain and symptom management frequently reassessed.
- Remember that open and honest communication between clinician and patient reassures the patient that these guidelines were established in his or her best interest.

Interacting with Patients in Recovery

As a final word, pain management with patients in recovery presents a unique challenge. Owing to fear of ostracism from some programs (e.g., Alcoholics Anonymous), some patients may be leery of taking opioids. Thus, the first choice with these patients should be to explore nonopioid therapies, which may require referral to a pain center (Parrino 1991). Alternative therapies may include the use of nonopioid or adjuvant analgesics, cognitive therapies, electrical stimulation, neural blockade, or acupuncture. If opioids are used as a therapy, it is necessary to structure their use with opioid management contracts, random urine toxicology screens, and occasional pill counts. If possible, attempts should be made to include the patient's recovery-program sponsor in order to garner his or her cooperation and assistance in successful monitoring of the condition.

References

American Society of Addiction Medicine (ASAM). ASAM public policy statement: The definition of addiction. Adopted April 12, 2011. www.asam.org/DefinitionofAddiction-LongVersion.html.

Bruera E, Moyano J, Seifert L, et al. The frequency of alcoholism among patients with pain due to terminal cancer. *J Pain Symptom Manage.* 1995;10(8):599–603.

Colliver JD, Kopstein AN. Trends in cocaine abuse reflected in emergency room episodes reported to DAWN. *Public Health Rep.* 1991;106(1):59–68.

Groerer J, Brodsky M. The incidence of illicit drug use in the United States, 1962–1989. *Br J Addict.* 1992;87(9):1345–1351.

Handelsman L, Stein JA, Bernstein DP, et al. A latent variable analysis of coexisting emotional deficits in substance abusers: alexithymia, hostility, and PTSD. *Addict Behav.* 2000;25(3):423–428.

Hay J, Passik SD. The cancer patient with borderline personality disorder: suggestions for symptom-focused management in the medical setting. *Psychooncology.* 2000;9(2):91–100.

Kirsh KL, Jass C, Bennett DS, Hagen JE, Passik SD. Initial development of a survey tool to detect issues of chemical coping in chronic pain patients. *Palliat Support Care.* 2007;5(3):219–226.

Lopez-Quintero C, Hasin DS, de Los Cobos JP, et al. Probability and predictors of remission from life-time nicotine, alcohol, cannabis or cocaine dependence: results from the National Epidemiologic Survey on Alcohol and Related Conditions. *Addiction.* 2011;106(3):657–669.

Parrino M. *State Methadone Treatment Guidelines.* TIPS 1 DHHS Publication No. (SMA) 93–1991. Washington, DC: US Government Printing Office, 1991.

Passik S, Schreiber J, Kirsh KL, et al. A chart review of the ordering and documentation of urine toxicology screens in a cancer center: do they influence patient management? *J Pain Symptom Manage.* 2000;19(1):40–44.

Passik SD, Kirsh KL, Webster L. Pseudoaddiction revisited: a commentary on clinical and historical considerations. *Pain Management.* 2011;1(3):239–248.

Portenoy RK, Lussier D, Kirsh KL, Passik SD. Pain and addiction. In Frances R, Miller F, Mack A, eds. *Clinical Textbook of Addictive Disorders.* 3rd ed. New York: Guilford, 2005; 367–395.

Savage SR, Kirsh KL, Passik SD. Challenges in using opioids to treat pain in persons with substance use disorders. *Addict Sci Clin Practice.* 2008;4(2):4–25.

Spiller H, Lorenz DJ, Bailey EJ, Dart RC. Epidemiological trends in abuse and misuse of prescription opioids. *J Addict Dis.* 2009;28(2):130–136.

Rinaldi RC, Steindler EM, Wilford BB, et al. Clarification and standardization of substance abuse terminology. *JAMA.* 1988;259(4):555–557.

Appendix 1

Sample AAPM Consent for Chronic Therapy

Consent for Chronic Opioid Therapy

A consent form from the American Academy of Pain Medicine

Dr_____ is prescribing opioid medicine. sometimes called narcotic analgesics, to me for a diagnosis of_____.
This decision was made because my condition is serious or other treatments have not helped my pain.

I am aware that the use of such medicine has certain risks associated with it, including, but not limited to: sleepiness or drowsiness, constipation, nausea, itching, vomiting, dizziness, allergic reaction, slowing of breathing rate, slowing of reflexes or reaction time, physical dependence, tolerance to analgesia, addiction and possibility that the medicine will not provide complete pain relief.

I am aware about the possible risks and benefits of other types of treatments that do not involve the use of opioids. The other treatments discussed included:

_____
_____
_____

I will tell my doctor about all other medicines and treatments that I am receiving.

I will not be involved in any activity that may be dangerous to me or someone else if I feel drowsy or am not thinking clearly. I am aware that even if I do not notice it. my reflexes and reaction time might still be slowed. Such activities include. but are not limited to: using heavy equipment or a motor vehicle, working in unprotected heights or being responsible for another individual who is unable to care for himself or herself.

I am aware that certain other medicines such as nalbuphine (Nubain™). pentazocine (Talwin™). buprenorphine (Buprenex™). and butorphanol (Stadol™). may reverse the action of the medicine I am using for pain control. Taking any of these other medicines while I am taking my pain medicines can cause symptoms like a bad flu. called a withdrawal syndrome. I agree not to take any of these medicines and to tell any other doctors that I am taking an opioid as my pain medicines and cannot take any of the medicines listed above.

I am aware that addiction is defined as the use of a medicine even if it causes harm, having cravings for a drug, feeling the need to use a drug and a decreased quality of life. I am aware that the chance of becoming addicted to my pain medicine is very low. I am aware that the development of addiction has been reported rarely in medical journals and is much more common in a person who has a family or personal history of addiction. I agree to tell my doctor my complete and honest personal drug history and that of my family to the best of my knowledge.

I understand that physical dependence is a normal, expected result of using these medicines for a long time. I understand that physical dependence is not the same as addiction. I am aware physical dependence means that if my pain medicine use is markedly decreased, stopped or reversed by some of the agents mentioned above. I will experience a withdrawal syndrome. This means I may have any or all of the following: runny nose, yawning large pupils, goose bumps, abdominal pain and cramping, diarrhea, irritability. aches throughout my body and a flu-like feeling. I am aware that opioid withdrawal is uncomfortable but not life threatening.

I am aware that tolerance to analgesia means that I may require more medicine to get the same amount of pain relief. I am aware that tolerance to analgesia does not seem to be a big problem for most patients with chronic pain. however, it has been seen and may occur to me. If it occurs, increasing doses may not always help and may cause unacceptable side effects. Tolerance or failure to respond well to opioids may cause my doctor to choose another form of treatment.

(**Males only**) I am aware that chronic opioid use has been associated with low testosterone levels in males. This may affect my mood, stamina, sexual desire and physical and sexual performance. I understand that my doctor may check my blood to see if my testosterone level is normal.

(**Females Only**) If I plan to become pregnant or believe that I have become pregnant while taking this pain medicine. I will immediately call my obstetric doctor and this office to inform them. I am aware that, should I carry a baby to delivery while taking these medicines. the baby will be physically dependent upon opioids. I am aware that the use of opioids is not generally associated with a risk of birth defects. However, birth defects can occur whether or not the mother is on medicines and there is always the possibility that my child will have a birth defect while I am taking an opioid.

I have read this form or have it read to me. I understand all of it. I have had a chance to have all of my questions regarding this treatment answered to my satisfaction. By signing this form voluntarily. I give my consent for the treatment of my pain with opioid pain medicines.

Patient signature _____ Date _____

Witness to above _____

Approved by the AAPM Executive Committee on January 14, 1999.

4700 W. Lake Avenue
Glenview, IL 60025-1485
847/375-4731
Fax 877734-8750
E-mail aapm@amctec.com
Web site www.painmed.org

Sample AAPM Agreement for Long-Term Controlled Substance Therapy for Chronic Pain

Sample for Adaptation and Reproduction on Physician Letterhead

PLEASE CONSULT WITH YOUR ATTORNEY
Long-term Controlled Substances Therapy for Chronic Pain

SAMPLE AGREEMENT

A consent form from the American Academy of Pain Medicine

The purpose of this agreement is to protect your access to controlled substances and to protect our ability to prescribe for you.

The long-term use of such substances as opioids (narcotic analgesics). benzodiazepine tranquilizers, and barbiturate sedatives is controversial because of uncertainty regarding the extent to which they provide long-term benefit. There is also the risk of an addictive disorder developing or of relapse occurring in a person with a prior addiction. The extent of this risk is not certain.

Because these drugs have potential for abuse or diversion, strict accountability is necessary when use is prolonged. For this reason the following policies are agreed to by you. the patient, as consideration for. and a condition of. the willingness of the physician whose signature appears below to consider the initial and or continued prescription of controlled substances to treat your chronic pain.

1. All controlled substances must come from the physician whose signature appears below or. during his or her absence, by the covering physician, unless specific authorization is obtained for an exception. (Multiple sources can lead to untoward drug interactions or poor coordination of treatment.)

2. All controlled substances must be obtained at the same pharmacy. where possible. Should the need arise to change pharmacies, our office must be informed. The pharmacy that you have selected is:

   _____ phone:_____.

3. You are expected to inform our office of any new medications or medical conditions, and of any adverse effects you experience from any of the medications that you take.

4. The prescribing physician has permission to discuss all diagnostic and treatment details with dispensing pharmacists or other professionals who provide your health care for purposes of maintaining accountability.

5. You may not share, sell, or otherwise permit others to have access to these medications.

6. These drugs should not be stopped abruptly, as an abstinence syndrome will likely develop.

7. Unannounced urine or serum toxicology screens may be requested, and your cooperation is required. Presence of unauthorized substances may prompt referral for assessment for addictive disorder.

8. Prescriptions and bottles of these medications may be sought by other individuals with chemical dependency and should be closely safeguarded. It is expected that you will take the highest possible degree of care with your medication and prescription. They should not be left where others might see or otherwise have access to them.

9. Original containers of medications should be brought in to each office visit.

10. Since the drugs may be hazardous or lethal to a person who is not tolerant to their effects, especially a child, you must keep them out of reach of such people.

11. Medications may not be replaced if they are lost, get wet. are destroyed, left on an airplane, etc. If your medication has been stolen and you complete a police report regarding the theft, an exception may be made.

12. Early refills will generally not be given.

13. Prescriptions may be issued early if the physician or patient will be out of town when a refill is due. These prescriptions will contain instructions to the pharmacist that they not be filled prior to the appropriate date.

14. If the responsible legal authorities have questions concerning your treatment, as might occur, for example, if you were obtaining medications at several pharmacies, all confidentiality is waived and these authorities may be given full access to our records of controlled substances administration.

15. It is understood that failure to adhere to these policies may result in cessation of therapy with controlled substance prescribing by this physician or referral for further specialty assessment.

16. Renewals are contingent on keeping scheduled appointments. Please do not phone for prescriptions after hours or on weekends.

17. It should be understood that any medical treatment is initially a trial, and that continued prescription is contingent on evidence of benefit.

18. The risks and potential benefits of these therapies are explained elsewhere (and you acknowledge that you have received such explanation).

19. You affirm that you have full right and power to sign and be bound by this agreement, and that you have read, understand, and accept all of its terms.

_____   _____

Physician Signature   Patient Signature

_____   _____

Date   Patient Name (Printed)

Approved by the AAPM Executive Committee on April 2, 2001.

AAPM
4700 W. Lake Avenue
Glenview. IL 60025-1485
847/375-4731   Fax 877/734-8750
E-mail aapm@amctec.com
Web site http://www.painmed.org

Appendix 3

Numerical Opioid Side Effect (NOSE) Assessment Tool

Not Present										As Bad As You Can Imagine
0	1	2	3	4	5	6	7	8	9	10
1. Nausea, vomiting, and/or lack of appetite	O	O	O	O	O	O	O	O	O	O
2. Fatigue, sleepiness, trouble concentrating, hallucinations, and/ or drowsiness/ somnolence	O	O	O	O	O	O	O	O	O	O
3. Constipation	O	O	O	O	O	O	O	O	O	O
4. Itching	O	O	O	O	O	O	O	O	O	O
5.nDecreased sexual desire/function and/ or diminished libido	O	O	O	O	O	O	O	O	O	O
6. Dry Mouth	O	O	O	O	O	O	O	O	O	O
7. Abdominal pain or discomfort/ cramping or bloating	O	O	O	O	O	O	O	O	O	O
8. Sweating	O	O	O	O	O	O	O	O	O	O
9. Headache and/or dizziness	O	O	O	O	O	O	O	O	O	O
10. Urinary retention	O	O	O	O	O	O	O	O	O	O

Smith HS. The Numerical Opioid Side Effect (NOSE) Assessment Tool. *Journal of Cancer Pain and Symptom Palliation*. 2005;1(3): 3–6.

Translational Analgesia Score (TAS)

For each of the following questions, respond by comparing your current state over the past month to your baseline status before you started your current treatment regimen by circling a number from zero to ten with zero being no improvement and ten being maximal improvements:

1) Over the past month, my pain treatment has improved my ability to do usual daily activities, including household work, work, school, and/ or social activities.

   0   1   2   3   4   5   6   7   8   9   10

2) Over the past month, my pain treatment has improved my ability to concentrate on work or daily activities.

   0   1   2   3   4   5   6   7   8   9   10

3) Over the past month, my pain treatment has improved the degree to which I feel too tired to do work (feeling that I could not get going and everything I do is an effort), or to tired to perform daily activities, and/or socialize because of my pain.

   0   1   2   3   4   5   6   7   8   9   10

4) Over the past month, my pain treatment has improved the degree to which I feel distress, restless, agitated, or could go and lie down and/or be alone because of my pain.

   0   1   2   3   4   5   6   7   8   9   10

5) Over the past month, my pain treatment has improved my mood or feelings of being depressed, frustrated, anxious, irritable, tense, hopeless, annoyed, or just plain fed up because of my pain.

   0   1   2   3   4   5   6   7   8   9   10

6) Over the past month, my pain treatment has improved my ability to sleep.

   0   1   2   3   4   5   6   7   8   9   10

7) Over the past month, my pain treatment has improved my ability to walk, sit, and/or stand for long periods.

   0   1   2   3   4   5   6   7   8   9   10

8) Over the past month, my pain treatment has improved my ability to go up stairs, and/or move or lift objects.

0   1   2   3   4   5   6   7   8   9   10

9) Over the past month, my pain treatment has improved the extent to which my pain interferes with optimal interpersonal relationships and/or intimacy.

0   1   2   3   4   5   6   7   8   9   10

10) Over the past month, to what degree have you, your significant other, your family, your coworkers, and/or your friends noticed any improvements in your socializing, recreational activities, physical functioning, concentration, mood, interpersonal relationships, activities of daily living, and/or overall quality of life?

0   1   2   3   4   5   6   7   8   9   10

Please write below specific examples of things you can now do or currently do frequently that you couldn't do or only did rarely when your pain was not controlled as well as it is now.

TAS = _____

The TAS is expressed as a number between 0 to 10 with a decimal being the average of the responses to the ten questions (or less; if the patient is paraplegic then they would not answer the questions regarding going up stairs, etc.).

As an example, a patient's response to the TAS tool is shown below:

1) Over the past month, my pain treatment has improved my ability to do usual daily activities, including household work, work, school, and/or social activities.

0   1   2   3   ④   5   6   7   8   9   10

2) Over the past month, my pain treatment has improved my ability to concentrate on work or daily activities.

0   1   2   ③   4   5   6   7   8   9   10

3) Over the past month, my pain treatment has improved the degree to which I feel too tired to do work (feeling that I could not get going and everything I do is an effort), or to tired to perform daily activities, and/or socialize because of my pain.

0   1   2   ③   4   5   6   7   8   9   10

4) Over the past month, my pain treatment has improved the degree to which I feel distress, restless, agitated, or could go and lie down and/or be alone because of my pain.

0   1   ②   3   4   5   6   7   8   9   10

5) Over the past month, my pain treatment has improved my mood or feelings of being depressed, frustrated, anxious, irritable, tense, hopeless, annoyed, or just plain fed up because of my pain.

0   1   2   3   ④   5   6   7   8   9   10

6) Over the past month, my pain treatment has improved my ability to sleep.

0   1   2   3   4   ⑤   6   7   8   9   10

7) Over the past month, my pain treatment has improved my ability to walk, sit, and/or stand for long periods.

0   1   ②   3   4   5   6   7   8   9   10

8) Over the past month, my pain treatment has improved my ability to go up stairs, and/or move or lift objects.

⓪   1   2   3   4   5   6   7   8   9   10

9) Over the past month, my pain treatment has improved the extent to which my pain interferes with optimal interpersonal relationships and/or intimacy.

0   ①   2   3   4   5   6   7   8   9   10

10)   Over the past month, to what degree have you, your significant other, your family, your coworkers, and/or your friends noticed any improvements in your socializing, recreational activities, physical functioning, concentration, mood, interpersonal relationships, activities of daily living, and/or overall quality of life?

0   1   ②   3   4   5   6   7   8   9   10

TAS = 2.6

Smith HS. Translational Analgesia and the Translational Analgesia Score (TAS). *Journal of Cancer Pain and Symptom Palliation.* 2005;1(3):15–19.

Clinical Guidelines for the Use of Chronic Opioid Therapy in Chronic Noncancer Pain: Opioid Treatment Guidelines (Chou et al. 2009)

Recommendations:

1. Before initiating COT, clinicians should conduct a history, physical examination and appropriate testing, including an assessment of risk of substance abuse, misuse, or addiction.
2. Clinicians may consider a trial of COT as an option if CNCP is moderate or severe, pain is having an adverse impact on function or quality of life, and potential therapeutic benefits outweigh or are likely to outweigh potential harms.
3. A benefit-to-harm evaluation including a history, physical examination, and appropriate diagnostic testing should be performed and documented before and on an ongoing basis during COT.
4. When starting COT, informed consent should be obtained. A continuing discussion with the patient regarding COT should include goals, expectations, potential risks, and alternatives to COT.
5. Clinicians may consider using a written COT management plan to document patient and clinician responsibilities and expectations and assist in patient education.
6. Clinicians and patients should regard initial treatment with opioids as a therapeutic trial to determine whether COT is appropriate.
7. Opioid selection, initial dosing, and titration should be individualized according to the patient's health status, previous exposure to opioids, attainment of therapeutic goals, and predicted or observed harms.
8. Methadone is characterized by complicated and variable pharmacokinetics and pharmacodynamics and should be initiated and titrated cautiously, by clinicians familiar with its use and risks.
9. Clinicians should reassess patients on COT periodically and as warranted by changing circumstances. Monitoring should include documentation of pain intensity and level of functioning, assessments of progress toward achieving

therapeutic goals, presence of adverse events, and adherence to prescribed therapies.

10. In patients on COT who are at high risk or who have engaged in aberrant drug-related behaviors, clinicians should periodically obtain urine drug screens or other information to confirm adherence to the COT plan of care.

11. In patients on COT not at high risk and not known to have engaged in aberrant drug-related behaviors, clinicians should consider periodically obtaining urine drug screens or other information to confirm adherence to the COT plan of care.

12. Clinicians may consider COT for patients with CNCP and history of drug abuse, psychiatric issues, or serious aberrant drug-related behaviors only if they are able to implement more frequent and stringent monitoring parameters. In such situations, clinicians should strongly consider consultation with a mental health or addiction specialist.

13. Clinicians should evaluate patients engaging in aberrant drug-related behaviors for appropriateness of COT or need for restructuring of therapy, referral for assistance in management, or discontinuation of COT.

14. When repeated dose escalations occur in patients on COT, clinicians should evaluate potential causes and reassess benefits relative to harms.

15. In patients who require relatively high doses of COT, clinicians should evaluate for unique opioid-related adverse effects, changes in health status, and adherence to the COT treatment plan on an ongoing basis, and consider more frequent follow-up visits.

16. Clinicians should consider opioid rotation when patients on COT experience intolerable adverse effects or inadequate benefit despite dose increases.

17. Clinicians should taper or wean patients off of COT who engage in repeated aberrant drug-related behaviors or drug abuse/diversion, experience no progress toward meeting therapeutic goals, or experience intolerable adverse effects.

18. Clinicians should anticipate, identify, and treat common opioid-associated adverse effects.

19. As CNCP is often a complex biopsychosocial condition, clinicians who prescribe COT should routinely integrate psychotherapeutic interventions, functional restoration, interdisciplinary therapy, and other adjunctive nonopioid therapies.

20. Clinicians should counsel patients on COT about transient or lasting cognitive impairment that may affect driving and work safety. Patients should be counseled not to drive or engage in potentially dangerous activities when impaired or if they describe or demonstrate signs of impairment.

21. Patients on COT should identify a clinician who accepts primary responsibility for their overall medical care. This clinician may or may not prescribe COT, but should coordinate consultation and communication among all clinicians involved in the patient's care.

22. Clinicians should pursue consultation, including interdisciplinary pain management, when patients with CNCP may benefit from additional skills or resources that they cannot provide.
23. In patients on around-the-clock COT with breakthrough pain, clinicians may consider as-needed opioids based upon an initial and ongoing analysis of therapeutic benefit versus risk.
24. Clinicians should counsel women of childbearing potential about the risks and benefits of COT during pregnancy and after delivery. Clinicians should encourage minimal or no use of COT during pregnancy, unless potential benefits outweigh risks. If COT is used during pregnancy, clinicians should be prepared to anticipate and manage risks to the patient and newborn.
25. Clinicians should be aware of current federal and state laws, regulatory guidelines, and policy statements that govern the medical use of COT for CNCP.

Guidelines based on the best available evidence and developed by multidisciplinary panels of experts are an important resource for promoting the effective and safe use of COT for CNCP. An expert panel convened by APS and AAPM concludes that COT can be an effective therapy for carefully selected and monitored patients with CNCP (Chou et al. 2009). However, opioids are also associated with potentially serious harms, including opioid-related adverse effects and outcomes related to the abuse potential of opioids (Chou et al. 2009).

Twenty-one of the 25 recommendations of the panel were strongly recommended and are here in Appendix 5. Although these guidelines are based on a systematic review of the evidence on COT for CNCP, the panel identified numerous research gaps. The evidence was very limited and the panel did not rate any of its 25 recommendations as supported by high quality evidence. Only four recommendations were viewed as supported by even moderate quality evidence (Chou et al. 2009).

Chou R, Fanciullo GJ, Fine PG, Adler JA, Ballantyne JC, Davies P, Donovan MI, Fishbain DA, Foley KM, Fudin J, Gilson AM, Kelter A, Mauskop A, O'Connor PG, Passik SD, Pasternak GW, Portenoy RK, Rich BA, Roberts RG, Todd KH, Miaskowski C; American Pain Society-American Academy of Pain Medicine Opioids Guidelines Panel. Clinical guidelines for the use of chronic opioid therapy in chronic noncancer pain. J Pain. 2009;10(2):113–30.

Index

"f" indicates material in figures and "t" indicates material in tables.